3965

830.

A.

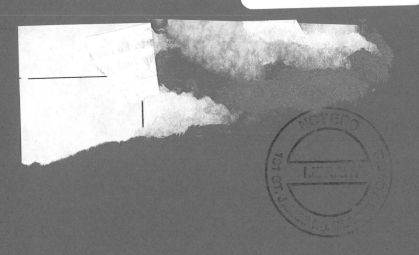

Fractures of the Hand and Wrist

Editorial Advisory Board

Douglas W. Lamb FRCS Chairman
Princess Margaret Rose Orthopaedic Hospital
Fairmilehead, Edinburgh, UK

Nicholas Barton FRCS
Department of Hand Surgery, University Hospital,
Queen's Medical Centre, Nottingham, UK

W. Bruce Connolly FRCS FRACS FACS
Hand Unit, Sydney Hospital, Macquarie Street,
Sydney, New South Wales, Australia

Lee W. Milford Jr BS MS MD
The Campbell Clinic, Madison Avenue,
Memphis, Tennessee, USA

Volumes already published

The Interphalangeal Joints
William H. Bowers

The Paralysed Hand
Douglas W. Lamb

Unsatisfactory Results in Hand Surgery
R. M. McFarlane

Volumes in preparation

The Thumb
James W. Strickland

Microsurgical Procedures
Viktor E. Meyer and Michael J. M. Black

Joint Replacement in the Upper Limb
William A. Souter

Congenital Malformations of the Hand and Forearm
Dieter Buck-Gramcko

Skin Cover in the Injured Hand
David M. Evans

Dupuytren's Disease
R. M. McFarlane, D. A. McGrouther and M. L. Flint

Fractures of the Hand and Wrist

EDITED BY

Nicholas Barton MB BChir FRCS(Eng)

Consultant Hand Surgeon,
Nottingham University Hospital and Harlow Wood Orthopaedic Hospital, Nottinghamshire, UK;
Civilian Consultant in Hand Surgery to the Royal Air Force

CHURCHILL LIVINGSTONE
EDINBURGH LONDON MELBOURNE AND NEW YORK 1988

CHURCHILL LIVINGSTONE
Medical Division of Longman Group UK Limited

Distributed in the United States of America by Churchill
Livingstone Inc., 1560 Broadway, New York, N.Y. 10036, and
by associated companies, branches and representatives
throughout the world.

First published 1988

ISBN 0–443–03366–8
ISSN 0269–4743; v. 4

British Library Cataloguing in Publication Data
Fractures of the Hand and Wrist.—(The Hand and upper
    limb, ISSN 0269-4743; v .4)
    1. Hand—Fractures   2. Wrist—Fractures
    I. Barton, N. J.   II. Series
    617'.157   RD559

Library of Congress Cataloging in Publication Data
    Fractures of the Hand and Wrist
    (The Hand and upper limb, ISSN 0269-4743; v .4)
    Includes index.
    1. Hand—Fractures   2. Wrist—Fractures
I. Barton, Nicholas J.   II. Series.   [DNLM: 1.
Fractures. 2. Hand Injuries. 3. Wrist Injuries. WE 830 F798]
RD559.F73   1988   617'.157   87-23839

Typeset, printed and bound in Great Britain by
William Clowes Limited, Beccles and London

D
617.575
FRA

Foreword

It is a privilege to write a foreword to this impressive book. Some of us can remember the days when the care of fractures of the hand was commonly delegated to recently qualified doctors who had received no special training in the subject, a practice that still holds in some less favoured countries. Even after the 'Report of Committee on Fractures' was published in 1935 by the British Medical Association and which led to the establishment of organized clinics in the UK, there was little concern shown at first for injuries of the hand. It is of interest to observe that the great masters Böhler (1935), Scudder (1938) and Watson-Jones (1943) used a mere 59, 62 and 65 pages respectively in their textbooks to discuss fractures of the wrist and hand. This contrasts with 24 chapters in the present volume to cover the same ground. This is a measure of the progress made in treatment and the options open to the surgeon of today, particularly in the techniques of internal (and external) skeletal fixation.

Conservative measures remain the 'best buy' for the great majority of fractures in the hand, though the advantages of accurate reduction and sound fixation are manifest for intra-articular fractures, unstable phalangeal and metacarpal fractures, certain carpal injuries, disruptions and replanta-tions. Operative techniques demand precision surgery, the necessary facilities and instrumentation and their use is not devoid of complications. This book offers a choice of treatment and this is surely good. Rigid adherence to a particular form of treatment is undesirable; the surgeon should be familiar with the available techniques and be ready to use the one that best suits the circumstances.

Nicholas Barton, whose leadership of a large hand service at the University Hospital, Nottingham, and the editorship of the British volume of the Journal of Hand Surgery fit him admirably for the task, has chosen his team well. Here is a galaxy of talent, surgeons of unrivalled experience and original thought whose contributions to the literature are well known. The international scholarship that is represented gives to the work the mark of powerful authority. This is a book written by experts for experts; for those who possess authority themselves yet still feel the need to consult the wealth of experience that can be found in these pages.

This book is the leader in its field and is likely to remain so.

Guy Pulvertaft

Preface

Fractures of the hand and wrist have been Cinderella subjects neglected by both orthopaedic and hand surgeons who gave their attention to other types of fracture or hand injury which they considered more important. There are many parts of the world where this still applies, often because doctors and facilities are limited. In some developing countries there are hand surgeons, but they are spending a great deal of time on replantation surgery which would be better spent in running an out-patient clinic for common hand injuries.

Such neglect is wrong for two reasons. In the first place, these fractures are very common. How common?

Dr Peter Meiring has analysed the attendances at the Adult Fracture Clinic of the Nottingham University Hospital, which serves a total population of about 750 000, for the month of January 1986. Of the total attendances, 46.4% were for fractures of the hand or wrist. This proportion was even higher than we expected, and we thought that perhaps January had been an abnormal month because it did include a period of snowfall when many people slipped and fell onto their outstretched hands.

The survey was therefore repeated in June 1986, when the total number of fractures was almost as great (and June has a day less than January) but the proportion of hand and wrist fractures was less, being 40.7%. These figures were then added together and multiplied by six to give estimated numbers for one year (Fig. 1). It is true that this includes a number of patients with suspected scaphoid fractures which were not confirmed, but it does *not* include fractures of distal half of the distal phalanx, which are treated in the Accident

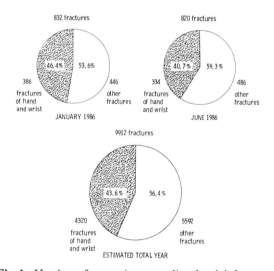

Fig. 1 Numbers of new patients attending the adult fracture clinics at Nottingham University Hospital

and Emergency Department, as are most soft-tissue injuries.

Analysis of the location of fractures within the hand and wrist showed that the snow probably did have an effect, because in January fractures of the distal end of the radius and ulna comprised 45.3% of the wrist and hand fractures, whereas in June these were only 35.3%, with a greater proportion of all other types and especially phalangeal fractures (Fig. 2).

Children with fractures are treated in a separate children's fracture clinic, and not included in the figures above. In 1981 there were 826 new attendances, of which 35.8% were fractures of the distal forearm (mostly greenstick fractures of the lower radius, above the level of a Colles fracture and not

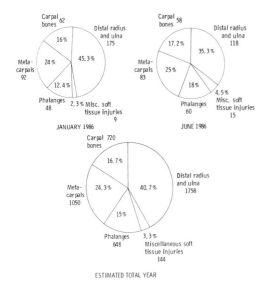

Fig. 2 Number of fractures affecting different parts of the hand and wrist in adults

strictly within the sphere of this book) and 14.7% were fractures of the carpus or hand (Worlock & Stower 1986a) though again most fractures of the distal phalanx are not included. A detailed analysis of the type and pattern of these carpal and hand fractures has also been published (Worlock & Stower, 1986b).

Thus each year our hospital treats about 1750 distal forearm fractures in adults and 300 in children, and 2560 fractures of the carpus and hand in adults and 270 in children. This adds up to a lot of fractures and, although we serve an unusually large population, it is clear that fractures of the hand and wrist are very common indeed and for this reason alone would demand much time and resources.

In the second place, while it is true that some of these fractures can be treated as minor injuries, and need little or no treatment, many fractures of the hand and wrist do cause lasting disability, which could usually have been prevented by proper treatment soon after the injury. Perceptive surgeons have always realized that these injuries can present just as great a challenge as fractures of larger bones: Sir Reginald Watson-Jones, in his book on fractures which was so influential throughout the world, said 'An open fracture of a phalanx is no less worthy of the skill of an expert than an open fracture of the femur'.

In recent years the truth of this has been widely appreciated by surgeons faced with the problems resulting from poor initial treatment of fractures of the hand and wrist. Simultaneously, the development of new methods of splintage and of internal and external fixation of fractures in general has made it possible to achieve satisfactory results after injuries which would previously have been hopeless, and these advances can be applied to severe fractures of the hand and wrist with great benefit.

In this volume, I have been fortunate enough to gather the experience and opinions of distinguished hand surgeons from all over the world; indeed, seven of them have been President of their national Hand Society.

Naturally, the emphasis throughout the book is on the difficult problems and the more complex methods of treatment, though in everyday practice most fractures of the phalanges, for example, will and should be treated by the simple conservative methods described in Chapter 3, and most Colles's fractures, to take another example, by the well-tried techniques described in Chapter 20. These methods, however, are not quite as simple as they seem, and will only achieve good results if they are applied with care and attention to detail. The hand surgeon may not always carry out the primary treatment of all these fractures himself, but it is his duty to make sure it is done properly and to supervise the follow-up of the patient.

Amongst the hundreds of fractures of the hand and wrist is a small proportion where more complicated methods of treatment are the only way in which a good result can be obtained, and other chapters give detailed accounts of these techniques.

In planning the volume, I was torn between having chapters on different types of fracture or on different types of treatment. The table of contents will show that I have settled for a compromise between these two: the book is essentially arranged by sites and types of fractures, but on particularly controversial subjects, differing approaches are described by different authors and there is, inevitably, disagreement between them. For example, the authors of Chapters 16 and 17 differ not only about treatment but even on such a basic matter as the likely result of conventional treatment: this reflects our continuing ignorance of many of the key facts and the need for further research.

Kirschner wires are mentioned many times, but are available in many different shapes and sizes so I decided to include an appendix about them.

I am grateful to all the authors for finding the time in their busy lives to contribute to this book and thus give it such a broad range of experience and attitudes. Mr R. G. Pulvertaft very kindly wrote the foreword; indeed, it must have been among the last things he did, as he died about two weeks later. Everybody who knew him will miss him. Tragically, his former pupil, Dr Richard Smith, whose chapter is a model of clarity as one would expect from such an outstanding teacher of hand surgery, also died before it was printed. It appealed to his sense of humour to write on Smith's and Barton's fractures in a book edited by Barton.

I also thank Mrs Doreen Beesley, Miss Lisa Dawes, and Miss Janet Parkin for much secretarial work behind the scenes.

Nottingham, 1987　　　　　　　　　　　　　N.J.B.

REFERENCES

Worlock P H, Stower M J 1986a Fracture patterns in Nottingham children. Journal of Pediatric Orthopedics 6: 656–660

Worlock P H, Stower M J 1986b The incidence and pattern of hand fractures in children. Journal of Hand Surgery 11B: 198–200

Acknowledgements

The following illustrations are reproduced by kind permission of the original authors and publishers:
Figures 3.9, 16.2D, 16.4 and 17.5, and Tables 16.1 and 16.2 from the *Journal of Bone and Joint Surgery*.
Figures 3.2, 7.17, 7.19, 12.4, 12.5, 12.6 and 12.7 from *The Hand*.
Figures 9.1, 9.3A, 9.5A, 9.7A, 9.8A, D, E and F, 9.9, 9.11, 9.12, 9.14A, 9.15, 10.3, 18.8 and 18.10 from the *Journal of Hand Surgery*.
Figure 8.10 from the *Journal of Trauma*.
Figures 17.6, 17.7 and 17.12 from *Clinical Orthopaedics and Related Research*.
Figure 6.2 from Surgery of the hand by H E Kleinert, in *A Textbook of Surgery*, A P Monaco (ed) 1985 (MacMillan).
Figure 6.6 from Tendon injuries by J E Kutz and D L Bennett, in *Methods and Concepts in Hand Surgery*, N A Watson, R J Smith (eds) (Butterworth).
Figure 8.11 from Multipurpose unilateral external fixator for hand surgery by M Rousso in Volume 2 of *The Hand*, R Tubiana (ed), 1985 (W B Saunders).
Figure 8.13 from the 2nd Edition of *The Small Fragment Set Manual*, U F A Heim, K M Pfeiffer (eds) 1982 (Springer Verlag).
Figures 10.12, 10.20, and 24.13A, B, and C from Fractures and joint injuries of the hand by N J Barton in *Watson-Jones Fractures and Joint Injuries*, 6th Edition, J N Wilson (ed), 1982 (Churchill Livingstone).
Figure 10.16 from Fractures by D W Lamb in *The Practice of Hand Surgery*, D W Lamb, K Kuczynski (eds), 1981 (Blackwell Scientific).
Figure 17.4 from *The Herbert Screw Bone Screw System* by T J Herbert, 1982 (Technical Publications, Zimmer Inc, Warsaw, Indiana).
Figures 23.1 and 23.3 from *Injuries and Infections of the Hand* by R H C Robins, 1961 (Edward Arnold).
The charts for Hand Assessment which form Figure 23.2 appear by kind permission of the British Orthopaedic Association.

Contributors

N. J. Barton MB BChir FRCS(Eng)
Consultant Hand Surgeon, Nottingham University Hospital and Harlow Wood Orthopaedic Hospital, Nottinghamshire; Civilian Consultant in Hand Surgery to the Royal Air Force

M. R. Belsky MD
Assistant Professor of Orthopaedic Surgery, Tufts Medical School; Attending Hand Surgeon, Newton Wellesley Hospital, New England Baptist Hospital, New England Medical Center, St Elizabeth's Hospital, Wellesley Hill, MA, USA

S. L. Biddulph MB BCh(Rand) FCS(S.A.) FRCS(Edin) FRCS(Eng)
Hand Surgeon, Orthopaedic Department, Johannesburg Hospital and University of the Witwatersrand; Hand Surgeon, Natalspriut Hospital, Alberton, South Africa

F. D. Burke MB BS FRCS
Consultant Hand Surgeon, Derbyshire Royal Infirmary, Derby and Harlow Wood Orthopaedic Hospital, Notts, UK

G. A. Buterbaugh MD
Clinical Instructor of Orthopaedic Surgery, University of Pittsburgh School of Medicine; Attending Orthopaedic Surgeon, Allegheny General Hospital, Pittsburgh, PA, USA

W. P. Cooney MD MS
Associate Professor of Orthopaedic Surgery, Mayo Medical School and Mayo Graduate School of Medicine, Rochester, MN, USA

R. A. Dickson MA ChM FRCS FRCSE
Professor and Head of Orthopaedic Surgery, University of Leeds; Consultant Orthopaedic Surgeon, St James's University Hospital and General Infirmary, Leeds, UK

J. H. Dobyns MD
Professor of Orthopaedic Surgery, Mayo Medical School; Consultant in Orthopaedic Surgery and Surgery of the Hand, Mayo Clinic; Attending Staff in Orthopaedic Surgery and Surgery of the Hand, Rochester Methodist Hospital and St Mary's Hospital, Rochester, MN, USA

R. G. Eaton BS MD
Professor of Clinical Surgery, Columbia College of Physicians and Surgeons; Director, Hand Surgery Center, St Luke's-Roosevelt Hospital Center, New York, NY, USA

W. E. Floyd III MD
Orthopaedic and Hand Surgeon, Macon Orthopaedic Associates, Macon, Georgia, USA

H. Hastings II MD
Clinical Assistant Professor, Department of Orthopaedics, Indiana University Medical Center, Indianapolis, Indiana, USA

T. J. Herbert FRCS FRACS
Consultant Orthopaedic Surgeon, Hand Unit, Sydney Hospital, Sydney, NSW, Australia

J. I. P. James MS FRCS(Edin) FRCS(Eng) Hon FRACS
Emeritus Professor of Orthopaedic Surgery, University of Edinburgh, Edinburgh, UK

J. E. Kutz MD
Associate Clinical Professor of Surgery, University of Louisville School of Medicine, Louisville, Kentucky, USA

D. W. Lamb MB FRCS(Edin)
Consultant Orthopaedic Surgeon, Princess Margaret Rose Orthopaedic Hospital, Fairmilehead, Edinburgh, UK

G. D. Lister FRCS
Professor of Surgery and Chief, Division of Plastic Surgery, University of Utah, Salt Lake City, UT, USA

J. D. Matiko MD
Instructor of Orthopaedic Surgery, Loma Linda University Medical Center; Orthopaedic Staff Surgeon, San Bernardino County Medical Center, San Barnardino, CA, USA

E. C. McElfresh MD MS
Clinical Professor, Department of Orthopaedics, University of Minnesota Medical School; Chief of Hand Surgery, Minneapolis Veterans' Administration Hospital, Minneapolis, MN, USA

P. Y. Milliez MD
Surgeon, Department of Traumatology, Hôpital Charles Nicolle, Rouen, France

J. R. Moore MD
Associate Professor, Department of Orthopaedic Surgery, Johns Hopkins University School of Medicine, Baltimore, MD, USA

P. J. Mulligan MD ChB FRCS(Glas) FRCS(Eng)
Consultant Orthopaedic Surgeon, Birmingham General Hospital and Royal Orthopaedic Hospital, Birmingham, UK

J. Noble MB ChM FRCSE
Consultant Orthopaedic Surgeon, University of Manchester, Manchester, UK

A. K. Palmer MD
Professor of Orthopaedic Surgery, State University of New York, Upstate Medical Center, Syracuse, NY USA

H. Potts MB ChB FRCS(Glas)
Registrar in Orthopaedic Surgery, Hope Hospital and Royal Manchester Children's Hospital, Manchester, UK

R. H. C. Robins MA MB BChir FRCS
Consultant Orthopaedic Surgeon, Royal Cornwall Hospital, Truro, UK

M. E. Ruff MD
Clinical Instructor of Orthopaedic Surgery, Ohio State University, Columbus, Ohio, USA

G. Segmüller MD
Head, Section of Hand Surgery, Clinic of Orthopaedic Surgery, Kantonsspital, St Gallen, Switzerland

R. J. Smith MD
Late Clinical Professor of Orthopaedic Surgery, Harvard Medical School; Chief of Hand Surgery Service, Department of Orthopaedic Surgery, Massachusetts General Hospital, Boston, MA, USA

W. M. Steel FRCS
Consultant Orthopaedic Surgeon, North Staffordshire Hospital Centre, Stoke-on-Trent, UK

J. M. Thomine MD
Professor of Orthopaedics and Head, Department of Orthopaedics and Traumatology, Hôpital Charles Nicolle, Rouen, France

H. J. R. Ulson MD
Formerly Assistant Professor, Department of Hand Surgery, Sta Casa de São Paulo Medical School; Postgraduate Course (Orthopaedics and Plastic Surgery), Escola Paulista de Medicina, São Paulo, Brazil

A. J. Weiland MD
Professor, Department of Orthopaedic Surgery, Division of Plastic Surgery and Department of Emergency Medicine; Chief, Division of Upper Extremity Surgery, Johns Hopkins University School of Medicine, Baltimore, MD, USA

G. M. White MD
Jewett Orthopaedic Clinic, Winter Park, Florida, USA

T. J. Wilton MB BS
Senior Orthopaedic Registrar, Derbyshire Royal Infirmary, Derby and Harlow Wood Orthopaedic Hospital, Notts, UK

Contents

SECTION

Hand fractures

1

Fractures of the phalanges

Sydney L. Biddulph

1   **Fingertip fractures**

Injuries to the small distal phalanx account for half of all bony injuries of the hand. Crush and avulsion injuries are most frequently encountered. Crush injuries are often compound and generally restricted to the tuft, but when severe can involve the whole bone. Avulsion fractures are almost never compound and are restricted to the base of the phalanx.

CLASSIFICATION

Fractures of the distal phalanx may be divided into four groups (Fig. 1.1). Fractures can involve the tuft: single or comminuted; the shaft: transverse, oblique, longitudinal or comminuted; base: dorsal avulsion, volar avulsion, lateral avulsion or longitudinal, and articular—any of above; and epiphyseal fractures. Each of these may be stable or unstable, displaced or undisplaced, simple or compound.

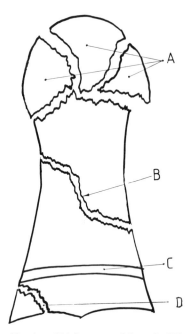

Fig. 1.1 Classification: (A) fractures of the tuft; (B) fractures of the shaft; (C) epiphyseal fractures; and (D) basal fractures

TUFT FRACTURES

Whether the fracture is single or comminuted, there is generally very little displacement. The injuries are often compound and soft tissue damage may be severe. In these cases, soft tissue repair and prevention of infection takes precedence over the bony injury. The fragments are usually stable within the surrounding periosteum and the dense fibrous bands that anchor the pulp to the bone. Unstable fractures are impossible to splint or fix because the fragments are so small.

With compound fractures, small widely separated fragments may be excised completely whilst performing a debridement of the wound. Care must be taken however not to remove too much bone as this will result in a loss of support to the nail bed with subsequent disturbance in nail growth. I do not think it is at all warranted to open a non-compound fracture in order to remove a widely splayed fragment.

However, tuft fractures usually unite without complication (Smith & Rider 1935). Widely splayed fragments may result in some cosmetic disfigurement of the finger tip. Very occasionally a fragment may not unite, but no treatment is required. Haematoma formation within the pulp or beneath the nail may lead to a build-up of pressure and produce severe pain. These haematomata should be drained immediately to give relief of symptoms. Drainage can be effective up to 48 h following the injury.

FRACTURES OF THE SHAFT

These fractures are usually minimally displaced. In addition, because of the paucity of subcutaneous tissue and the nature of the injury, the fractures are often compound. They are generally the result of a crush injury in an industrial or domestic situation.

Fixation

Fractures of the shaft may be comminuted, transverse, oblique or longitudinal. Irrespective of the type of fracture, any significant displacement should be reduced. If the fracture is stable following reduction, no treatment other than splinting the injured digit to a neighbouring digit is indicated. On the other hand, if it remains unstable some form of fixation is necessary. In my experience this is most easily and effectively achieved by the use of Kirschner wires (Fig. 1.2). Usually a single longitudinal wire will suffice. With midshaft fractures it is not necessary to immobilize the distal interphalangeal joint. Fractures close to the base cannot be stabilized without immobilizing the distal joint as well.

It is advisable to use a sturdy Kirschner wire. A thin wire is liable to be deflected volarly or dorsally by the wedge-shaped tip of the phalanx. Driving a Kirschner wire along the dorsal surface of the phalanx may result in damage to the root of the nail and subsequent distorted growth. Persistent wide separation of the fragments on X-ray should make one suspect the possibility of soft tissue interposition between the fragments; even the nail bed has been found to be entrapped between the fragments (Rockwood & Green 1984). This constitutes an indication for open reduction of the fracture and repair of the nail bed.

Comminuted and longitudinal fractures are

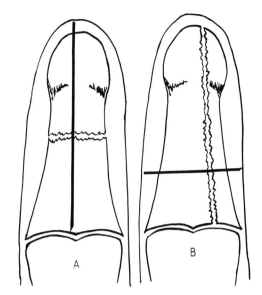

Fig. 1.2 (A) Internal fixation of transverse fracture of the shaft using a single longitudinal Kirschner wire. Note that the distal joint should not be immobilized and the wire may be cut short so that the end is buried. (B) Longitudinal fractures are fixed using a transverse Kirschner wire

more difficult to control. It may be impossible to achieve stability using a Kirschner wire. The only alternative is an external device such as a Stack mallet finger splint (Stack 1969) or an aluminium splint. Occasionally one may be obliged to accept a degree of instability but this should not affect the process of union.

Longitudinal fractures not infrequently extend through the joint surface at the base of the distal phalanx. As with all fractures involving joint surfaces, an attempt should be made to achieve perfect reduction. This can often be achieved by closed manipulation. The reduction may be maintained by inserting a transverse Kirschner wire. Usually one wire will suffice. Circlage wiring should not be used, as the insertion will damage the nail bed.

These fractures are usually sufficiently united to permit mobilization after three weeks.

As with fractures involving the tuft, repair of skin and nail bed is important and may take precedence over the treatment of the underlying fracture.

Skin defects are best covered by simple split-skin grafting. When a fracture is associated with loss of distal pulp tissue it may be impossible to get adequate skin cover. Under these circumstances a local flap (Fig. 1.3) may be useful to restore pliable yet durable skin, with sensation, to the tip of the digit (Biddulph 1979).

It is known that accurate repair of the nail bed at the time of the injury results in the least disturbance of subsequent nail growth (Zook et al 1984). It is therefore rewarding to spend time accurately piecing together a fragmented nail bed. When there has been actual tissue loss, the defect can be made up by taking a free graft of a nail bed from a toe. (Shepard 1983, Saito et al 1983). The nail, if available, should not be discarded. If completely detached it should be cleaned and replaced under the nail fold after repair of the nail bed has been accomplished. It may be necessary to remove a partially detached nail before repairing the nail bed. It should then be replaced. The nail bed should be repaired with 0/6 catgut.

Malunion

The effect of the profundus tendon on the unstable fracture is to produce volar angulation. Persistent

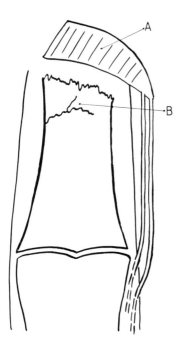

Fig. 1.3 Skin defects over the fractured bone (B) may be covered using a variety of flaps (A)

volar angulation will impart a drooping effect on the distal phalanx similar to a mallet finger deformity. Lateral angulation and splaying of the fragments will result in a broad or distorted nail. It is doubtful whether the cosmetic appearance warrants surgical correction.

Non-union

A small percentage of cases, usually of the transverse variety, result in non-union (Read 1982). A common cause is the interposition of soft tissues. Radiological evidence of union often lags many months behind sound clinical union. Therefore these cases are best assessed using clinical criteria such as the absence of pain and local tenderness.

Non-union leads to an unstable fingertip which prejudices the patient's pinch. Clinically the type of pinch resembles the unstable pinch seen in arthritis where the distal joint has been destroyed. In these cases open reduction, internal fixation and bone graft are indicated.

FRACTURES AT THE BASE

These fractures are almost invariably of the avulsion type. Occasionally a longitudinal fracture may involve the joint surface. An avulsion fracture is indicative of joint instability when a collateral ligament or volar plate is involved, and tendon imbalance when the extensor tendon is avulsed.

The most common fracture at the base is due to avulsion of the extensor tendon. This usually results from stubbing the finger as one does when receiving a hard ball. However, it can even follow such everyday activities as shaking hands or dressing. The fragment may vary from pin-head size to one which involves more than half of the articular surface. In the latter case, the distal interphalangeal joint may become unstable and permit volar subluxation (Fig. 1.4).

Lateral avulsion fragments are usually small and due to disruption of the collateral ligaments. Volar avulsion fragments may be associated with rupture of the volar plate which is attached to the base of the phalanx. As with extensor tendon avulsion, the size of fragment varies from very small up to one which involves half of the base. Joint instability

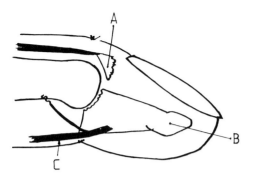

Fig. 1.4 Large dorsal avulsion fractures (A) may allow volar subluxation of the distal phalanx (B) by the Profundus tendon (C)

and dorsal subluxation may accompany large fractures (Fig. 1.5).

The profundus tendon attaches more distally along the shaft of the phalanx and is rarely associated with a fracture. The radiological position of the fragment left attached to a tendon serves as a useful guide to the degree of tendon retraction.

Treatment

It is of cardinal importance to diagnose any tendon or ligamentous disruption early.

Undisplaced fragments

Undisplaced fragments should be managed conservatively by adequate splinting for six weeks. An external device or a Kirschner wire introduced percutaneously can be used but the latter is preferred. It is important that the joint remain in extension at $0°$. Hyperextension of the distal interphalangeal joint may cause ischaemia of the dorsal skin surface and must be avoided.

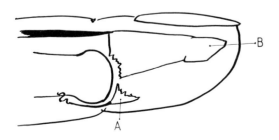

Fig. 1.5 Large volar avulsion fractures (A) may allow dorsal subluxation of the distal phalanx (B)

Small displaced fragments

Very small displaced fragments are best discarded (Fig. 1.6) and the associated extensor tendon, volar plate or collateral ligament re-inserted into the base of the distal phalanx. Any existing flexion or extension contracture of the joint must be corrected prior to repair of the tendon. This is generally achieved by physiotherapy or splintage but occasionally a surgical release may be necessary.

Large displaced fragments

Larger displaced fragments need accurate reduction because the articular surface is involved. If the joint is subluxed, it should be reduced before replacement of the avulsion fragment in its correct position.

In all cases, the joint should be stabilized in full extension at $0°$ using a longitudinal Kirschner wire (Fig. 1.7 & 1.8). The splintage should be main-

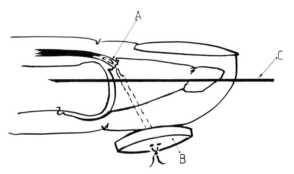

Fig. 1.6 Very small fragments may be discarded and the extensor tendon (A) reinserted into the distal phalanx. It is held in place by a pull-out suture tied over a button (B). The repair is protected for six weeks using a Kirschner wire (C)

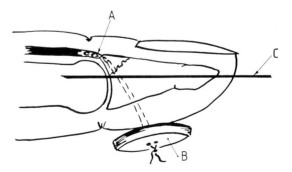

Fig. 1.7 Large dorsal fragments (A) should be accurately replaced and are most easily secured using a pull-out suture tied over a button (B). Any instability of the distal phalanx and the repair should be supported using a Kirschner wire (C)

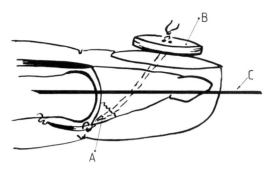

Fig. 1.8   Large volar fragments (A) should be accurately replaced and secured using a pull-out suture tied over a button (B). The repair is supported and any subluxation fixed by a Kirschner wire (C)

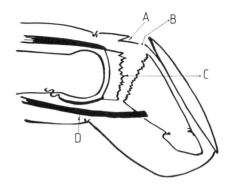

Fig. 1.9   Epiphyseal fractures (C) are most commonly volarly angulated by the Profundus tendon (D). These fractures are often compound through the nail bed (B) after the nail has been avulsed from under the nail fold (A)

tained for six weeks following which gentle mobilization should be commenced. When the joint has been grossly distorted, for example by a depressed basal fracture, it would be more economical to perform a primary arthrodesis of the joint in a straight position.

EPIPHYSEAL FRACTURES

These fractures obviously only occur in the young, prior to fusion of the epiphysis. The type of injury is usually a blunt crush and the lesion falls into Salter's Group II (Salter & Harris 1963). Neither fractures with minimal displacement nor those that are angulated volarly are usually accompanied by severe soft tissue injury. On the other hand, severe dorsally angulated fractures are frequently compound through the nail bed (Fig. 1.9). The nail is avulsed from its bed in its posterior third, the root being pulled out from under the cuticle (Barton 1979).

Management consists of thorough cleansing of the wound and reduction of the dorsally angulated

fracture. The nail bed should be accurately repaired in the older child, but in the very young patient it is not necessary. The nail should never be discarded but replaced under the nail fold to provide stability for the fracture (Seymour 1966). If necessary, additional stability may be provided by use of a Kirschner wire (Fig. 1.10), though this is seldom required. The fracture is usually sufficiently healed after 4 weeks to allow removal of the Kirschner wire.

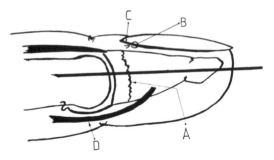

Fig. 1.10   Treatment of epiphyseal fractures consists of the reduction of the fracture (A), accurate repair of the nail bed (B) and replacement of the nail under the nail fold (C). Occasionally, as shown here, a Kirschner wire may be needed to provide stability

REFERENCES

Barton N J 1979 Fractures of the phalanges of the hand in children. The Hand 2:134–143
Biddulph S L 1979 The neurovascular flap in finger tip injuries. The Hand 2:59–63

Read L 1982 Non-union in a fracture of the shaft of the distal phalanx. The Hand 14:85–88
Rockwood C A, Green D P 1984 Fractures in Adults, 2nd ed. J B Lippincott, Philadelphia, p 317

Saito H, Suzuki Y, Fujino K, Jajima T 1983 Free nail bed graft for treatment of nail bed injuries of the hand. Journal of Hand Surgery 8:171–178

Salter R B, Harris W R 1963 Injuries involving the epiphyseal plate. The Journal of Bone and Joint Surgery 45A:587–622

Seymour N 1966 Juxta-epiphyseal fracture of the terminal phalanx of the finger. The Journal of Bone and Joint Surgery 48B:347–349

Shepard G H 1983 Treatment of nail bed avulsions with split-thickness nail bed grafts. Journal of Hand Surgery 8:49–54

Smith F L, Rider D L 1935 A study of the healing of one hundred consecutive phalangeal fractures. Journal of Bone and Joint Surgery 17:91–109

Stack H G 1969 Mallet finger. The Hand 1:83–99

Zook E G, Roxanne J G, Russell R C 1984 A study of nail bed injuries. Causes, treatment and prognosis. Journal of Hand Surgery 9A:247–252

2

Epiphyseal fractures

INTRODUCTION

Epiphyseal fractures comprise a significant proportion of fractures in the paediatric hand. Barton (1979 & 1984) reported a 28.7% incidence of epiphyseal fractures in his series of 454 phalangeal fractures. More specifically in the children, Leonard and Dubravcik (1970) reported a 41% incidence of epiphyseal fractures in their series of 263 paediatric phalangeal fractures. Hastings and Simmons (1984) have indicated epiphyseal injuries of the hand occur 34% more commonly than elsewhere in the skeleton.

Appropriate treatment of most of these epiphyseal fractures produces good functional results, but effective treatment is dependent on a thorough knowledge of the developmental and functional anatomy, fracture patterns, and the pitfalls of specific methods of treatment.

DEVELOPMENTAL ANATOMY

The phalanges, like the long bones of the child, have epiphyses located at both the proximal and distal ends (Ogden 1982). However, unlike the long bones, only one epiphysis in each phalanx forms a secondary ossification centre. In the phalanges, this secondary ossification centre forms at the proximal epiphysis of each phalanx. The majority of the longitudinal growth occurs at this end of the phalanx. In contrast, the secondary ossification centre in the metacarpals forms distally, except in the thumb where it is proximal. In both the phalanges and metacarpals, at the end opposite the secondary ossification centre, the epiphyseal

cartilage is rapidly replaced by endochondral ossification until only a thin layer of cartilage exists. This layer comprises articular cartilage, germinal epiphyseal cartilage, and a slow-growing, spherical physis that contributes little to longitudinal growth but allows continued hemispherical growth of the end of the bone as the joint enlarges (Ogden 1984).

In boys, secondary ossification in the epiphysis of the *proximal phalanx* begins at 15 to 24 months and the epiphysis fuses with the shaft at 16 years. In girls, it starts at 10 to 15 months and fuses at 14 years.

The secondary ossification centres of the *middle and distal phalangeal* epiphyses appear six to eight months later and fuse to the shaft at the same time as those of the proximal phalanx (Greulich & Pyle 1959). The epiphyses of the phalanges of the little finger appear significantly later than those of the index, middle, and ring fingers (O'Brien 1984). In some individuals the epiphyses may remain open for longer, and they can thus fracture through the closing epiphysis (Fig. 2.1) up to the age of 17 (Hastings & Simmons 1984).

FUNCTIONAL ANATOMY

Knowledge of the tendinous and ligamentous anatomy of the phalanges is important in understanding the varied patterns of epiphyseal fractures and planning proper treatment. In the metacarpophalangeal joint (MCP) of the finger, the cord portion or true collateral ligament takes origin from the metacarpal epiphysis and inserts directly into the epiphysis of the proximal phalanx. The fan portion or accessory collateral ligament

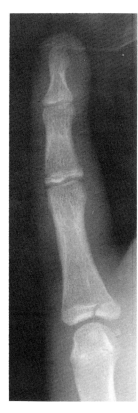

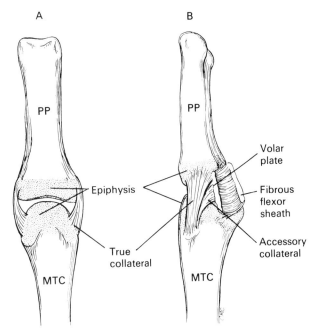

Fig. 2.2 Ligamentous anatomy of the metacarpophalangeal joint. (A) dorsal view. (B) lateral view

Fig. 2.1 Radiograph shows a 17-year-old male who suffered a fracture through a closing epiphysis of the proximal phalanx

inserts into the lateral edge of the volar plate. In maximum flexion, the collateral ligaments are under the greatest length and tension because of the eccentric origin of the ligament on the metacarpal and the flare of the metacarpal head, producing a cam effect. The volar plate is only loosely attached to both the metacarpal and phalangeal epiphyses and is quite mobile, allowing lateral laxity and some hyperextension of the MCP joint (Fig. 2.2).

The ligamentous anatomy in the proximal interphalangeal (PIP) joint is quite different. The PIP joint is a hinge joint without significant lateral motion. The cord portion of the collateral ligament inserts not only into the epiphysis of the middle phalanx but also into the periosteum of the metaphysis. The volar plate is less mobile and is firmly attached to the base (epiphysis) of the middle phalanx (Fig. 2.3). The attachment of the volar plate to the proximal phalanx, however, is

loose, allowing the volar plate to fold on itself like an accordion. The collateral ligaments of the PIP joints are under greatest tension (length) in approximately 15° of flexion when the fibres are tented over the lateral aspect of the condyle of the proximal phalanx. This is the best position for immobilization of this joint. Immobilization of the PIP joint in excessive flexion results in contracture of the checkrein ligament of the volar plate, often leading to a fixed flexion contracture (Watson et al 1979).

The extensor tendon insertion of the central slip and terminal band is into the epiphyses of the dorsal aspect of the middle and distal phalanges respectively as shown in Figure 2.3. The flexor digitorum superficialis and the flexor digitorum profundus tendons insert into the volar surfaces of the middle and distal phalanges, respectively, just distal to the physis (Fig. 2.3A).

Variability in the insertions of the collateral ligaments, volar plate, and flexor and extensor tendons of the MCP and PIP joints explains several clinical observations. Salter-Harris Type III (Salter & Harris 1963) (see Fig. 2.4) physeal fractures are seen most commonly in the proximal phalanx and less commonly involve the middle or distal

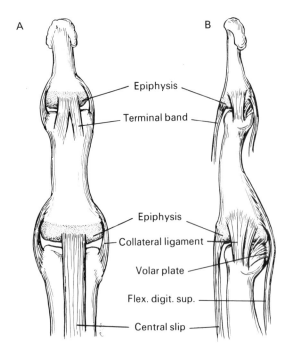

Fig. 2.3 Ligamentous and tendinous anatomy of the proximal and distal interphalangeal joints. (A) dorsal view. (B) lateral view

phalanx. These fractures in the proximal phalanx are usually avulsions of the collateral ligaments and are orientated sagittally; these fractures in the middle and distal phalanges are usually avulsions of either the volar plate or extensor mechanism insertion and are oriented coronally. Furthermore, the difference in the level of insertion between the extensor and flexor tendon into the distal and middle phalanx accounts for the characteristic flexion deformities seen with the Salter-Harris Type I or II (Salter & Harris 1963) physeal fractures of these bones. The significance of these anatomical relationships and their role in epiphyseal fractures of the phalanges will be elaborated in the discussion of specific fractures.

GENERAL CONSIDERATIONS

Incidence

Epiphyseal fractures of the phalanges occur most commonly during adolescence and more often in boys (Barton 1979, Hastings & Simmons 1984).

However, Barton found that this male predominance applied only in older children. In his series of 130 epiphyseal fractures, 73 fractures occurred in children 11 years of age or younger; of these 45 were girls and 28 boys. Of 57 fractures in children 12 years of age or older, 47 were in boys and only 10 in girls. Most authors (Hastings & Simmons 1984; Leonard & Dubravcik 1970) report equal involvement of the right and left hands, but closer analysis of epiphyseal fractures of the phalanges only may indicate some predominance of the right hand (Barton 1979), especially in injuries caused by falling onto the outstretched hand.

The little finger and thumb were most commonly fractured and are associated with more fracture displacement in the series of Hastings and Simmons (1984). However, Leonard and Dubravcik (1970), while agreeing that it is most commonly the little finger that is involved, found the thumb to be the least commonly involved digit. The ring and middle fingers are next most commonly fractured and the index finger least. In general, when the central digits are involved, the fractures are less displaced and easier to treat (Hastings & Simmons 1984).

Salter–Harris Type II (Salter & Harris 1963) fractures are the most common epiphyseal fractures; Types III and IV are less common, and Types I and V the least common (Fig. 2.4). The proximal phalanx is involved twice as often as either the middle or distal phalanx. Fractures of the distal phalanx are slightly more common than fractures of the middle phalanx.

In adults, industrial accidents account for the majority of phalangeal fractures (O'Brien 1984). In children, falls, crushing injuries, and direct blows account for most of the epiphyseal injuries of the phalanges. In Barton's series (1979) of 130 epiphyseal fractures, falls accounted for 48% of fractures; crushing injuries, 16% (predominantly in toddlers and caused by doors or gates); and direct blows for 14% of fractures. In Hastings and Simmons's series (1984) of 354 paediatric hand fractures, torque and angulation forces accounted for 34% of fractures; crush injuries, 21%; direct blows, 10%; and axial compression, 9.5% of fractions. In general, angular and rotatory deformities resulting from torque or angulation forces were seen more proximally in the digit, whereas

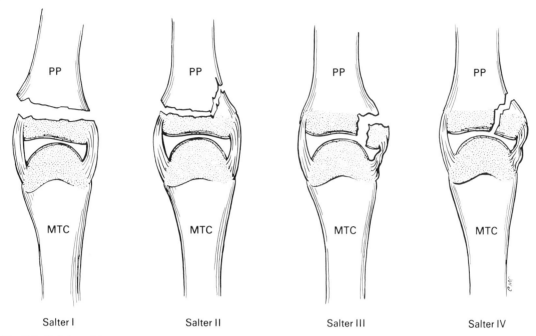

Salter I   Salter II   Salter III   Salter IV

Fig. 2.4 Epiphyseal fractures of the proximal phalanx showing Salter classification of fracture type

crush injuries predominantly involved the distal end of the digit.

Clinical and radiographic evaluation

A thorough, detailed, and systematic clinical examination should precede radiographic evaluation and should be correlated with the mechanism of injury whenever possible. Swelling, ecchymosis, and deformity are the most common findings. Bony tenderness and tenderness over the collateral ligaments (especially the origin and insertion) is often helpful diagnostically. In younger children, co-operation is usually more difficult, but persistent limitation of motion of the joint or digit usually implies significant injury. A local anaesthetic is often helpful before testing stability of the interphalangeal and metacarpophalangeal joints, which should be tested in both flexion and extension. Excessive hyperextension of the joint indicates injury to the volar plate. Collateral ligament and volar plate injuries associated with epiphyseal fractures are common following dislocations of the interphalangeal and metacarpophalangeal joints. Simple dislocations in the absence of epiphyseal fractures are extremely rare in children.

Postero-anterior and lateral X-rays are essential to evaluate epiphyseal fractures. Oblique X-rays can be particularly useful in evaluating subtle or intra-articular fractures. The most common pitfall in treating epiphyseal fractures of the phalanges is failure to obtain a true lateral X-ray of the injured finger due to overlap of the adjacent fingers. Tomograms may occasionally be necessary, particularly with epiphyseal fractures of the proximal phalanx. Stress views can be useful in differentiating ligamentous instability from instability due to epiphyseal fracture.

Several non-traumatic entities may be confused with trauma to the phalangeal epiphyses. Kirner's deformity is a spontaneous palmar and radial curving of the terminal phalanx of the little finger observed between the ages of 8 and 14 years (Dykes 1978). Differentiation of Kirner's deformity from trauma is made by the clubbed appearance of the affected finger, the narrowed and curved appearance of the diaphysis, and the bilaterality of the deformity (O'Brien 1984). Frostbite and other ischaemic insults to the digit can result in necrosis of the physis and epiphysis of the digits. Angulation and lateral growth deformities can occur and are associated with premature closure of the physis.

Thiemann's disease (osteochondrosis of the epiphysis of the phalanges) is a rare, hereditary entity characterized by narrowing and fragmentation of the epiphysis predominantly of the middle and distal phalanges (Cullen 1970). Resolution of Thiemann's disease and healing of the phalanx is the rule, but permanent joint deformity can occur.

Principles of treatment

The primary focus in the treatment of epiphyseal injuries is usually the fracture, and more subtle and significant soft tissue injuries may be overlooked. Both open and closed injuries must be examined for injury to adjacent tendons, nerves, and blood vessels.

The majority of paediatric hand fractures can be treated by closed methods, but immobilization of a child's hand can be challenging. Well-fitted plaster casts or splints are the best treatment for older children but are more difficult to apply and can be dangerous in a younger child in whom bulky, soft dressings may provide more appropriate immobilization. Skin or skeletal traction is rarely indicated. Splints or casts should be applied in the 'intrinsic plus' position to maintain maximum length of the collateral ligaments and to prevent extension or flexion contractures of the MCP and PIP joints. Immobilization of a single digit in a child has been associated with an increased incidence of angulation and rotational deformity and should be avoided.

Immobilization with or without closed reduction is satisfactory for the majority of closed epiphyseal fractures of the phalanges. Open reduction is sometimes necessary for displaced intra-articular fractures (Salter-Harris Type III and IV) unable to be satisfactorily reduced by closed methods, and is often useful in the treatment of open injuries. In Leonard and Dubravcik's (1970) series of 263 phalangeal fractures in children, 75% were treated by simple external immobilization, 15% by closed reduction under anaesthesia followed by external immobilization, and 10% required open reduction and internal fixation. Hastings and Simmons (1984) were able to treat 80% of their children's hand fractures by external immobilization alone. Bora et al (1976) required K-wire fixation for 20% of their epiphyseal fractures in the hand. However,

Barton (1979) suggested this may not have been necessary in all cases.

Regional or general anaesthesia is usually necessary to achieve a satisfactory closed or open reduction of displaced fractures. Either digital block or ulnar and median nerve blocks at the wrist, depending on the location of the fracture, may be appropriate. More extensive nerve blocks are difficult in children, and general anaesthesia may be necessary in younger children.

Immobilization for three weeks following closed reduction of epiphyseal fractures is usually satisfactory and can often be shortened to two weeks for younger children. Open reduction has, however, been associated with diminished blood supply to the fracture fragments and may contribute to delayed healing. In this situation, immobilization for six weeks has been recommended (Leonard & Dubravcik 1970). This may be true for diaphyseal fractures but rarely is more than three weeks' immobilization required for epiphyseal fractures of the phalanges (Salter & Harris 1963).

Pulvertaft (1966) has stated that hand fractures which unite with angulation '... will usually correct with growth provided the angulation is in the same plane as the joint movement. Where angulation is in the opposite plane, i.e., ulnar or radial deviation or rotational, the malposition will persist.' Barton (1979), however, has pointed out that most epiphyseal fractures of the phalanges occur at the base of the proximal phalanx close to the metacarpophalangeal joint which is not a true hinge but allows some side-to-side movement. Epiphyseal fractures in this location will remodel to some extent in both the flexion/extension and radial/ulnar planes. Most authors (Barton 1979; Hastings & Simmons 1984; Jones & Jupiter 1985; Leonard & Dubravcik 1970; O'Brien 1984) agree that rotational deformities do not spontaneously correct and are associated with the most significant functional impairments. Careful attention to rotatory alignment in the splint is mandatory to prevent rotational deformity and is best assessed by studying the planes of the fingernails, comparing the injured digit to the adjacent normal fingers and to the orientation of the corresponding digit orientation in the opposite hand. Malrotation of the thumb is more difficult to assess but is less important to correct during treatment (Ogden 1982).

Formal and supervised rehabilitation is rarely required following the closed treatment of epiphyseal fractures of the phalanges. Physical and/or occupational therapy is usually reserved for those fractures requiring open reduction or associated with significant soft tissue injuries. Dynamic and static splinting can be useful adjuncts in the management of these more difficult fractures, and an appropriate programme of rehabilitation should be planned for each individual.

Residual deformity is the most common complication of children's hand fractures. In Hastings and Simmon's series (1984), malunion was most often associated with failure to obtain adequate true postero-anterior and lateral radiographs of the individual digits, failure to check rotational alignment of the injured finger after reduction in a position of full flexion, and was based on the sometimes erroneous assumption that growth would correct a deficient reduction. Displaced intra-articular fractures (Salter–Harris Type III and IV), Salter–Harris Type I distal phalangeal fractures (due to crushing injuries), and open fractures were especially prone to residual deformity and produced the majority of the poor functional results (Hastings & Simmons 1984).

EPIPHYSEAL FRACTURES OF THE DISTAL PHALANX

Epiphyseal fractures of the distal phalanx can result from either crush injuries or hyperflexion forces applied to the end of the digit.

Crush injuries

Crush injuries more commonly involve the younger child, and the fractures are often comminuted. Longitudinal split fractures often result in a bifid distal phalanx (cloven hoof fracture) which is of little clinical significance. Significant soft tissue injuries including 'bursting' skin lacerations and nail-bed injuries are frequent. The majority of these injuries are open fractures and require irrigation and cleansing with appropriate debridement, prior to the reduction and splinting. Sutures should be used sparingly and only to reapproximate loose skin flaps. Nail-bed injuries should be

meticulously repaired with a 6/0 chromic or polydioxanone suture (PDS; Ethicon) using magnification. Only sufficient nail should be removed to allow repair of the nail bed. The eponychial fold should be splinted with petroleum gauze, silastic, or the removed nail.

Hyperflexion injuries

Fractures resulting from hyperflexion injuries occur most commonly in the pre-adolescent or adolescent, and the fracture pattern varies depending on the child's age (Fig. 2.5).

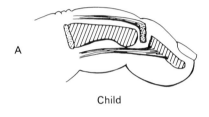

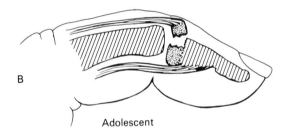

Fig. 2.5 Hyperflexion injuries to the distal phalanx epiphysis vary with age. (A) shows a child, (B) shows an adolescent

Pre-adolescent injury

In the pre-adolescent injury, the fracture is usually an open Salter-Harris Type I or II and is commonly mistaken for an open dislocation of the distal interphalangeal joint. In this injury, the epiphysis with its extensor insertion remains extended while the remainder of the phalanx is acutely flexed by the unopposed pull of the flexor profundus tendon. The displaced metaphysis protrudes dorsally, avulsing the nail from its proximal nail bed at the level of the eponychial fold (Fig. 2.6A). Seymour (1966) called attention to the temptation to remove the partially avulsed nail. In his series, six patients

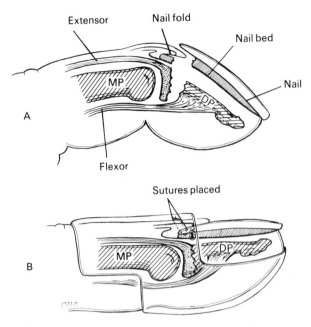

Fig. 2.6 Seymour fracture with nail-bed avulsion (A) and maintenance of the reduction by preservation of the nail (B)

had the nail removed, and difficulty in maintaining the reduction of the distal phalanx was often encountered. Three of these six patients developed infections of the nail bed. However, the meticulous repair of the nail-bed laceration, replacement of the nail under the proximal nail fold, after irrigation, and application of a slight hyperextension force to the distal phalanx by a volar splint for 2 weeks was successful in maintaining a good reduction in all his other patients (Fi.g 2.6B). He felt that Kirschner wire fixation was unnecessary, and three of the five cases in his series treated with Kirschner wires became infected, one infection necessitating amputation of the finger. Infection can be particularly devastating in this fracture, and Enger and Glancy (1978) have pointed out that infection will often result in further damage to both the nail bed and the growth plate. If infection occurs, the detached nail should then be removed, the wound debrided and irrigated, the fracture splinted, and the patient treated with appropriate antibiotics. Pollen (1973) believes leaving the nail predisposes to infection and recommends its removal. Barton (1979) found results from the treatment of this fracture were only fair because of persistent mallet deformity.

Adolescent injury

In the adolescent hyperflexion injury, the fracture is usually a Salter–Harris Type III (avulsion of the extensor insertion) and is a true mallet finger fracture (Fig. 2.7A). Application of a hyperextension splint will often allow satisfactory reduction of the fracture. Splinting is required for 3–4 weeks. If an anatomical reduction cannot be achieved by closed manipulation then open reduction and Kirschner wire fixation may be necessary. Curtis (personal communication) has advocated more aggressive open reduction (Fig. 2.7B) of these fractures to minimize dorsal deformity (bump) and extensor lag, but Wehbé and Schneider (1984) reported no difference in the incidence of dorsal deformity, functional impairment, or union rate between surgical and closed (splint) treatment. However, mallet-type epiphyseal fractures with volar subluxation of the distal phalanx should be treated by open reduction and Kirschner wire fixation.

EPIPHYSEAL FRACTIONS OF THE MIDDLE PHALANX

The middle phalanx is the least common of the phalanges to be fractured. Once fractured, however, the resulting deformities are easily explained by the musculotendinous forces acting at this level (*see* Fig. 2.8). The central slip inserts into the epiphysis dorsally, whereas the flexor digitorum superficialis tendon inserts volarly along the shaft distal to the epiphysis. The volar plate of the PIP joint is securely attached to the epiphysis, and the insertion of the collateral ligaments of the PIP joint extends distal to the epiphysis onto the metaphysis.

Salter–Harris *Type II* and, less commonly, *Type I* fractures usually result from excessive extension or flexion deformities that would cause a dislocation in the adult. Characteristically, the central slip extends the epiphysis and proximal phalanx, while the flexor superficialis flexes the distal fragment producing angulation convex dorsally of the fragments (Fig. 2.8A). These fractures may be missed in the young child. They must be reduced and splinted in complete extension (Fig. 2.8B); 3 weeks of immobilization is usually adequate.

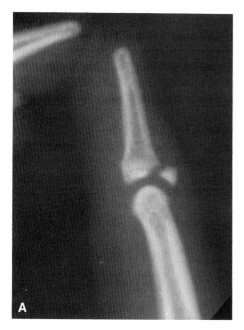
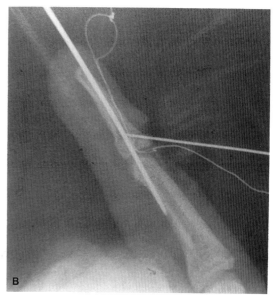

Fig. 2.7 Adolescent type hyperflexion injury to epiphysis of distal phalanx. Before (A) and after (B) open reduction

Blair and Marcus (1981) have described a Salter–Harris Type II fracture of the middle phalanx with a condylar fracture of the proximal phalanx and dorsal extrusion of the entire PIP joint. Open reduction achieved a satisfactory result.

Hyperflexion injuries of the PIP joint may result in a *Type III* avulsion fracture of the central extensor tendon insertion (Fig. 2.8C). Associated disruption of the triangular ligament and volar subluxation of the lateral bands can produce a typical boutonniere deformity. Volar Salter–Harris Type III injuries occur from hyperextension injuries and avulsion of the insertion of the volar plate (Fig. 2.8D). Dorsal Type III injuries should be immobilized in extension. If satisfactory reduction is not obtained, open reduction and Kirschner wire fixation may be necessary. Volar Type III fractures are best treated in an extension block

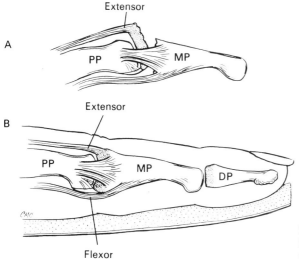
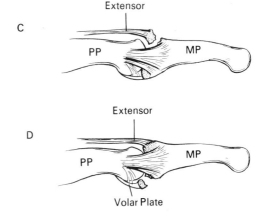

Fig. 2.8 Epiphyseal fractures of the middle phalanx and immobilization of a Salter–Harris Type I fracture in extension (A–D)

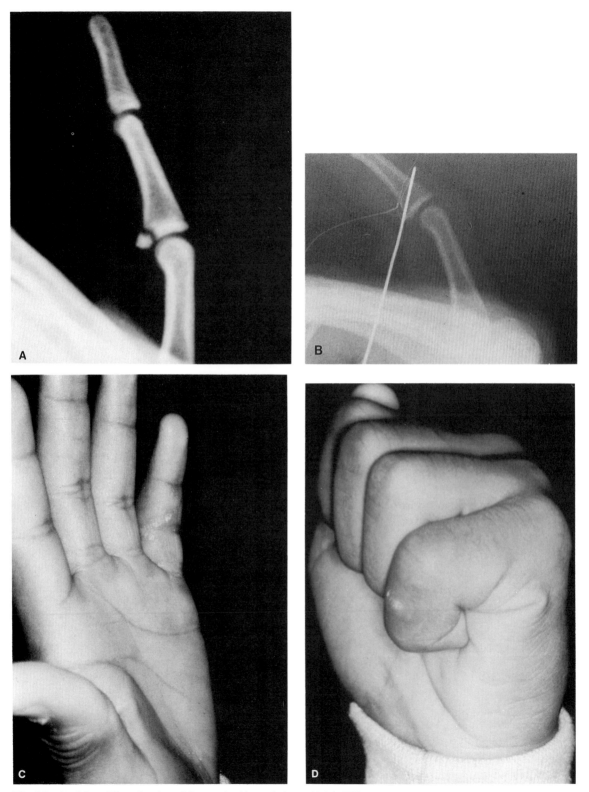

Fig. 2.9 Avulsion of the volar plate of the proximal interphalangeal joint (PIP) requiring open reduction (A & B) with final PIP joint range of motion (C & D)

splint to allow reattachment of the volar plate and preserve PIP joint motion. Open reduction and Kirschner wire fixation may be required for either volar Type III injuries or for dorsal injuries (Fig. 2.9A–D). Radial or ulnar Salter–Harris Type III fractures of the middle phalanx are uncommon due to extension of the collateral ligament insertion onto the metaphysis.

Simple dislocations (with no fracture) of the PIP joint are extremely rare in children. Dislocations combined with epiphyseal fractures do occur and are best treated by closed reduction of the dislocation and appropriate treatment of the epiphyseal fracture. Jones and Jupiter (1985) have reported an irreducible palmar dislocation of the PIP joint associated with an epiphyseal fracture of the middle phalanx.

EPIPHYSEAL FRACTURES OF THE PROXIMAL PHALANX

The proximal phalanx is the most common site of epiphyseal fractures in the hand.

Type II fractures

Salter–Harris Type II fractures (*see* Fig. 2.4A) are the most frequent; they result from twisting or hyperextension forces and most commonly affect the little and ring fingers and the thumb. This type of fracture often leaves not only the classic Thurston-Holland metaphyseal fragment attached to the epiphysis but also a transverse plate of the metaphyseal subcondylar bone (Werenskiold fragment).

Rang (1983) has coined the term *extra octave fracture* for the common Salter–Harris Type II fracture of the little finger with ulnar deviation (Fig. 2.10). Closed reduction will usually correct the rotational and angular malalignment. However, problems with this specific fracture occur because the epiphysis lies proximal to the web space and it is difficult to get purchase on the proximal fragment while manipulating the distal fragment.

Wood (1976) and Sandzen (1979) have advocated the use of a pencil between the fingers, as a fulcrum over which the diaphysis can be levered

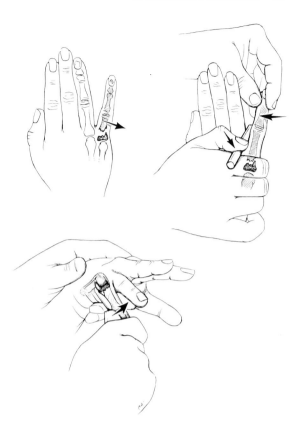

Fig. 2.10 'Extra-octave' fracture showing two methods of reduction

(Fig. 2.10). Green (1977) and Rang (1983) have advocated flexing the metacarpophalangeal joint to stabilize the proximal fragment by tightening the collateral ligaments and then abducting and rotating the finger to correct the angulation and rotation deformities (Fig. 2.10). The little finger should then be strapped to the ring finger, and protection of the reduction in an ulnar gutter splint for 3 weeks is usually sufficient. These fractures tend to drift and become redisplaced due to the pull of the abductor digiti minimi muscle. Irreducible fractures requiring open reduction have been encountered occasionally, due to fibrous tissue or flexor tendon interposition between the fracture fragments (Cowan & Kronick 1975).

Type III fractures

Salter-Harris Type III physeal fractures of the proximal phalanx represent ligamentous avulsions due to the exclusively bony insertions of the collateral ligaments into the epiphysis. They result from abduction or adduction stress on the digit and, although they are frequently displaced, joint stability is rarely compromised (O'Brien 1984). Treatment usually consists of strapping the injured finger to the bordering, uninjured finger. If closed treatment fails to achieve an anatomical reduction, open reduction and Kirschner wire fixation may be necessary.

Type IV fractures

Salter–Harris Type IV fractures of the proximal phalanx are quite rare; Barton (1979) reported only two cases in his series of 203 phalangeal fractures. They occur in older children and result from a combination of longitudinal compression and rotation forces.

Impacted fractures of the proximal phalanx

Coonrad and Pohlman (1969) have reported 41 children with impacted fractures of the proximal third of the proximal phalanx, often involving the epiphysis. These basal fractures tend to occur in older children and angulate towards the palm due to flexion of the proximal fragment by the intrinsic muscles and shortening by axial pull of the extrinsic

extensors. If the displaced or angulated fracture is allowed to heal in $22°$ or more angulation, the extensor tendon and its expansion over the proximal phalanx became shortened preventing full flexion. Furthermore, the altered and relatively elongated course of the flexor tendons around the increased angle at the fracture site further limits flexion and prevents full extension. The most common cause of an angular deformity in this fracture is immobilization of the digit in insufficient flexion at the MCP and PIP joints. This is one of the few indications for the immobilization of the PIP joint in flexion. A true lateral X-ray is mandatory to assess accurately the presence of angulation. If an angular malunion occurs, an opening wedge osteotomy of the proximal phalanx can correct the deformity and resultant functional limitations. In younger children, since angulation occurs in the plane of motion of the joint, significant remodelling can occur.

CONCLUSION

Epiphyseal fractures of the phalanges present many unique problems, but careful attention to detail is rewarded by good functional and cosmetic results. A thorough understanding of the functional and developmental anatomy allows rational treatment and will prevent many of the deformities which occur with these sometimes difficult fractures.

REFERENCES

Barton N J 1979 Fractures of the phalanges of the hand in children. Hand 11(2):134–143
Barton N J 1984 Fractures of the hand. Journal of Bone and Joint Surgery 66B:159–167
Blair W F, Marcus N A 1981 Extrusion of the proximal interphalangeal joint: a case report. Journal of Hand Surgery 6:146–147
Bora F W, Ignatius P, Nissembaum M 1976 The treatment of epiphyseal fractures in the hand. Journal of Bone and Joint Surgery 58A:286–291
Bora F W, Nissenbaum M, Ignatius P 1976 The treatment of epiphyseal fractures of the hand. Orthopaedic Digest 5:11–17
Coonrad R W, Pohlman M H 1969 Impacted fractures in the proximal portion of the proximal phalanx of the finger. Journal of Bone and Joint Surgery 51A:1291–1296
Cowan N J, Kronick A D 1975 An irreducible juxtaepiphyseal fracture of the proximal phalanx. Clinical Orthopaedics and Related Research 110:42–3

Cullen J C 1970 Thiemann's disease. Osteochondrosis juvenilis of the basal epiphyses of the phalanges of the hand. Report of two cases. Journal of Bone and Joint Surgery 52B:532–534
Dykes R G 1978 Kirner's deformity of the little finger. Journal of Bone and Joint Surgery 60B:58–60
Enger W D, Glancy W G 1978 Traumatic avulsion of the fingernail associated with injury to the phalangeal epiphyseal plate. Journal of Bone and Joint Surgery 60A:713
Green D P 1977 Hand injuries in children. Pediatric Clinics of North America 24:903–918
Greulich W W, Pyle S I 1959 Atlas of bone growth. Stanford University Press, Stanford
Hastings H, Simmons B P 1984 Hand fractures in children. Clinical Orthopaedics and Related Research 188:120–130
Jones N F, Jupiter J B 1985 Irreducible palmar dislocation of the PIP joint associated with an epiphyseal fracture of the middle phalanx. Journal of Hand Surgery 10A:261–267
Leonard M H, Dubravcik P 1970 Management of fractured

fingers in the child. Clinical Orthopaedics and Related Research 73:160–168

O'Brien E T 1984 Fracture of the hand and wrist region. In: Rockwood C A, Wilkins K E, King R E (eds) Fractures in children, J B Lippincott Company, Philadelphia

Ogden J A 1982 Skeletal injury in the child. Lea and Febiger, Philadelphia

Ogden J A 1984 Uniqueness of growing bones in fractures in children. In: Rockwood C A, Wilkins K E, King R E (eds) Fractures in children, J B Lippincott Company, Philadelphia

Pollen A G 1973 Fractures and dislocations in children. Williams and Wilkins, Baltimore

Pulvertaft R G 1966 Internal fixation in the treatment of hand fractures. Proceedings of the Second Hand Club Meeting, pp 385–388 (published in 1975 by The British Society for Surgery of the Hand)

Rang M 1983 Children's fractures. J B Lippincott Company, Philadelphia

Salter R B, Harris W R 1963 Injuries involving the epiphyseal plate. Journal of Bone and Joint Surgery 45A:587–622

Sandzen S C 1979 Atlas of wrist and hand fractures. PSG Publishers, Littleton, Massachusetts

Seymour N 1966 Juxta-epiphyseal fracture of the terminal phalanx of the finger. Journal of Bone and Joint Surgery 48B:347–349

Watson H K, Light T R, Johnson T R 1979 Checkrein resection for flexion contracture of the middle joint. Journal of Hand Surgery 4:67–71

Wehbé M A, Schneider L H 1984 Mallet fractures. Journal of Bone and Joint Surgery 66A:658–669

Wood V E 1976 Fractures of the Hand in Children. Orthopaedic Clinics of North America 7:527–542

J. I. P. James

3 Fractures of the shafts of the phalanges: conservative treatment

INTRODUCTION

Fractures of the phalanges are very common. Over two decades, more than 2000 patients were seen with this injury at the Hand Clinic at the Royal Infirmary, Edinburgh. A number of these involved the articular ends of the phalanges and their management lies outside this chapter's ambit. However a majority of this common fracture involve the shaft.

Most fractures of the phalanges are the result of industrial injuries, the usual mechanism being crushing and trapping of fingers in machinery with considerable force. A smaller number occur from traffic accidents. As one would expect from these sources, a very large majority occur in men.

Though essentially simple, their treatment needs meticulous attention to detail to obtain a good functional result. To restore full function to the hand of a highly trained man who has suffered this injury demands all the skills of even the most experienced hand surgeon. Though in recent years it has improved, it must be said that too often the outcome of their care in a casualty department or in a general orthopaedic clinic is a tremendous loss of function and working skill. This becomes clear if the subsequent evaluation of hand function is detailed, prolonged and skilful; frequently, because of a lack of trained evaluation, it is not realized how poor the average result is. There are few injuries which are commonly treated as badly as finger fractures. However, this should no longer be accepted as there are efficient methods which can be relied upon to give good results.

There are several reasons for this unsatisfactory state of affairs. Primarily it is because the difficulties are not appreciated, so that often these injuries are left to junior casualty officers and others with no training or experience in dealing with a type of injury which can tax the most experienced hand surgeon.

Whereas metacarpal fractures rarely cause difficulty, even when incorrectly treated, there is no such margin of safety in the finger. The metacarpals support each other and are sheathed by interosseous muscles, whereas the fractured finger is unstable, with no supporting soft tissues. Minor degrees of malalignment or malrotation are common and may be serious as they can cause great loss of function. The soft tissue in the finger, tendon, nerve, artery and skin are very vulnerable to injury at the same time as the fracture, a complication of peculiar difficulty. Finally, the metacarpophalangeal and interphalangeal joints lose function with extraordinary speed, as the result of what might seem to be minor errors and omissions. Elsewhere in the body, such minor errors of detail would not matter overmuch, but in the hand they inevitably cause loss of function. The prevention of joint stiffness is indeed the most important factor in the care of these injuries and will be discussed very fully later.

TYPES OF FRACTURE

These shaft fractures can be classified by their position in the phalanx (base, mid-shaft or neck), by the shape of the fracture (transverse, spiral, oblique or comminuted), or by which phalanx is affected. More than one finger may be involved and they may each have different types of injury. The displacement of the transverse mid-shaft fracture is an extreme forward angulation, almost at right angles. This is obvious clinically; but in transverse basal fractures an almost equal forward angulation can easily be missed: clinically because of the dorsal soft tissue swelling and radiologically because of the difficulty of taking satisfactory lateral radiographs of the four fingers and of interpreting them (Fig. 3.1). Oblique fractures are prone to lateral deviation and shortening. Spiral fractures are frequently rotated.

The majority of phalangeal shaft fractures are closed injuries but because of the minimal soft-tissue covering they are also quite often compound, with marked soiling of the bones and remaining soft-tissue. In cutting and crushing injuries, damage to digital nerves, arteries, extensor and flexor tendons can be a major complication. These structures must be carefully examined when the patient is first seen.

Though the treatment of the soft tissue injury is not the subject of this chapter, a comment is indicated. When the injury is compound, routine excision of the wound is indicated to prevent infection. Closure is made more difficult by the inelasticity of the skin; there is none to spare. Skin excision must therefore be minimal. Primary closure may be contraindicated if there is more than minimal swelling and this may have to be delayed or require split-skin grafting. Damage to vessels, nerves and tendons may add up to an indication for amputation. This is determined by the soft-tissue injuries; the fracture is rarely a factor in such a decision unless there is gross loss of phalangeal shaft substance.

Fractures of the shafts of the proximal and middle phalanges

The proximal and middle phalanges are usually injured by similar mechanisms and may present similar problems (Lamb 1981) but this is dependent upon whether the fracture is basal, mid-shaft or the neck. The way in which the bone breaks depends upon the injuring force, particularly whether it is direct or indirect. There are three typical patterns of fracture: transverse, oblique, or spiral (Fig. 3.2), and each has somewhat different problems of treatment. In addition, there is a further group consisting of comminuted fractures, which are considered in Chapter 8.

Transverse fractures

These usually occur in the mid-shaft and show a typical forward angulation which may be almost $90°$ (Fig. 3.3). The periosteum is intact on the concavity of the fracture and this periosteal hinge facilitates and guides reduction by closed methods. As already noted, the proximal phalanx, when transversely fractured near the base, may have marked angulation, yet this is easily overlooked (Coonrad & Pohlman 1969).

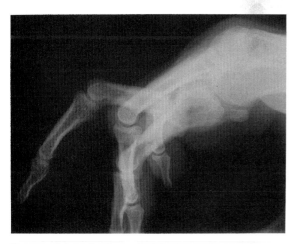

Fig. 3.1 A lateral radiograph of the fingers showing the difficulty of seeing a basal shaft fracture though it may be markedly angulated. In this case, there is such a fracture with about $50°$ of angulation convex forwards

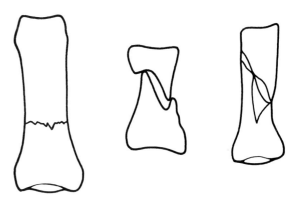

Fig. 3.2 Tracings of X-ray films showing typical patterns of fracture of the shafts of the phalanges: left to right, transverse, oblique, spiral

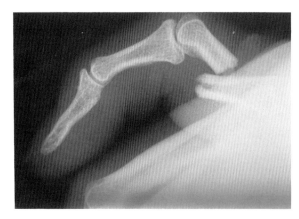

Fig. 3.3 A displaced transverse fracture with marked displacement and angulation convex forwards

Oblique fractures

Caused by an angulatory force, these often split the condyles and may allow shortening. The degree of shortening is partly dependent on the degree of soft tissue injury, particularly of the periosteum.

Spiral fractures

Caused by a rotational force, these are not usually displaced far, though they may be malrotated. The lack of displacement is a consequence of the minimal periosteal damage in this type of injury.

Fracture of the shaft of the distal phalanx

These are rarely significantly displaced but often grossly comminuted from a crushing injury. In general terms, shaft fractures of this phalanx cause no problems; the difficulties all arise from the associated soft tissue injuries of the pulp. Fractures of the distal phalanx are discussed in more detail in Chapter 1.

TREATMENT

Stable phalangeal fractures

Surprisingly, many phalangeal fractures are undisplaced, stable, and require neither reduction nor

splintage. The essential reason for stability is an intact periosteum. This is seen in fissure fractures from direct injury (Fig. 3.4). Transverse fractures with little or no displacement are also often stable (Fig. 3.5) and oblique and spiral frequently so. Some experience is required to recognize these injuries, but something like 30–40% of phalangeal fractures do not need reduction and splintage (James 1962a & b).

However, though reduction and splintage of the fracture is not necessary in these cases, the patient does require treatment. Mobilization is the third component of fracture treatment and its neglect

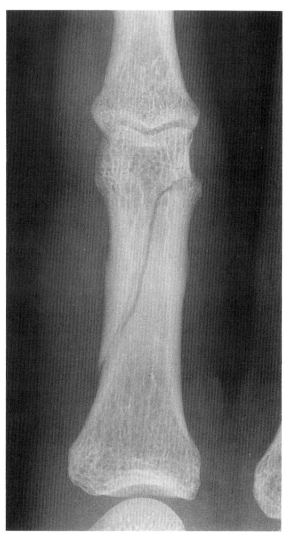

Fig. 3.4 Undisplaced fissure fracture. This is a stable fracture and does not need to be immobilized

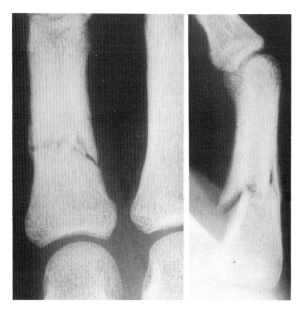

Fig. 3.5 This fracture, essentially transverse and with little displacement, was stable. It was treated by early mobilization and, as can be seen, united satisfactorily without any increase in deformity

can lead to catastrophic and permanent stiffness, even in minor injuries of the fingers. In this sense, there are no 'minor' injuries of the hand; even the most trivial-seeming injury can cause severe permanent disability if treated wrongly or neglected (Borgeskov 1967).

Although correct splintage of the fingers for up to 3 weeks probably causes minimum harm, in practice, in the majority of casualty departments and sadly in many orthopaedic clinics, splints are *not* applied correctly and cause immense problems from stiffness and contractures, both usually permanent. Splints which are not essential should always be avoided.

It is essential to encourage active movement of the interphalangeal and metacarpophalangeal joints from the beginning (James & Wright 1966) and to advise the patient against resting it or using a bandage or finger-stall. Mobilization should at first be supervised and is conducted by the methods detailed later. However, in the majority of these cases there is no loss of function even in the first week or two. If in doubt of the stability, the injured finger can be strapped to a normal digit (Fig. 3.6), and put through a full range.

Unstable fractures

In general, these shaft fractures present no difficulty in reduction if treated within a few hours. Delay beyond 12–24 hours causes many of these fractures to be irreducible because of the induration caused by haemorrhage and oedema. This is the main reason why open reduction is sometimes necessary. However, if delay is avoided, most cases can be treated by closed methods.

Closed reduction

Though local anaesthesia can be used, it is somewhat unsatisfactory in producing complete analgesia; because the amount of fluid in the finger is increased, reduction is made more difficult and the circulation might even be threatened. Light general anaesthesia is ideal, as also is local anaesthesia distal to a tourniquet: the Bier technique.

Transverse fractures. When anaesthesia is complete, the finger is gently manipulated with slight traction and flexion of the distal digit beyond the fracture (Mansoor 1969). The periosteal hinge permits and guides full correction but checks movement beyond this point. Reduction is generally complete (Fig. 3.7). The finger is then splinted.

Spiral fractures. The main deformity is rotatory though this may be complicated by angulatory deformity. The fracture is usually stable and easy to reduce by reversing the rotation which tightens the periosteum. Reduction is followed by splintage.

Oblique fractures. These are the most difficult to reduce closed (Lamphier 1957) but if fresh the angulatory deformity can often be corrected with ease. It is splinted whilst trying to force it into over-correction. The periosteal hinge will not permit excessive correction but stretching the periosteum to its full length overcomes shortening which is the main problem.

Conclusion. In summary, therefore, reduction of all three types of shaft fracture consists of reversing the direction of injury and using the intact periosteal hinge as the mechanism by which reduction is controlled. In transverse fractures correction of the $90°$ anterior angulation by gentle longitudinal traction and then flexing the distal fragment to align it with the proximal fragment is both easy and successful. Spiral fractures are

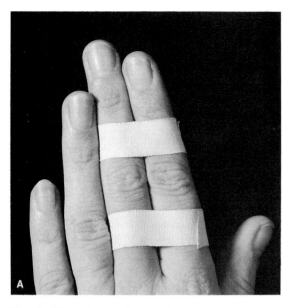 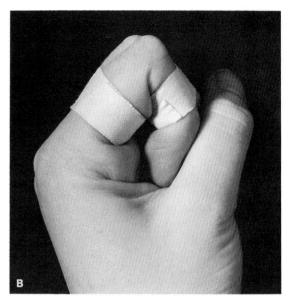

Fig. 3.6 These photographs show the method of strapping an injured finger to its normal neighbour which allows full movement. The strapping should go round the centres of the phalanges (A) and leave the joints free (B). (If any material is placed between the fingers to absorb sweat, it must be soft and flexible so that it does not restrict movements at all.)

reduced by reversing the direction of rotational injury to correct malrotation of the distal fragment rotation and checking that it has been corrected by looking at the nail. Overcorrection is prevented by the intact periosteum. Oblique fractures may be difficult unless treated very early but, if angulation and shortening are corrected by longitudinal

traction, they are often stable, though shortening may recur and require internal fixation.

Splintage

Splintage must hold the reduced fractured phalanx straight. The usual splint is an aluminium strip. The commercial pattern is too soft and the patient can bend and straighten it. Either a thicker metal strip must be used or the edges of the commercial strip turned over to make it rigid. The splint is applied to the volar surface of the finger after reduction, and fixed with adhesive strips as shown in Figure 3.8. For stable middle phalangeal fractures, the splint may be applied to the volar surface of the finger, not extending to the palm. In proximal phalangeal fractures it must include the metacarpophalangeal joint and palm but should not cross the wrist, because if it does the splint will be pushed up and down during wrist movement. The pulp and nail must always be visible. The nail is the sole visible guide also as to whether there is rotational deformity. In addition, the colour of the pulp-tip and nail show whether circulation is impaired, as it may be.

Whilst the function of the splint is to keep the

Fig. 3.7 Radiographs showing transverse fracture of the shaft of the middle phalanx after reduction and splintage. The position of the fracture is excellent but the PIP joint is unacceptably flexed

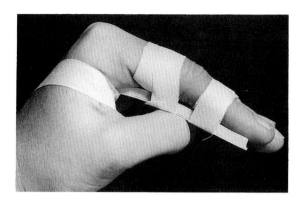

Fig. 3.8 A fractured finger correctly positioned on an aluminium splint, with the MCP joint flexed and the interphalangeal joints straight. The fingertip is left uncovered so that it can be inspected end-on to check that rotation is correct.

fracture reduced and immobilize the finger, the position in which the finger is splinted is a factor of supreme importance in the avoidance of stiffness, the most common and serious consequence of a finger fracture. The position to be used is determined by the peculiar properties of the finger-joints when immobilized. Each has a position of safety and also a position of danger, the latter will almost invariably lead to stiffness that is often irreversible.

The metacarpophalangeal joint. The metacarpophalangeal (MCP) joint is extremely sensitive to incorrect positioning. Its dangerous position is in *extension* (Koch 1935). If this joint is splinted straight for as little as 2 weeks it can become permanently stiffened, causing much loss of function of the hand. The anatomical reason for this is clear. The antero-posterior diameter of the metacarpal head is greater than its height. In extension the collateral ligament is relaxed and takes up a sinuous shape; in flexion it is stretched taut. The anatomical purposes are to permit abduction and adduction of the fingers at the MCP joint of the open hand and to give a firm base to the fingers in the flexed, cupped hand.

If the MCP joint is immobilized in extension the ligament relaxes and becomes inelastic; also, in the injured or dependent hand, oedema accumulates around the ligament which soon becomes infiltrated with fibroblasts and then becomes fixed in that position so that it is too short to flex over the metacarpal head. There is then an extension contracture, often virtually complete, causing effective ankylosis of the joint.

The proximal interphalangeal joint. If this joint is held flexed for as little as three weeks, or even less when there is haemorrage and oedema from a fracture, there will be a permanent flexion contracture which is likely to be irreversible, however treated. It is essential to prevent this and the anatomical reason for its development must be understood (Fig. 3.9). The collateral ligament is taut in both flexion and extension to retain lateral stability of the finger in all positions and does not become shortened when held in flexion. The anterior palmar plate is attached proximally by a thin membrane and in contracted fingers it can be shown not to be the cause of contracture as its division does not relieve the condition. However, anterior to the collateral ligament, but posterior to the palmar plate there is a small ligamentous structure, the accessory collateral ligament (Kuczynski 1968). It is this which becomes shortened in the contracted interphalangeal joint. A flexion contracture of the interphalangeal joint is the constant danger in an immobilized finger and must be prevented by splinting the interphalangeal joints in *full* extension. *Flexion* is the position of danger. Stiffness in extension can occur due to the extensor expansion becoming adherent to the fracture site, but is rare and can often be relieved by vigorous flexion exercises when the fracture has healed.

Distal interphalangeal joint. The distal interphalangeal joint should be splinted in almost full extension. It may become stiff in either extension or flexion, but as it is used in extension or near this position, some loss of flexion is not very disabling. In contrast, a flexion contracture is very disabling.

It is clear, therefore, that splinting must maintain the phalangeal fracture in alignment and correct rotation, with the interphalangeal joints extended fully and the metacarpophalangeal joint flexed to $90°$ or near that position (James 1970). This is easily achieved using an aluminium splint (*see* Fig. 3.8). It must be remembered that the metacarpophalangeal joint is at the level of the distal palmar crease and the right-angle bend of the splint must be applied at this point, not more distally as is all too common. If positioned distally, it will cause the exact opposite of the desired

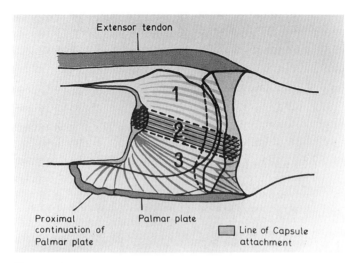

Fig. 3.9 Schematic representation of the ligamentous anatomy of the proximal interphalangeal joint. The components of the lateral capsule are 1: the upper area, 2: the collateral ligament and 3: the accessory collateral ligament, where most contracture occurs

position (Fig. 3.10) and lead to contractures which may well be permanent.

Although the safe position can be held for several weeks without danger, 3 weeks is sufficient for phalangeal fractures to unite enough for mobilization to be allowed after this time (Wright 1968). Callus may not be visible in the radiograph at this time, but the fracture is rigid on examination.

In multiple finger fractures, and in those associated with severe skin and soft tissue damage, splinting may be difficult. An excellent alternative is the 'boxing glove' bandage of the hand in which the hand is bandaged over fluffed gauze with the interphalangeal joints extended, the metacarpophalangeal flexed and the thumb abducted to keep the first web space stretched. The term 'boxing glove bandage', though frequently used, needs some clarification. When the bandage is finished it does bear a resemblance, perhaps somewhat fanciful, to a boxing glove (Fig. 3.11b). However, within it, the thumb is abducted and the interphalangeal joints extended: the opposite of their positions in a true boxing glove.

This bandaging is invaluable in many hand injuries and procedures. It not only holds the hand in the correct position but gently compresses it, preventing or reducing oedema and haemorrhage, the arch-enemies of hand function.

Although the bandage is an essential part of the treatment of many injured hands, it is not easy to learn how to do it correctly. It is so important that the surgeon should apply it himself. The hand is held upright by an assistant's hand on the forearm. With the wrist in about 20° dorsiflexion, the thumb

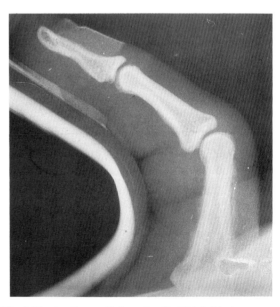

Fig. 3.10 A splint applied too distally. This holds the metacarpophalangeal joint extended and the interphalangeal joint flexed: just what is *not* wanted

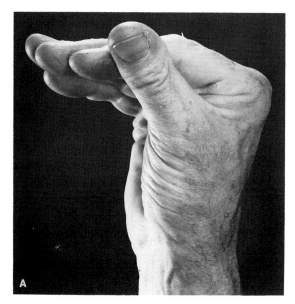
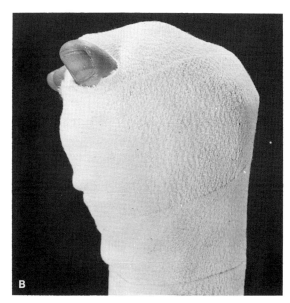

Fig. 3.11   The position of the hand before bandaging (A). The completed 'boxing-glove' bandage (B)

is widely abducted, the metacarpophalangeal joints flexed to 90° and the interphalangeal joints fully extended (Fig. 3.11A). Fluffed gauze is placed in the palm to fill the concavity; an adequate quantity is important. The hand and wrist are then wrapped in soft plaster wool (such as Orthoband) while maintaining the position. Finally it is bandaged firmly but not tightly with a crepe bandage still maintaining the position of thumb and fingers (*see* Fig. 3.11B). The finger tips are left exposed. If the wrist is kept extended and the palm well filled the bandage will be correct. The bandaged hand can be suspended to further control oedema.

Reduction and maintenance of reduction in phalangeal fractures must be meticulous. The criteria are much more rigorous than in other bones. If there is lateral or medial angulation or malrotation (Fig. 3.12), then on flexion the damaged finger will cross over and overlie or underlie one of the other fingers, grossly interfering with making a fist or grasping an object in the palm. As the flexor tendon glides within the fibrous flexor sheath, the posterior wall of which is the periosteum of the phalanx, malalignment or incomplete apposition may seriously impair or even totally prevent finger flexion. In addition to these errors of reduction and immobilization, stiffness of joints from failure to hold rigorously the safe

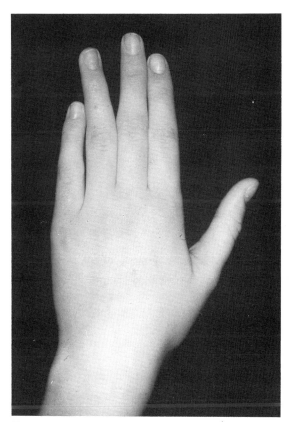

Fig. 3.12   Rotary malunion after a fracture of the proximal phalanx. At the time of reduction, the fingers must be inspected end-on to check rotation

causes serious loss of function in many injured fingers. When the whole hand is immobilized incorrectly, not a rare occurrence, stiffness of uninjured fingers is often seen.

Conservative management of phalangeal shaft fractures is appropriate for the great majority of these injuries. This emphasis on the value of closed management is because it is nearly always easy and successful, whereas most hand surgeons have found open reduction and fixation difficult and often followed by stiffness. However, malposition of these fractures cannot be accepted, because the late correction of malunion of phalangeal fractures is notoriously more difficult and frequently unsuccessful.

Therefore, if the position of the fracture proves irreducible by closed methods or is subsequently lost or the patient seen late, open correction and/or internal fixation is essential. These procedures are described in Chapters 5 and 6.

Mobilization and rehabilitation

The ever-present difficulty in the management of fractures of the phalanges is stiffness of the hand and unceasing care and meticulous attention to detail are essential if acceptable results are to be obtained. If the methods outlined here have been observed, in particular the correct positioning of the joints when splinted or bandaged, difficulties will be minimal. If treatment has been less skilled and there are flexion contractures of the proximal interphalangeal joints or extension contractures of the metacarpophalangeal joints, restoration of function will be difficult, prolonged and often ineffective. An additional adverse factor is the presence of severe soft tissue trauma with haemorrhage.

The well-managed hand

At the end of three weeks of splintage the fracture will be clinically united and ready for active movement. The metacarpophalangeal joint which has been held in $90°$ of flexion will extend and flex through a full range almost immediately. The interphalangeal joints may have limited flexion because of adhesions between the extensor tendons and the periosteum and subcutaneous tissues. On the flexor aspect, the tendons may be adherent within the sheath at the site of fracture or over a wide area because of haemorrhage. The surgeon must show the patient how to hold the metacarpophalangeal joint straight and immobile using his other hand and then to carry out active flexion at the interphalangeal joints. This must be done for some 5–10 minutes every hour, if the patient requires it, initially under the supervision of a physiotherapist trained in the management of hands. Within a week, the patient should attempt physical work and soon after he should be persuaded to do the hardest physical labour he can find to do. 'Massaging' the indurated hand by gripping the handle of a fork, spade or hammer and using it is the best possible treatment. Rehabilitation is completed by an early return to work. With this regime the hand which has been well managed from the beginning will be normal in 6 months or less. There is little improvement after this time.

The neglected hand

This is a totally different problem, requiring very prolonged treatment and with frequently disappointing results. At first, the main problem is likely to be that the interphalangeal or metacarpophalangeal joints are stiff, and probably contracted (Fig. 3.13). The problem may be complicated by malunion. At 3 weeks it is essential to remove all dressings, if possible, and all splints. The patient is taught an intensive programme of active finger exercises which he does at home for 10 minutes in each hour every day. These concentrate on metacarpophalangeal flexion and interphalangeal extension and flexion. In some cases the shoulder will have been allowed to stiffen and this too is actively mobilized. Active and hard manual work is resumed as early as possible and is probably the single most important element in the recovery.

Injured hands of this type are often indurated. The soft tissues have been distended with blood from haemorrhages and with oedema, and by this

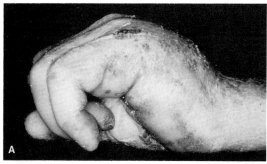

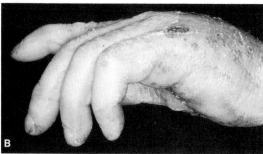

Fig. 3.13 A minor injury (note the healed laceration) was incorrectly bandaged for 10 days. On attempting flexion (A) the metacarpophalangeal joints only flex some 20°–30°. On extension (B) there is a 40° interphalangeal joint contracture. The thumb was also adducted. The hand is oedematous. (The patient was admitted, the hand elevated and hourly exercises maintained. He recovered function except for the interphalangeal joint contracture which showed no change. This is the typical result of erroneous positioning, a serious problem in this man even though the error was corrected after 10 days.)

stage there is an ingrowth of fibroblasts into these fluid exudates. Early compression bandaging, elevation and (best of all) active exercises are used to prevent these; in the later stages they are used in an attempt to get rid of the oedema and prevent recurrence, but by then they are frequently ineffective.

It is tempting to manipulate stiff and contracted finger joints but this must *never* be done. The consequent tearing of adhesions and soft tissue always makes these joints worse.

In the late stage knuckle-duster splints with an elastic band may occasionally help the stiff, extended metacarpophalangeal joints. The safety pin or Capener splint may be used in an attempt to overcome interphalangeal joint flexion contracture. When improvement with these measures has stopped, and it is often very limited, surgical excision of the contracted ligament is occasionally beneficial.

Fractures of the phalanges are one of the commonest injuries to the hand. Well managed treatment along the lines outlined in this chapter can give excellent and consistent results. Neglect of any detail, particularly joint position if the hand is immobilized, can result in an appallingly stiff hand and loss of skilled function.

There are no trivial injuries to the hand, least of all a fractured finger.

REFERENCES

Borgeskov S 1967 Conservative therapy for fractures of the phalanges and metacarpals. Acta Chirurgica Scandinavica 133:123–130

Coonrad R W, Pohlman M H 1969 Impacted fractures in the proximal portion of the proximal phalanx of the finger. Journal of Bone and Joint Surgery 51A:1291–1296

James J I P 1962a Fractures of the proximal and middle phalanges of the hand. Acta Orthopaedica Scandinavica 32:401–442

James J I P 1962b Common simple errors in the management of hand injuries. Proceedings of the Royal Society of Medicine 63:69–71

James J I P 1970 The assessement and management of the injured hand. Hand 2:97–105

James J I P, Wright T A 1966 Fractures of metacarpals and proximal and middle phalanges of the finger. Abstract, Journal of Bone and Joint Surgery 48B:181–182

Koch S 1935 Deformities of hand resulting from loss of joint function. Journal of the American Medical Association 104:30–35

Kuczynski K 1968 The proximal interphalangeal joint. Journal of Bone and Joint Surgery 50B:656–663

Lamb D W 1981 Fractures. In: Lamb D W, Kuczynski K (eds) The practice of hand surgery. Blackwell, Oxford, London, Edinburgh, pp 206–208

Lamphier T A 1957 Improper reduction of fractures of the proximal phalanges of fingers. American Journal of Surgery 94:926–930

Mansoor I A 1969 Fractures of the proximal phalanx of fingers: a method of reduction. Journal of Bone and Joint Surgery 51A:196–198

Wright T A 1968 Early mobilisation of fractures of the metacarpals and phalanges. Canadian Journal of Surgery 11:491–498.

4 Fractures of the shafts of the phalanges: treatment by functional bracing

INTRODUCTION

This chapter describes a system of functional bracing designed for the treatment of displaced fractures of the shaft of the proximal phalanx of the fingers. The method aims to retain reduction of the fracture while simultaneously allowing early active mobilization of the proximal interphalangeal (PIP) joint of the involved finger because it appeared to us that stiffness at the proximal interphalangeal joint remains the main residual impairment after correct conservative treatment of such fractures.

According to Barton (1979), fractures of the shaft of the proximal phalanx are amongst the most frequent fractures of the finger bones. In our in-patient orthopaedic department (Thomine et al 1981), they accounted for 40.6% of a series of 177 fractures of proximal and middle phalanges which we had to treat.

Problems in conventional treatment

It is well-known that malunion of such fractures can lead to functional impairment, but this can be avoided by correct reduction and retention. After conventional splinting, our own series showed that residual bone deformity was rare but there was a high incidence of severe stiffness of the PIP joint, though the metacarpophalangeal (MCP) joint remained normal. Likewise, James (1962) noticed that in 75 displaced fractures of the proximal (58 cases) and middle (17 cases) phalanx treated by reduction and plaster for only three weeks, some flexion contracture and loss of flexion at PIP level occurred in about three cases out of four. Although only one case out of four was compound, only one out of eight was associated with intra-articular injury, and only one out of 12 associated with tendon laceration. He found that 58 fingers developed PIP stiffness though only seven had appreciable malunion. In this series, splinting was done with 70° of flexion at MCP level and 20° at PIP level; James emphasizes that no contracture of MCP joint occurred, but that flexion contractures of PIP joint have been a continuing problem despite the decreased flexion used.

Although the severity of soft-tissue damage must influence the frequency of stiffness, there is nothing we can do about this. In contrast, we can vary the type and duration of splintage. Wright (1968) demonstrated that the duration of immobilization definitely influences function after phalangeal fractures, whatever the kind of injury sustained. He stated that, in crush fractures, immediate mobilization, when allowed by stability, ended in full function (including a full range of articular movement) in 77% of cases; but immobilization, even short, sharply decreased this percentage of good results to only 32.3% after three weeks of splinting. Even in less serious trauma, without crushing, good results decreased from 85% after mobilization to 68.8% with three weeks of immobilization. For both kinds of lesion, immobilization for longer than three weeks is correlated with significantly fewer good results (18.7% after crushing and 57.2% after non-crushing injuries).

Wright's statements have been fully confirmed in the specific field of proximal phalangeal shaft fractures in our own series. Review of 41 such lesions (excluding the thumb) treated conservatively with protracted immobilization for a mean of 50 days showed that less than one out of four fractured fingers regained a satisfactory range of movement at the PIP joint (i.e. full flexion and less than $30°$ lack of extension); only seven PIP joints regained full active motion and 17 did not reach the minimal useful range of between $30°$ and $70°$ (Thomine et al 1981).

In addition to this risk of stiffness, correct permanent reduction of displacement is mandatory to obtain a normal hand function. Fingers overlapping in grasp will occur as a consequence of malunion if there remains any malrotation or lateral inclination. Persistence of the characteristic dorsal angulation will simultaneously impair total active flexion of the involved finger and active extension of its PIP joint. Closed manipulation after passive flexion of the MCP joint usually achieves reduction of any deformity, but as stressed by Barton (1984) any fracture which has needed reduction will also need immobilization to maintain that reduction until it becomes stable. However secondary displacement remains frequent up to the end of the third week during conservative treatment; in our series about a quarter of them occurred between the 15th and the 20th day (Thomine et al 1981).

Finally, if early mobilization can prevent stiffness at the PIP joint, it can only be easily achieved in undisplaced or slightly displaced stable fractures. Displaced fractures need a time of immobilization which cannot be shorter than three weeks: that is, enough to allow adhesion to form, specially when the original injury involved direct trauma or had a crushing component.

It could be assumed that internal fixation is able to convert unstable fractures into stable ones and thus allow early mobilization, but most authors have been disappointed by the results of such procedures in fingers. Heim and Pfeiffer (1982), though they have advocated a rather extensive use of internal fixation in other hand fractures, state cautious and limited indications for open fixation for this kind of fracture. They also emphasize the technical difficulties which can be encountered in its realization. Osteosynthesis may be harmful to the soft-tissues and may itself contribute to stiffness, either by pinning soft-tissue to bone when percutaneous Kirschner wires are used or through the surgical scarring in open reduction with internal fixation of whatever type. This supplementary risk of adhesions cannot always be prevented by intensive physiotherapy care, even in the most skilled hands (Merle et al 1981).

Wide agreement appears to limit the use of oesteosynthesis to irreducible fractures and to those which are demonstrated as definitely unstable despite correct splinting.

THEORETICAL BASIS OF FUNCTIONAL BRACING

The technique we describe aims to reconcile the necessity of early mobilization as stressed by Wright, and that of correct retention of the bone fragments despite this mobilization (Thomine et al 1983).

In the main it is designed to treat displaced fractures of the proximal phalanx which have needed initial closed reduction; but this technique can also be useful to allow, at an early stage, a large range of active mobilization in less severe stable fractures, when pain or local consequences of direct trauma hinder spontaneous motion.

The two main principles of its realization are permanent full flexion of MCP joints and temporary non-surgical 'syndactylization' of all four fingers.

Fracture retention

Fracture retention is necessary to oppose any tendency of the fracture towards recurrent displacement that early mobilization might cause.

Retention in the sagittal plane

This method must resist the muscular imbalance and other forces that cause the usual backward bending deformity. Continued maintenance of the MCP joints in strong flexion acts against this deformity by slackening the intrinsic muscles. At the same time this position acts against stiffening of the MCP joints, as in the conventional splinting position (Fig. 4.1).

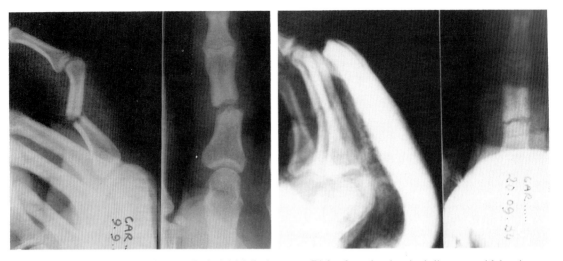

Fig. 4.1 Transverse mid-shaft fracture. Left: initial displacement. Right: frontal and sagittal alignment with bracing

Retention in the frontal plane

Frontal plane retention must oppose lateral and medial deviation of the distal fragment. Continuous 'syndactylization' of the adjacent fingers allows the adjacent sound diaphysis to act as a splint for the fractured diaphysis.

Axial stabilization

The aim of axial stabilization is to prevent rotational malunion which is the main cause of finger overlapping during flexion. It is easy to check at the start, with the fingers in extension, that the plane of the finger nail of the fractured finger is normally orientated by comparison with the opposite hand. Besides, 'syndactylization' with neighbouring fingers ensures that correct position will be maintained during active flexion; indeed when the PIP joints are flexed together, it automatically maintains a correct axial position by forcing the fractured finger to take part in the convergence of fingers which accompanies flexion.

Active mobilization

The principal purpose of functional bracing is to allow early active mobilization of the PIP joint of a fractured finger to the fullest possible extent. As stressed by James (1962), immobilization in flexion, even prolonged, of sound MCP joints does not result in stiffness. This fact has been confirmed by our retrospective study of fractures of the proximal phalanx treated by traditional methods (Thomine et al 1981).

If mobilization is restricted to early active motion of the PIP joint, there is a problem of muscular power. Indeed a discrepancy between the local soft-tissue resistances (aggravated by oedema) and the muscular forces disposable in the fractured finger exists, even before adhesions have formed; loss of active mobility after simple oedematous swelling of a sound finger is an everyday occurrence. 'Syndactylization' of the four fingers increases considerably the available strength by adding that of the sound fingers to that of the fractured fingers. It is thus possible to obtain assisted active mobility of the PIP joint involved over its entire range, as well as activation of the tendons of the injured finger. 'Syndactylization' particularly helps full extension (Fig. 4.2) which otherwise is difficult to achieve due to the relative weakness of the extensor mechanism.

To obtain this result it is necessary to put the mechanical axis of the four PIP joints into a single line; this alignment must be maintained by bracing since it does not exist in normal opening and closing movements of the hand.

Full flexion of the MCP joints suppresses the discordance between digital rays (due to inequality in the length of metacarpals) which appears in

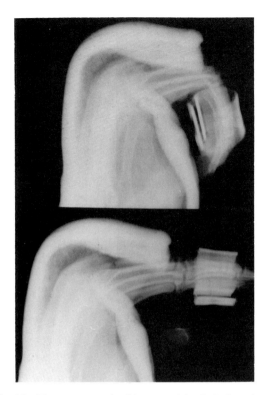

Fig. 4.2 Transverse proximal fracture of the shaft: lateral radiograph showing reduction maintained during active motion of PIP joints through an almost complete range of movement. (Note particularly the full active extension at the PIP joints.)

extension. In addition any difference in length between the proximal phalanges must also be compensated for. This can be eliminated by using the sagittal mobility of carpometacarpal joint. Flexion at the fourth and fifth carpometacarpal joints allows the PIP joints of the ring and little fingers to be advanced and in this way to be aligned with those of the index and middle fingers which are normally at almost the same level (Fig. 4.3).

PRACTICAL REALIZATION OF FUNCTIONAL BRACING

The bracing is done only after emergency reduction of the fracture by the usual manoeuvres.

It can be applied on the first day, or , more often, after some days of standard immobilization— valuable in relieving pain and eliminating oedema.

The brace is made of two plaster-of-paris splints, one palmar and the other dorsal, united by circular plaster bands. They have to provide stabilization of the wrist, retention of the metacarpal arch in the position that aligns PIP joints, and maintenance of the MCP joints in flexion.

Marked extension of the wrist (Fig. 4.4) appears necessary for several reasons. First, in order to help active flexion, it compensates for the slackening of the flexors caused by the flexion of MCP joints. Secondly, it compensates for the tension in the extensors resulting from the MCP joint flexion, which would otherwise be likely to restrict flexion at the PIP joint, especially in the index. Finally, this wrist position keeps the MCP joints from escaping into extension during efforts to extend the fingers, as has been seen when bracing has been made too straight. The MCP joints can thus be maintained at $90°$ flexion, providing both relaxation of interossei muscles and the possibility of aligning the axes of flexion of the four PIP joints.

Method of application

Extension of the wrist

Extension of the wrist is maintained by the palmar splint which comprises a short forearm segment and a palmar segment which *must* stop at the palmar flexion crease: this is essential to leave later flexion at the MCP joints entirely free. This section

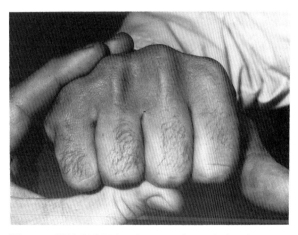

Fig. 4.3 With MCP joints flexed, flexion at the fourth and fifth carpometacarpal joints allows alignment of the axis of the PIP joints

is put in place first and while it is drying, the hollow of the metacarpal arch from flexion of the ulnar two carpometacarpal joints must be carefully preserved (Fig. 4.4).

Application of dorsal splint

The dorsal piece is then applied; it extends from the forearm to the heads of the proximal phalanges. While it is drying, the MCP joints are kept in $90°$ of flexion. It is moulded on the dorsal aspect of the metacarpals to keep the 4th and 5th metacarpals in flexion (Fig. 4.4). This will bring the PIP joints of all four fingers into line with each other.

Union of palmar and dorsal sections

Next, the palmar and dorsal pieces are united by circular bands of plaster around the palmar and forearm segment, the thumb column remaining free.

Bracing completion

Finally, the bracing is completed by 'syndactylization' of all four fingers using a malleable metal or plastic splint which is bent to form a tranverse loop around the fingers (Fig. 4.5). Its sponge-rubber covering protects the skin and prevents it

slipping out of place. It is placed distal to the PIP joints, the metallic splint for syndactylization encasing the middle phalanges and, if necessary in short fingers, the proximal part of the distal phalanges, but it should leave the pulp and nails free so their vascularization and orientation can be checked. It should not abut against the palmar plaster section during finger flexion because this would then be blocked.

After-care

With the functional brace in place, the patient can, without mechanical aids or physiotherapy, undertake active mobilization of the fingers, which will be the only physical therapy possible until the bracing is removed. The latter is continued until the stability of the fracture and the mobility of the fingers are satisfactory. This takes about 5 weeks. During this period, there must be both clinical and radiological supervision and readjustment of the brace if necessary. It is particularly important to check on the metacarpophalangeal flexion which can decrease as oedema decreases; a felt pad under the plaster covering the phalanges will restore the correct level of flexion at MCP joints.

Exact antero-posterior and lateral radiographs—with the beam perpendicular to the shafts of the proximal phalanges—has to be done weekly for the

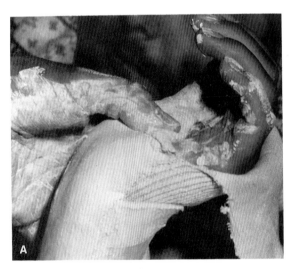
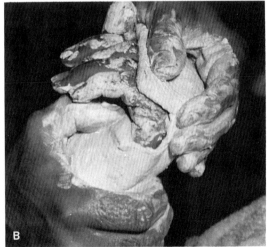

Fig. 4.4 Moulding of the plaster spints. (A): the volar part, put in place at first, maintains wrist extension. It must allow full flexion of MCP joints and flexion at carpometacarpal level. (B): the dorsal part covers proximal phalanges and maintains MCP joints flexion. Its moulding insures carpometacarpal flexion

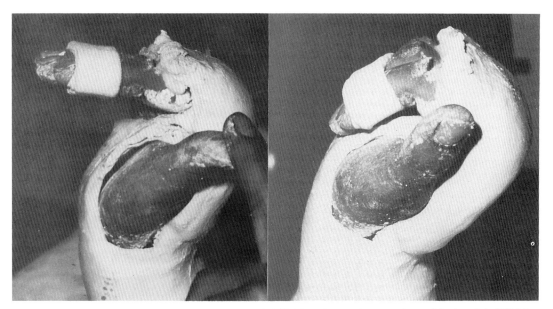

Fig. 4.5 'Syndactylization' of all four fingers distal to the PIP joint allows active extension and flexion of the PIP joints

first three weeks, after which time displacement is unusual.

After removal of bracing, final rehabilitation is left to spontaneous activity.

RESULTS OF FUNCTIONAL BRACING

Material

Among 24 fractures treated by functional bracing, 22 have a sufficient follow-up (35 days to 6 months) and will be considered.

There were 18 men and four women; their ages range from 19 to 69 years, so there are no children or teenagers in this series.

The finger involved was the index in nine, middle in six, ring in four and little in three, with no predominance of either hand.

There were 11 transverse or short oblique fractures (Fig. 4.6), eight long oblique fractures (Fig. 4.7) and three comminuted fractures (Fig. 4.8). Fractures of the base and neck of the phalanx and articular fractures of the head of the proximal phalanx were excluded.

Crushing injury was identified in nine cases. Seven fractures were compound and two of these were associated with a partial laceration of extensor tendon. In such cases, wound suture was performed before closed reduction, conventional splinting, and further bracing.

Four fractures were braced without preliminary reduction because they were only slightly displaced; in the remaining 18 cases, reduction was performed under regional or general anaesthesia. The shortest bracing time has been 21 days and the longest 80 days; the usual duration was about 45 days.

Results

No infection was observed. All fractures united but one refracture occurred at the 50th day; this nevertheless united without stiffness after new immobilization and bracing.

Anatomical results

Examples are illustrated in Figures 4.6, 4.7 and 4.8.

Residual deformity in the frontal plane was observed in five cases; in each it consisted of ulnar deviation which was 10° in two cases and less than 10° in three cases.

Residual deformity in the sagittal plane was observed in nine cases. One had united in 25° of volar flexion. In eight, some permanent backward

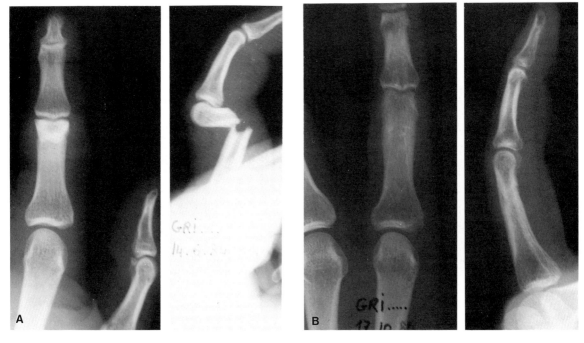

Fig. 4.6   Transverse distal fracture of index finger. (A): initial displacement. (B): appearance four months later, when the PIP joint had a range of motion from 10° to 100°

bending remained; it comprised between 10 and 15° in three patients and less than 10° in four. The recurrent fracture healed with about 25° of residual backward bending which did not prevent a normal range of motion at the PIP joint (0° to 90°).

Malrotation was observed in only one case; it was a 10° radial rotation which did not cause serious functional impairment. Figure 4.9 shows how the rotational deformity shown in Figure 4.7 has been corrected.

Range of motion

No stiffness at the MCP joint or distal interphalangeal joint was observed.

The criterion for assessment of the functional results has been the active mobility of the PIP joint at the end of the treatment. These results are presented in Table 4.1 and an example is shown in Fig. 4.9.

Loss of extension was observed in 16 cases but

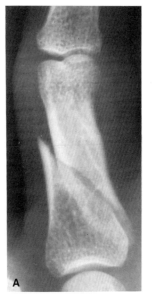
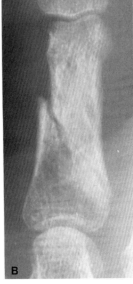

Fig. 4.7   Long oblique fracture of ring finger. (A): initial displacement. (B): immediately after removal of the cast-brace, the orientation of the phalangeal condyles shows correction of original rotational deformity

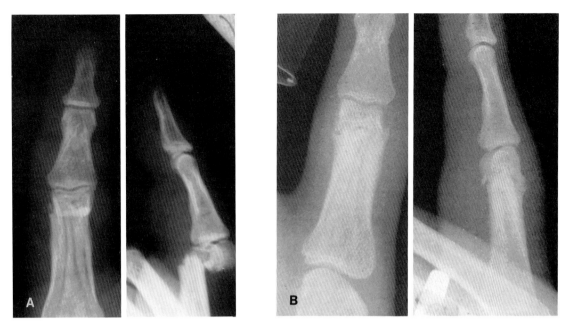

Fig. 4.8 Compound comminuted fracture of shaft of proximal phalanx of index finger. (A) : original displacement. (B) : Radiograph after $2\frac{1}{2}$ months, when PIP motion was between $0°$ and $80°$

Table 4.1 Active range of motion at PIP joint of fractured finger after functional bracing.

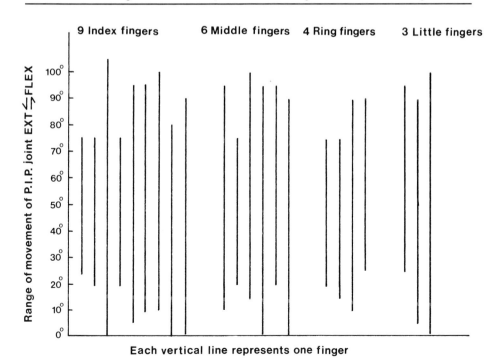

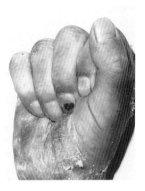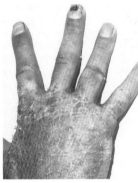

Fig. 4.9 This is the hand of the patient with the fracture of ring finger whose radiograph is shown in Figure 4.7. The picture is taken 43 days after the injury. The cast-brace has just been removed and the range of active movement is demonstrated. (Note also that there is no rotational deformity.)

was never more than $25°$ and was $10°$ or less in six cases.

Flexion was never less than $75°$ and reached $90°$ or more in 15 cases.

Using the criteria developed at the 1980 Symposium of the 'SOFCOT' on Finger Stiffness (De La Caffinière and Mansat 1981), the following results were recorded:

1. 12 cases were rated 'good' with a range of motion equal or superior to a sector beginning at $10°$ and going to $80°$;
2. 10 cases were rated 'fair' with a range of motion equal or superior to a sector beginning at $25°$ and going to $75°$; and
3. there were no 'bad' results, since all the PIP joints affected recovered at least a range of motion superior to the so-called 'useful' sector which begins at $30°$ and goes to $70°$.

CONCLUSION

The results found in the review of the present series show that, using this method, all cases regained more than the 'useful' mobility at the PIP joint.

Mobilization did not impede consolidation and only two significant malunions ($25°$ of backward bending and $25°$ of volar flexion) can be attributed to it.

Functional bracing requires attention to detail, but can be applied without special equipment or facilities, so may be a valuable aid in the treatment of proximal phalangeal fractures.

REFERENCES

Barton N J 1979 Fracture of the shaft of the phalanges of the hand. Hand 11:119–133
Barton N J 1984 Fractures of the hand. Journal of Bone and Joint Surgery 66B:159–167
Caffinière J Y De La, Mansat M 1981 Raideur post traumatique des doigts longs. Symposium à la 55ème réunion annuelle de la SOFCOT 1980. Revue de Chirurgie Orthopédique et Réparatrice de l'Appareil Locomoteur 67:515–571
Heim U, Pfeiffer K M 1982 Small fragment set manual. Springer Verlag, Berlin
James J I P 1962 Fractures of the proximal and middle phalanges of the fingers. Acta Orthopaedica Scandinavica 32:401–412

Merle M, Foucher G, Mole D, Michon J 1981 Résultats fonctionnels des fractures ostéosynthésées de la première phalange des doigts longs. Annales de Chirurgie 35:765–770
Thomine J M, Bendjeddou M S, Gibon Y, Biga N 1981 Les fractures diaphysaires de la première phalange. Résultats du traitement. Annales de Chirurgie 35:759–764
Thomine J M, Gibon Y, Bendjeddou M S, Biga N 1983 L'appareillage fonctionnel dans le traitement des fractures diaphysaires des phalanges proximales des quatre deniers doigts. Annales de Chirurgie de la Main 2(4):298–306
Wright T A 1968 Early mobilisation in fractures of the metacarpal and phalanges. Canadian Journal of Surgery 11:491–498

M. R. Belsky and R. G. Eaton

5

Fractures of the shafts of the phalanges: percutaneous wire fixation

Displaced shaft fractures of the phalanges and the metacarpals occur frequently. Successful treatment of these fractures provides excellent hand function in a high percentage of cases with a minimum of complications. Because these fractures are usually quite unstable, inadequate treatment may lead to persistent malrotation and angulation of the digit which can prevent the return of satisfactory hand function and appearance.

Closed reduction followed by percutaneous wire fixation is an effective technique in treating these fractures. It was described by Vom Saal in 1952 and has been the standard approach of the Roosevelt Hospital Hand Service in New York City since 1969. This technique has proved successful in a high percentage of cases in treating displaced shaft fractures of the phalanges (Belsky et al 1984). It has also been applied to fractures of the metacarpals with good results (Belsky & Eaton 1982).

Most shaft fractures will reduce using a satisfactory anaesthetic and longitudinal traction if treated within five days of the injury. Our method of anaesthesia, reduction of the fracture, placement of the wires, and postoperative care is described in this chapter.

TECHNIQUE

Wrist block anaesthesia

A wrist block provides excellent anaesthesia of the digits, while allowing the patient to move the fingers through a range of motion. This is the most sensitive method of assessing anatomical reduction and stability and of avoiding rotatory deformity.

The drug of choice for this block is 2% mepivacaine because of its rapid onset and duration of 2–4 hours. An appropriate combination of the four peripheral nerves at the wrist (median, ulnar, dorsal sensory branch of the ulnar, and superficial radial nerves) is blocked to anaesthetize the injured finger.

Wrist block anaesthesia can also be used for metacarpal fractures but there may be some discomfort as the wire reaches the base of the metacarpal.

Reduction of the displaced fracture

The proximal phalangeal fracture is reduced by applying gentle longitudinal traction on the finger with the joints in slight flexion. The remaining intact periosteum, the flexor sheath, and even the partially encircling extensor mechanism serve to guide the fragments back into anatomical position during the traction–flexion manoeuvre. Reduce any angular or rotational deformity.

Once the fracture is reduced, the finger is held still while a percutaneous wire is inserted to maintain reduction.

Percutaneous Kirschner wire fixation

The method of wiring involves passing Kirschner wires across the fracture. The wires may be directed either longitudinally or transversely (Fig. 5.1). The choice is determined by the type of shaft fracture being treated.

Transverse or short oblique fractures

For transverse or short oblique fractures of the neck, midshaft, or base, one longitudinal Kirschner

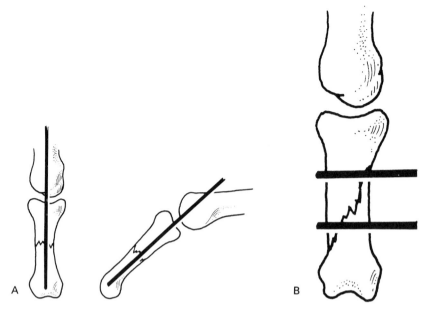

Fig. 5.1 Percutaneous K-wire fixation of proximal phalangeal factures: (A) longitudinal and (B) transverse

wire is used (Fig. 5.2). With proper sterile technique the wire is passed to one side of the extensor tendon, through the metacarpal head and down the medullary canal of the proximal phalanx (Fig. 5.3). The wire is drilled as far as the subchondral bone in the condyle. The K-wire is passed with either a T-handle Jacob's chuck device or a power-driven wire inserter. The former allows

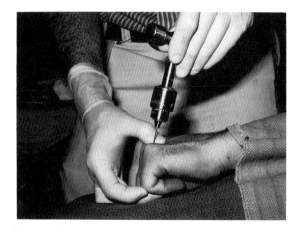

Fig. 5.2 The wire is inserted to one side of the extensor tendon, through the metacarpal head and down the medullary canal of the proximal phalanx to the subchondral bone in the condyle. The T-handle Jacob's chuck device facilitates insertion

very sensitive control of the wire, leaving one hand free to hold the finger in the reduced position. The chuck device is also less expensive, making it more available for the emergency room outpatient setting.

The choice of wire size varies with fracture location and bone size. For most fractures in adults, size 0.035 inch (0.9 mm) or 0.045 inch (1.1 mm) in diameter is adequate. The occasional distal neck fracture is adequately stabilized with two or three very fine 0.028 inch (0.7 mm) K-wires used together for intramedullary fixation (Fig. 5.4). This smaller wire is also used for single longitudinal wire fixation in shaft fractures in young children.

Spiral or long oblique fractures

Spiral or long oblique fractures are treated differently. Reduction is obtained in a similar manner but maintained with transversely placed parallel K-wires. An image intensifier and a power-driven wire inserter facilitate fixation of these fractures. A fracture clamp or towel clip temporarily maintains the reduction and mark the location for K-wire insertion. Two or three 0.028 inch (0.7 mm) K-wires are inserted parallel and as far apart as possible while still engaging both cortices and both

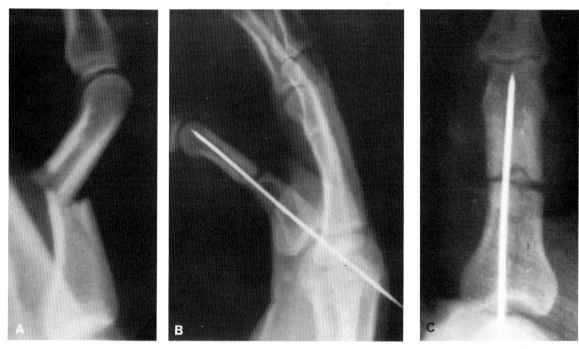

Fig. 5.3 Radiographs of a displaced unstable proximal phalangeal fracture. (A) typical collapse deformity of a midshaft fracture. (B and C) following reduction and percutaneous K-wire fixation (prior to trimming the wires)

fracture fragments as shown in Figure 5.5 (Arzimangolou & Skiadaressis 1952).

The patient is now asked to flex the interphalangeal joints as much as he can manage to confirm satisfactory alignment of the digits.

Dressing and plaster cast

After insertion, all wires are trimmed to project 2 or 3 mm outside the skin. If the finger is particularly swollen, and likely to continue to swell significantly because of the severity of injury, it is better to leave the wire projecting a little further outside the skin. This prevents a potential source of pain likely as the skin contracts down over the projecting tip as the swelling recedes. The transverse wires in the border digits (index and little fingers) are left projecting on the side opposite to the adjacent finger. For the long and ring fingers, the wire ends are carefully padded to protect the adjacent finger. Joshi (1976) prefers to bury the end of the wire just beneath the skin.

After reduction and fixation, the hand is dressed and protected in a rigid short-arm plaster cast. Care is taken to immobilize the fracture adequately

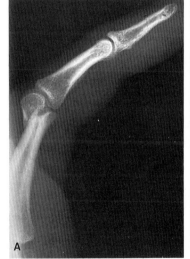
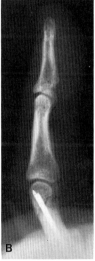

Fig. 5.4 A displaced fracture of the neck of the proximal phalanx treated with two or three fine 0.028 inch (0.7 mm) K-wires inserted longitudinally in a 'stacked' fashion. (A) Dorsal displacement of this unstable fracture. (B) The fracture after closed fixation and internal fixation

and also the adjacent digit distal to the PIP joint. If the fracture is significantly unstable or distal, immobilization is extended to the distal phalanx.

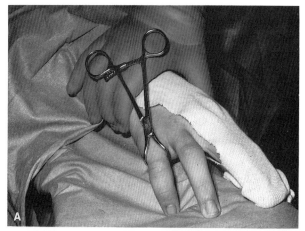

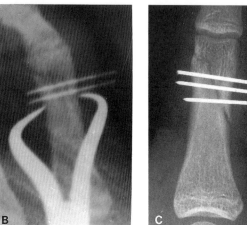

Fig. 5.5 Fixation with transverse parallel K-wires for an oblique fracture. (A) Following reduction, a fracture clamp is applied. (B) Under the image intensifier, using the clamp acts as a marker for accurate placement of the K-wires. (C) Final placement of the wires (prior to dressing and plaster cast)

motion exercises while still protecting the pin site and preventing MCP joint motion.

AFTER-CARE

The cast remains on for 3 weeks in most cases. The cast is then removed and the fracture and pin sites are examined (Fig. 5.6). Usually the fracture is not tender and the pin sites are dry and clean. A longitudinal wire is removed at this time by gentle traction with needle-nosed pliers. Transverse wires can be left in for one additional week while active PIP joint motion begins (Fig. 5.7). Anaesthesia is

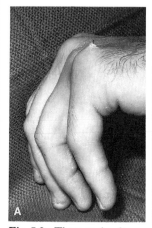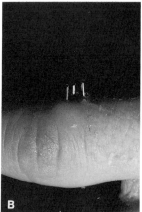

Fig. 5.6 Three weeks after surgery, the cast and dressings are removed. (A) The pin site is dry and clean and the longitudinal wire will now be removed. (B) These transverse wires, not crossing a joint, remain in for one more week

It is particularly important to bandage the pin sites properly and protect exposed wires from contact with the cast or adjacent fingers. *The snug-fitting rigid cast is a necessary part of this technique and can not be obviated with a partial cast or splint.* Motion inside the cast can cause pain as well as inflammation where the pin passes through the skin.

Each patient is seen during the first week after reduction to assure proper cast fit. A radiograph is obtained to verify that the reduction of the fracture and the position of the wire have been maintained. The cast often loosens by the first week and is remade. For the proximal, more stable, fractures the cast is fabricated to allow active PIP joint

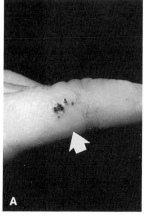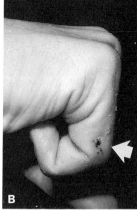

Fig. 5.7 Parallel wires remain in for one more week to allow (A) active extension, and (B) active flexion

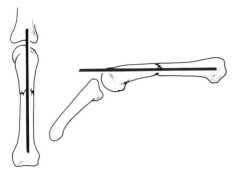

Fig. 5.8 Drawing demonstrates the location of a properly percutaneously placed K-wire after reduction of a displaced shaft fracture of the metacarpal

not necessary for removal of the wires. The patient is then instructed in range of motion exercises and told to massage the skin overlying the fracture. A forearm splint that supports the digits is given to the patient for one more week and removed for exercises. Progressive mobilization starting 3 weeks after reduction of the fracture prevents significant adhesion of the tendons and joint capsules and encourages maturation of fracture callus. With exercises three to five times each day and weekly visits to the surgeon, a co-operative patient's motion is often fully restored over the next 3 weeks.

RESULTS

In our prospective consecutive series of 100 displaced shaft fractures of the proximal phalanx treated by closed reduction and internal fixation, 90% had good or excellent results (Belsky et al 1984). Most of the excellent group, 55 of the 65 fractures, had no measurable loss of motion following treatment. Only a few had some loss of motion at the PIP or MCP joints.

There were 10% that had poor results. This group had a number of complicating factors, most important of which was lack of patient compliance. Two patients had fractures that were never adequately reduced and should therefore not have been treated in that position.

DISCUSSION

Joshi (1976) reported satisfactory results in 55 of 61 fractures of the proximal phalanges treated by a similar method, though he started mobilization of the interphalangeal joints after a week. Six fingers had moderate to severe restriction of movements: three of these were attributed to insecure fixation of the distal fragment because the wire was too short, one to intra-articular protrusion of the distal end of the wire, and one to closed rupture of the flexor tendon—though the exact cause of this is not stated. Complications were most frequent in the little finger.

In this technique of *closed* reduction and internal fixation, it is fundamental that reduction be as nearly perfect as possible in order to restore equilibrium to the flexor and extensor forces that act across the phalanx. Excellent reduction can be obtained with a minimum of experience and insertion of the wires is not difficult to master.

Laboratory testing has shown that fixation provided by longitudinal smooth K-wires is not as secure as that provided by plates, screws, crossed oblique wires and certain circlage and intraosseous wiring techniques (Massengill et al 1982, Alexander et al 1981, Fyfe & Mason 1979, Lister 1978). However, the dressing placed on healing hand fractures does not require the maximum of rigid fixation. With a good reduction of the displaced fracture there is restoration of the balance between the flexor and extensor forces. This obviates the need for rigid fixation by plates and screws. However, failure to obtain a satisfactory closed reduction remains an indication for open reduction.

The major advantage of this closed technique is its simplicity. Reduction and fixation can be done without hospitalization, in the emergency room or surgeon's office, wherever radiographs are readily available. Such a system represents a major reduction in cost as well as significant savings in time.

REFERENCES

Alexander H, Langrana N, Massengill J B, Weiss A B 1981 Development of new methods for phalangeal fracture fixation. Journal of Biomechanics 14:377–87

Arzimanoglou A, Skiadaressis S M 1952 Study of internal fixation by screws of oblique fractures in long bones. Journal of Bone and Joint Surgery (Am) 34:219–23

Belsky M R, Eaton R G 1982 Displaced shaft fractures of the ring and little finger metacarpals. Presented to the American Academy of Orthopedic Surgeons, New Orleans, Louisiana Jan 1982

Belsky M R, Eaton R G, Lane L B 1984 Closed reduction and internal fixation of proximal phalangeal fractures. Journal of Hand Surgery 9A:725–29

Fyfe I S, Mason S 1979 The mechanical stability of internal fixation of fractured phalanges. Hand 11:50–4

Joshi B B 1976 Percutaneous internal fixation of fractures of the proximal phalanges. Hand 8:86–92

Lister G 1978 Intraosseous wiring of the digital skeleton. Journal of Hand Surgery 3:427–35

Massengill J B, Alexander H, Langrana N, Mylod A 1982 A phalangeal fracture model-quantitative analysis of rigidity and failure. Journal of Hand Surgery 7:264–70

Vom Saal F H 1953 Intramedullary fixation in fractures of the hand and fingers. Journal of Bone and Joint Surgery 35:5–16

6 Fractures of the shafts of the phalanges: open reduction and internal fixation

Fractures occur more commonly in the hand than in any other part of the skeleton. Fractures of the phalanges can vary from simple, undisplaced metaphyseal fractures to comminuted intra-articular fractures with associated tendon, ligamentous, neurovascular and other soft tissue injuries. The final result of treatment of such fractures depends upon a complex inter-relationship between the type of fracture, the accuracy of reduction, the nature of associated soft tissue injuries and the postoperative management and rehabilitation.

Anatomical considerations

Anatomically, the phalanges occupy a position between gliding tendon surfaces and contribute proximally and distally to very precise articulation. The challenge in treatment of phalangeal fractures is to provide stability to achieve union while at the same time preserving motion of the adjacent joint, maintaining a smooth surface for flexor tendon gliding, and allowing for extensor tendon movement proximally and distally for proper digital function and balance.

Displacement and angulation of phalangeal fractures is influenced by two factors: the mechanism of injury and the muscles acting as deforming forces on the fracture fragments (Green & Rowland 1984). Unstable fractures of the *proximal phalanx* typically present with volar angulation. The proximal fragment is flexed by the action of the interossei, while the distal fragment is pulled into extension by the action of the central slip on the middle phalanx (Fig. 6.1A).

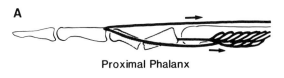

Proximal Phalanx

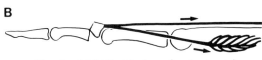

Proximal Middle Phalanx (metaphysis)

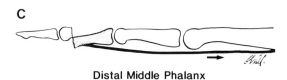

Distal Middle Phalanx

Fig. 6.1 Unstable fractures of the proximal phalanx typically present with angulation convex in a palmar direction (A). Proximal metaphyseal fractures may have angulation convex dorsally (B). Distal fractures of the middle phalanx have angulation convex towards the palmar surface (C)

Fractures of the *middle phalanx* have entirely different muscle forces acting upon them and can be angulated either volarly or dorsally depending upon whether the fracture is proximal or distal to the insertion of the flexor digitorum sublimis tendon. Proximal metaphyseal fractures will have a dorsal angulation, the proximal fragment being pulled into extension through the action of the central slip (Fig. 6.1B). Diaphyseal fractures may be angulated in either direction or neither. Distal fractures of the middle phalanx commonly show volar angulation due to the strong pull of the flexor sublimis tendon volarly on the proximal fragment and extension of the distal fragment by the terminal extensor tendon acting through the distal phalanx (Fig. 6.1C).

Closed versus open treatment

The methods used in the management of phalangeal fractures fall into one of three categories: non-operative treatment (*see* Chapters 3 and 4), closed reduction and percutaneous pinning (*see* Chapter 5), or open reduction and internal fixation. Choosing the proper method is not always easy. Certainly many patients will recover excellent function with little or no treatment, and elaborate surgical procedures would only be detrimental. However, the judicious use of operative methods can markedly improve the functional result in many complex fractures.

Closed reduction with external splint or cast immobilization remains the method of choice for most undisplaced fractures and for fractures in which a stable anatomical reduction can be achieved. After a short period of immobilization ($2\frac{1}{2}$–3 weeks), they should be protected by a removable splint while the digit is started on gentle range-of-motion exercises (Fig. 6.2).

Fractures that are displaced and difficult to reduce or hold in reduction by external immobilization may be fixed by percutaneous Kirschner wire fixation or, alternatively by open reduction and internal fixation. The percutaneous K-wire technique, where two or more smooth wires are passed transversely or obliquely across the fracture fragments or passed longitudinally to serve as an intramedullary device, has advantages over open reduction techniques because it obviates the need for soft tissue dissection. However, it is often difficult to obtain a complete and accurate reduction without visualizing the fracture. Also, the presence of the wire passing through the skin can tether soft tissue structures (Fig. 6.3) limiting early mobilization (Barton 1984).

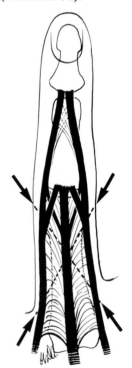

Fig. 6.3 Percutaneous K-wire technique

More complex fractures in which an adequate reduction cannot be achieved by either closed or percutaneous means, those with extensive comminution with or without bony loss, the majority of open fractures, those with associated nerve and tendon laceration and revascularization or replantation cases, are the most likely to need open reduction and internal fixation techniques. When internal fixation is desirable or necessary to maintain reduction, the advantages of providing stable internal fixation must be weighed against the soft

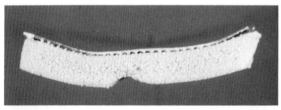

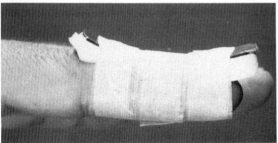

Fig. 6.2 Fractures should be protected by a removable splint when gentle range of motion of the digit is commenced

tissue injury which results from the surgical manoeuvre required to insert the device.

Stabilization versus rigid fixation

Internal fixation devices can provide either stabilization or rigid internal fixation. Internal fixation is rigid when the stress resulting from active but unresisted motion of adjacent joints causes no motion at the fracture interface (Meyer et al. 1981). The advantages of this method are that it ensures that anatomical reduction is maintained and eliminates the need for plaster or other external immobilization devices. Furthermore, it permits nearly immediate mobilization. Rigid immobilization can only be achieved when there is precise reduction of fragments with interfragmentary compression. The most common example of this method is the ASIF (Association for the Study of Internal Fixation) technique of interfragmentary compression using screws and plates.

More often, the site or shape of the fracture, the presence of comminution, bone loss or inability to achieve an exact reduction will require the use of a 'stabilization' technique. The most common example of such a technique is the use of Kirschner wires.

INDICATIONS

The indication for open reduction and internal fixation must be carefully defined to avoid overtreatment of those fractures better managed by non-operative methods. As in other areas of the skeleton, open reduction is indicated in those phalangeal fractures which are irreducible or in which reduction cannot be maintained by closed methods. Open methods are especially useful when phalangeal fractures occur in multiple adjacent digits or when a fracture cannot be held in a position of function in a splint. Widely displaced epiphyseal fractures, particularly involving the articular surface (Salter–Harris Types III and IV), require precise reduction.

Open fractures of the phalanges frequently enjoy certain advantages when managed by open reduction and internal fixation techniques. Digital injuries with open fractures are commonly the result of high energy trauma and often include injury to accompanying soft tissues. When internal fixation techniques are used, bulky plaster or dressings can be eliminated, and wound care is facilitated. More importantly, motion of adjacent joints can be started earlier. This concept is vitally important when there is a phalangeal fracture in the presence of an associated tendon laceration. Prompt anatomical reduction with stabilization leading to early joint mobilization gives the best chance for minimizing adhesions of the tendon to the fracture site.

Fractures of the phalanges have some unique characteristics not shared by larger bones. The most apparent is that small deviations (as little as $5°$) in rotational alignment can cause interference with function of other fingers and, thus, the whole hand. Generally, angular errors of alignment are less of a problem. Articular fractures in the phalanges require anatomical reduction with restoration at the joint surface to minimize the chance of post-traumatic arthritis. Finally, successful skeletal stabilization in cases of digital revascularization or replantation requires internal fixation which is secure and allows for adjacent neurovascular, tendon and soft tissue repair: this is considered in detail in Chapter 15.

Open reduction and internal fixation of the phalanges, when used in properly selected cases and performed skilfully, provides important advantages in fracture treatment and the functional result. Internal fixation in the hand enjoys the same advantages as in other areas of the skeleton; accurate reduction and secure fracture stabilization which allows early joint motion.

There has been a continuing effort to design more versatile techniques which provide secure fixation but at the same time minimize operative trauma. When internal fixation is required, the following techniques are useful.

METHODS OF OPEN REDUCTION AND INTERNAL FIXATION

Open reduction with Kirschner wire fixation

In spite of the recent introduction of new and varied techniques for fracture stabilization, the modification of the steel pins introduced by Martin Kirschner in 1909 remains a most versatile tool in the surgeon's armamentarium for internal fixation of fractures in the hand (Kirschner 1909). In 1953, Vom Saal expanded the application of Kirschner wires to include phalangeal fractures, describing a percutaneous technique (Vom Saal 1953). Subsequent innovations have included various open and percutaneous approaches using either single or multiple pins placed obliquely, transversely or longitudinally.

Open reduction and internal fixation using Kirschner wires can be employed for nearly any fracture configuration but is especially useful in fractures of the shafts of the phalanges where other more bulky devices, which require extensive exposure and may interfere with tendon gliding, would be disadvantageous.

Placement of Kirschner wires is largely dependent on the anatomy of the fracture. Oblique or spiral fractures are readily stabilized by two pins placed perpendicular to the fracture surface. Transverse fractures are best stabilized by a cross-pinning technique, and highly comminuted fractures can be held reduced by many small K-wires introduced at different angles (Fig. 6.4).

For isolated closed fractures of the proximal phalanx, a straight mid-lateral approach reflecting the neurovascular bundle and flexor tendons volarly is usually best, but this may need to be modified to expose and repair other associated soft tissue injuries. In the case of an open fracture, the incision has been determined by the injury.

Using subperiosteal dissection, the fracture fragments are exposed and reduced to an anatomical position. At least two K-wires, introduced with power equipment, are drilled across the fracture fragments. The use of two wires increases the stability of the fracture while preventing rotation which could occur around a single pin. When an oblique insertion is attempted, K-wires have a tendency to slide along the cortex. To avoid this, a powered drill should always be used. In addition, an appropriately sized hypodermic needle can be used as a guide for the K-wire (Fig. 6.5).

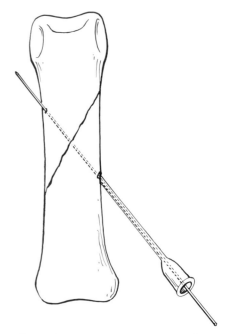

Fig. 6.5 K-wires have a tendency to slide along the cortex when oblique insertion is attempted. A hypodermic needle can be used as a guide for K-wire insertion

The outer parts of the wires are then cut off adjacent to the bone and the skin pulled over the cut end of the wire to produce a closed wound. For those fractures with limited access for pinning, retrograde placement of the K-wires (Fig. 6.6) is helpful in ensuring proper apposition of the fragments (O'Brien 1982).

In vitro analysis of Kirschner wire failure in phalangeal fractures has shown that pins placed

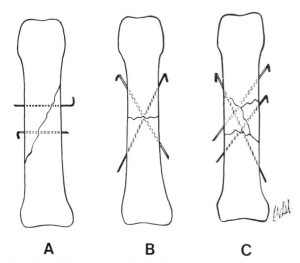

A   B   C

Fig. 6.4 (A) Transverse K-wire fixation for spiral fracture. (B) Transverse fracture stabilized by cross-pinning technique. (C) Comminuted fracture held by several small K-wires

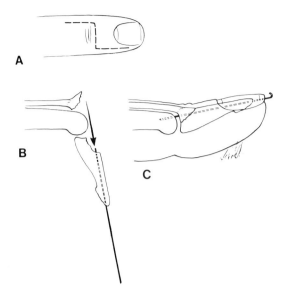

Fig. 6.6   A 0.035 inch (0.9 mm) K-wire is placed from proximal to distal through the distal phalanx, then retrograded across the fragment at the joint

dorsal to the central axis of the finger afford greater rigidity than those placed in the central axis (Massengill et al 1979).

As previously noted, a major advantage enjoyed by the K-wire technique over other methods of fracture stabilization is its versatility. Nearly any type of fracture, save for severely comminuted patterns, can be adequately stabilized by two or more K-wires. This technique places a minimal amount of metallic foreign body within the phalanx. The need for extensive dissection is eliminated. Furthermore, pins can be inserted in such a way that they do not interfere with tendon gliding, an important consideration when early mobilization is desirable.

It must be borne in mind that open reduction and K-wire fixation is a method of 'stabilization' of a fracture, as opposed to rigid fixation. This is due to the fact that exact anatomical reduction with inter-digitation of fragments is seldom achieved. Also K-wires themselves are unable to produce inter-fragmentary compression. The implications of this fact lie in the need for postoperative protective splinting (usually for $2\frac{1}{2}$–3 weeks) until there is sufficient intrinsic fracture healing to allow joint motion without loosening of the wires.

The potential problem of fracture instability with distraction of fragments using the closed K-wire technique, especially crossed oblique wires, is avoided by using pins of sufficient diameter and firmly compressing the fracture fragments when advancing the pins. Transfixion of soft tissue and potential pin tract infection are possible when pins are left protruding through the skin. This disadvantage appears to outweigh the benefit of easy removal of protruding pins, and we currently recommend cutting pins off adjacent to the bone.

Interosseous wiring

In an attempt to overcome some of the drawbacks of Kirschner wire fixation, such as distraction of fragments and transfixion of soft tissue, and to increase stability by adding interfragmentary compression, Robertson (1964) developed a method utilizing parallel wire loops between fragments to achieve interphalangeal arthrodesis. This technique was expanded by Lister (1978) by adding an oblique K-wire and was shown to be efficacious for use in transverse phalangeal fractures, intra-articular avulsion fractures and interphalangeal arthrodeses.

The use of interosseous wires to immobilize phalangeal fractures is indicated in those fractures not amenable to simpler forms of internal fixation. Specifically, for transverse phalangeal shaft fractures, the method obviates the possibility of distraction using crossed K-wires because the interosseous loop can provide a degree of interfragmentary compression and at the same time act to control rotation (Fig. 6.7A). Intra-articular condylar fractures too small for screw fixation lend themselves to interosseous technique by looping the wire through the fragment or, alternatively, by engaging the ligament or tendon attached to it.

Long oblique or spiral fractures are not appropriate for the technique and are better stabilized by two K-wires or interfragmentary screws (Fig. 6.7B). In addition, highly comminuted fractures or fractures with bone loss where adequate bone-to-bone contact cannot be achieved will not allow compression by the wire loop and are better treated with multiple K-wires.

When using this technique on a transverse phalangeal fracture, it is best to have incisions on both sides of the phalanx. A hole is then drilled

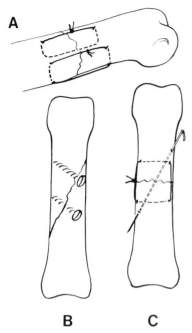

Fig. 6.7 (A) Use of interosseous wiring to provide interfragmentary compression and to control rotation of transverse phalangeal shaft fracture. (B) Spiral fractures are better stabilized by use of interfragmentary screws. (C) Stabilization of a transverse phalangeal fracture with interosseous wiring and oblique K-wire

using a 0.035 inch (0.9 mm) Kirschner wire in the midlateral axis of the bone parallel to the fracture surface in each fragment. Size No. 0 stainless monofilament wire is threaded through the holes. Before tightening the wire, a 0.035 inch (0.9 mm) K-wire is drilled obliquely across one fragment. The interosseous wire is tightened and the oblique K-wire is advanced across the second fragment. The interosseous wire acts to provide interfragmentary compression and control rotation, while the oblique K-wire adds stability and resists angulatory forces (Fig. 6.7C).

Biomechanical studies comparing crossed K-wires with interosseous wiring technique have verified that the interosseous loop is consistently more rigid, especially when supplemented with an oblique K-wire (Fyfe & Mason 1979). Recent studies comparing the relative strengths of internal fixation techniques have shown that two interosseous wires at 90° to each other are stronger than either a single interosseous wire or one with a supplementary K-wire (Vanik et al 1984).

The interosseous wiring technique, when applied to transverse fractures of the diaphyses of phalanges, provides the benefits of secure fixation with interfragmentary compression. The result of this is that little or no splinting is necessary after the immediate postoperative period. Active and passive range of motion is begun early which minimizes joint stiffness and improves the ultimate functional result.

Open reduction and internal fixation by ASIF (AO) techniques

The fundamental principle of the Swiss ASIF (Association for the Study of Internal Fixation, formerly called the Association for Osteosynthesis and abbreviated to AO) is to provide fracture stability by means of anatomical reduction and rigid internal fixation. Rigid internal fixation may be achieved in different ways but the fundamental aim is to provide interfragmentary compression. The development of the small fragment set has allowed these principles to be expanded to internal fixation of fractures in the hand (Heim & Pfeiffer 1982).

Currently, the most appropriate fractures for the use of interfragmentary screw compression are oblique or spiral fractures of the diaphysis of the proximal phalanx and intra-articular fractures with a large bony fragment.

A displaced spiral fracture of the proximal phalanx often results in permanent impairment of motion due to the close proximity of flexor and extensor tendons and adjacent joints. The use of K-wires or wire loops may provide insufficient stability to allow the early, vigorous exercise necessary for full functional recovery. In these circumstances, interfragmentary compression using two small ASIF 'mini' screws can provide the necessary rigidity for early aggressive range-of-motion exercises. The use of a plate and screws is very rarely indicated in phalangeal fractures because the bulk of the implant interferes with tendon gliding and the surgical exposure is more extensive. ASIF implants have little applicability in the treatment of open fractures.

The rationale of producing rigid interfragmentary compression allowing for early active motion during healing is appealing. However, even those most experienced with the use of such techniques point out their relatively limited indications in phalangeal fractures (Crawford 1976, Steel 1978). The technique is difficult and the margin for error is small (Heim & Pfeiffer 1982). The unavoidable soft-tissue dissection and damage to the periosteal blood supply must be weighed against the advantages of achieving rigid fixation.

OPEN REDUCTION WITH EXTERNAL FIXATION

The use of external fixation devices has enjoyed popularity in the treatment of severely comminuted fractures of the long bones of the extremities, especially when there is concomitant bone and soft tissue loss. The development of 'mini' external fixation components has expanded the applicability of this technique to its use in the phalanges. Matev was the first to utilize such a method when he applied the technique to distraction lengthening of the thumb metacarpal following amputation (Matev 1970). Subsequently, the method was extended to its use in the management of injured digits (Kessler et al 1979). Chapter 13 describes methods of external fixation in detail.

The advantage of external fixation is that the device acts to rigidly immobilize fracture fragments while at the same time maintaining proper length of the remaining soft tissue envelope. Associated tendon and neurovascular repairs can be carried out. Wound care is facilitated because no form of external splintage is required. Adjacent uninjured joints can be quickly mobilized. In cases of significant bone loss, the use of a silastic block spacer allows for later bone grafting in an acceptable soft tissue bed.

REHABILITATION

Nowhere in the skeleton is proper postoperative fracture care more important than following phalangeal fractures. Regardless of the method of fixation, appropriate rehabilitation of the hand is needed to prevent stiffness of adjacent joints and attain the optimum functional result.

Of utmost importance is timely clinical and radiographical examination during the period of fracture healing. In particular, patients allowed early active motion must be instructed and encouraged to perform specific exercises to minimize joint stiffness.

In all fractures but those with the most rigid fixation, plaster splints or other external immobilization will be required to protect the fragments from stress until healed. A variety of splinting techniques, from the application of postoperative dressings to more elaborate custom-made splints, may be required to achieve the best functional result.

Far too often the application of postoperative dressings and splinting is relegated to the least experienced member of the surgical team. The properly applied dressing is bulky and uniformly supportive but not constrictive. Of special importance is immobilization in the 'safe position', i.e. that position which has the least chance of leading to stiffening of the small joints. This position is defined by: (1) interphalangeal joint extension; (2) palmar abduction and extension of the thumb to maintain the web space; and (3) metacarpophalangeal joint flexion. This 'safe' position— discussed fully in Chapter 3—places the supporting ligamentous structures of the joints of the hand under maximum stretch.

There is a well-known lack of correlation between the radiographic and clinical signs of union of phalangeal fractures. Immobilization should *not* be continued until consolidation at the fracture line is visible on radiograph; motion should be initiated as soon as the fracture is clinically stable (usually $2\frac{1}{2}$–3 weeks).

Once mobilization of the digit has begun, the use of custom-made polyethylene splints which employ either static immobilization or dynamic splinting, or a combination of both, can provide localized splinting of the fracture while encouraging motion of the adjacent joints. Supervised physical therapy employing conventional modalities as well as more modern techniques of electrical muscle stimulation (Faradic) can improve the final functional result.

Rehabilitation is further considered in Chapter 23.

REFERENCES

Barton N J 1984 Fractures of the hand. Journal of Bone and Joint Surgery 66B: 159–167

Bilos Z J, Eskestrand T 1979 External fixator use in comminuted gunshot fractures of the proximal phalanx. Journal of Hand Surgery 4: 357–359

Crawford G P 1976 Screw fixation for certain fractures of the phalanges and metacarpals. Journal of Bone and Joint Surgery 58A: 487–492

Fyfe I S, Mason S 1979 The mechanical stability of internal fixation of fractured phalanges. The Hand 11: 50–54

Green D P, Rowland S A 1984 Fractures and dislocations in the hand. In: Rockwood C A, Green D P (eds) Fractures in Adults, J B Lippincott, Philadelphia

Heim U R S, Pfeiffer K M 1982 Small fragment set manual: technique recommended by the ASIF Group, 2nd edn, Springer-Verlag, New York

Kessler I, Hecht O, Baruch A 1979 Distraction lengthening of digital rays in the management of the injured hand. Journal of Bone and Joint Surgery 61A: 83–87

Kirschner M 1909 Uber Nagel extension. Beitrage zur Klinischen Chirurgie 64: 266

Kleinert H E 1985 Surgery of the hand. In: Monaco A P (ed) Textbook of Surgery, MacMillan Publishing Co., New York

Kutz J E, Bennett D L 1986 Tendon injuries. In: Smith R J, Watson N A (eds) The hand—affections, infections and injuries, Butterworths, London

Lister G D 1978 Intraosseous wiring of the digital skeleton. Journal of Hand Surgery 3: 427–435

Massengill J B, Alexander H, Parson J R, Schecter M J 1979 Mechanical analysis of Kirschner wire fixation in a phalangeal model. Journal of Hand Surgery 4: 351–356

Matev I B 1970 Thumb reconstruction after amputation at the metacarpophalangeal joint by bone lengthening. A preliminary report of three cases. Journal of Bone and Joint Surgery 52A: 957–965

Meyer V E, Chiu D T W, Beasley R W 1981 The place of internal skeletal fixation in surgery of the hand. Clinics in Plastic Surgery 8: 51–64

O'Brien E T 1982 Fractures of the metacarpals and phalanges. In Green D P (ed) Operative Hand Surgery. Churchill Livingstone, New York

Robertson D C 1964 The fusion of interphalangeal joints. Canadian Journal of Surgery 7: 433–437

Steel W M 1978 The AO small fragment set in hand fractures. Hand 10: 246–253

Vanik R K, Weber R C, Matloub H S, Sanger J R, Gingrass R P 1984 The comparative strengths of internal fixation techniques. Journal of Hand Surgery 9: 216–221

Vom Saal F H 1953 Intramedullary fixation in fractures of the hand and fingers. Journal of Bone and Joint Surgery 35A: 5

7 Articular fractures

Loss of motion and deformity are the two major complications of phalangeal fractures. These problems are particularly troublesome in those fractures involving the joint surfaces. This should occasion no surprise since intra-articular fractures of any long bone are prone to joint stiffness and the joints between the miniature long bones are no exception.

In major long bone fractures with articular involvement, preservation of motion and prevention of secondary arthrosis have been achieved by precise reduction of the fracture at open operation and by the use of internal fixation devices to maintain accurate restoration of the joint surfaces. By such means, the high incidence of post-traumatic arthrosis at the ankle, knee, and elbow has been greatly reduced. There has been a tendency to extrapolate these techniques to the finger joints in the belief that careful reduction and fixation of intra-articular fractures would prevent secondary problems such as stiffness, deformity and arthrosis. However, before advocating these difficult and demanding procedures, the natural history of articular fractures of the phalanges should be studied. It will then become evident, in at least some fractures, that their behaviour is not quite what might be expected and that a favourable outcome can be achieved without surgery.

It has become very clear that inexpert surgery in the major joints can result in imperfect restoration of joint surfaces, unstable fixation and secondary stiffness of the joint, a situation which may well be worse than the result from conservative management. It is all the more important, therefore, that unnecessary surgery should be avoided. Where open reduction is appropriate, the demands on the operator's skill are much greater in the tiny confines of the interphalangeal joints than in the major joints. There is therefore a need for a review of the outcome of intra-articular fractures so that treatment may be planned in a rational fashion and unnecessary operations avoided.

A study of intra-articular fractures presenting to the hand injury clinic in Stoke-on-Trent over a period of eight years has provided valuable information regarding the classification and behaviour of these injuries.

Material and methods

The records were reviewed of patients presenting with articular fractures of the digits, but excluding avulsion fractures. Between 1972 and 1980, 159 cases were identified and an attempt was made to review them all. Seventy-five patients were traced and re-examined at intervals varying from six months to seven years after injury. Although there was insufficient information in the notes of 47 others to determine the outcome, the type of fracture, aetiology and management could be assessed from the records.

At the review examination the range of motion in the joints of the injured digit was measured and expressed as a percentage of the movement in the normal finger of the other hand. Function, measured by a simple grip-testing dynamometer, was also compared to the uninjured side. Radiographs were taken to evaluate the state of the affected joints. The patient was questioned as to the presence of pain and any change in occupation as a direct result of the injury was recorded. To assess the final outcome of these injuries four parameters, namely pain, deformity, motion and function, were measured and to each a possible score of 100 was given. For motion and function the measured percentage of the normal side was used. Pain was scored by the patient between zero and five; this was then multiplied by 20 so that absence of pain scored 100 and extreme pain zero. Angulatory or rotational deformity, if present but less than $15°$, scored 75, whereas a greater deformity was scored zero. A total score of 400 was considered an 'excellent' result, 350 as 'good', 300 as 'fair' but less than this 'poor'.

AETIOLOGY

Table 7.1 details the causative factors found in this series. It is often difficult for a patient to describe exactly the mechanism of injury, but an attempt was made to segregate the fractures into those resulting from a direct blow, a crushing injury or a twist. Domestic injuries accounted for 52 of the fractures studied and these were mainly simple blows received in housework or the results of falls in the home. Industrial accidents accounted for most of the crushing injuries. Road traffic accidents were few, but sports injuries frequent. Most of the sporting accidents were caused by a blow on the end of the finger in cricket, football or other ball games; knocks from hockey-sticks and rackets were not unusual. Whilst domestic, industrial and road accidents were evenly distributed between basal and condylar fractures, there is a striking preponderance of sports injuries in the basal group (Table 7.2).

INCIDENCE

Barton (1977), in an unselected series of 100 fractures of the fingers, found joint involvement in

Table 7.1 Aetiological factors in articular fractures

Mechanism of injury	Accident type				Total
	Domestic	Industrial	RTA*	Sport	
Blow	34	17	10	41	102
Crush	9	20	2	2	33
Twist	9	4	2	9	24
Total	52	41	14	52	159

* RTA = Road traffic accident

Table 7.2 Causative factors in basal and condylar fractures

Accident type	Fracture type	
	Basal	Condylar
Domestic	27	25
Industrial	21	20
RTA*	7	7
Sport	39	13
Total	94	65

* RTA = Road traffic accident

one third. In a later review (Barton 1984) of 454 phalangeal fractures, 18.5% were articular injuries. Lee (1963), reporting from Oxford, found that over a period of $4\frac{1}{2}$ years, 1225 patients attended the accident service with fractures of the phalanges and of these 225 or 19% had articular involvement. It seems likely, therefore, that articular fractures account for slightly less than 20% of all phalangeal fractures. Since this figure includes many minor avulsion injuries, corner or chip fractures, mallet fractures and undisplaced articular fractures, it follows that serious intra-articular fractures and fracture–dislocations are not common injuries and will be seen only sporadically even in large accident centres. It is therefore difficult to collect large series of individual fractures and this is reflected in the paucity of cases reported in the literature where intricate operative procedures are often recommended on the basis of a handful of treated cases. Many hand surgeons are not involved in the primary treatment of fractures in the accident and emergency department and may only see selected cases referred by the accident and emergency staff or as late referrals by the general practitioner. The more common articular fractures may then become rarities to the super-specialist.

DIAGNOSIS

The diagnosis of an intra-articular fracture depends on clinical awareness, careful examination and accurate radiographs of the involved digits. The presence of swelling, bruising or deformity in the region of a joint should immediately alert the examiner to the possibility of articular injury. Careful and gentle examination will elicit tenderness over the site of injury and, more importantly, will reveal instability. Whenever dislocation, subluxation or ligamentous injury is suspected, the inter-phalangeal joints should be gently examined, applying medial and lateral stress to determine the presence of instability of the collateral ligaments. Stable fractures and joint injuries may be accompanied by a range of movement little short of normal whilst, in contrast, unstable fractures or fracture-dislocations will be accompanied by considerably more stiffness and pain on motion.

In busy accident units with inexperienced staff, clinical examination is often brief and too much reliance is placed on radiographs. If these are correctly requested, the diagnosis may be evident but two errors are frequently made. Firstly, views of the hand may be requested and these are seldom of diagnostic value in injuries of interphalangeal joints, especially if the fingers are flexed. In digital injuries fingers should be radiographed individually. Secondly, it is important by accurate centring to obtain true antero-posterior and lateral views of the digits. If this is difficult with conventional X-ray film, dental film may be placed between the fingers. In no circumstances should one rely only on antero-posterior and oblique films.

The presence of avulsion fractures should alert the examiner to the possibility of ligamentous injury and further examination of the integrity of the collateral and volar ligaments should be undertaken. If there is doubt, stress radiographs may be of value. Where a dislocation has occurred, check radiographs after reduction are important to note the position of any small fragment.

CLASSIFICATION

Intra-articular fractures may be classified into basal, condylar and avulsion groups (Fig. 7.1). There is clearly an overlap when considering fractures of the joint margins, but the avulsion group has been taken to include those small bony fragments which are associated with sprains or tendon avulsions.

Basal fractures

These have been subdivided into three types (Fig. 7.2). Type I—undisplaced marginal fractures; Type II—comminuted fractures where the articular surface has been driven into the phalanx; and

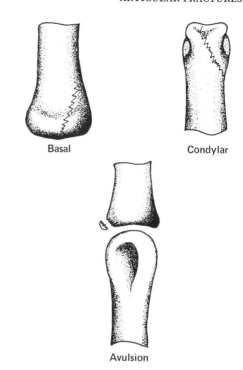

Basal   Condylar

Avulsion

Fig. 7.1 Classification of articular fractures

Type III—displaced fractures of either the dorsal or volar margin, commonly associated with joint subluxation or dislocation. Table 7.3 shows the distribution of basal fractures of the three types in

Table 7.3 The distribution of basal fractures

	Fracture type	Terminal phalanx	Middle phalanx	Proximal phalanx
I	Undisplaced	9	3	13
II	Comminuted	7	5	10
III	Marginal	27	9	6

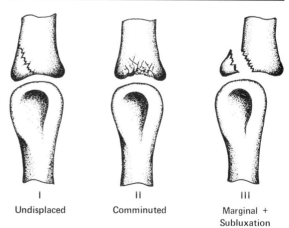

I   II   III
Undisplaced   Comminuted   Marginal + Subluxation

Fig. 7.2 Classification of basal fractures

the three phalanges. It will be noted that comminuted fractures were found most often at the base of the proximal phalanx, whilst the Type III fracture of the joint margin was seen most often in the terminal phalanx. Further subdivision of the marginal fractures according to the percentage of the joint involved is important; it is customary to divide the articular surface into thirds, thus making three subgroups.

Condylar fractures

Condylar fractures were found to follow a similar pattern to that described by London (1971) and his classification has been followed (Fig. 7.3). Type

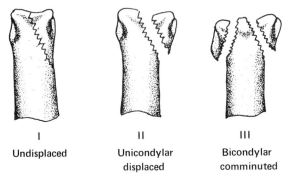

I	II	III
Undisplaced	Unicondylar displaced	Bicondylar comminuted

Fig. 7.3 Classification of condylar fractures

I are stable fractures without displacement, Type II unicondylar unstable fractures, and Type III bicondylar or comminuted fractures. Table 7.4 shows the distribution of these types in the middle and proximal phalanges. There is a preponderance of comminuted fractures at the terminal interphalangeal joint, reflecting the vulnerability of this region to crush injuries.

Table 7.4 The distribution of condylar fractures

	Fracture type	Middle phalanx	Proximal phalanx
I	Undisplaced	1	13
II	Unicondylar	10	9
III	Comminuted	10	4

Avulsion fractures

Avulsion fractures have not been broken down into any formal classification. Their behaviour reflects the extent of the tendinous or ligamentous injury and, whilst they have been included in this chapter

as articular fractures, the diagnosis and management of these injuries should properly be considered as ligament and tendon avulsions.

INJURIES OF THE TERMINAL INTERPHALANGEAL JOINT

Basal fractures

These have been divided into the three types shown in Figure 7.2. Table 7.3 shows that, of the total of 43 fractures, nine were undisplaced, seven were comminuted and 27 were displaced marginal fractures. The large number of marginal fractures reflects the frequency of blows on the fingertip caused by cricket balls, netballs and footballs as well as simple falls. Comminuted fractures may also be caused by sporting injuries where the articular surface of the terminal phalanx is driven straight into the head of the middle phalanx.

Of the 33 patients who could be reviewed (Table 7.5) 23 were excellent or good. It is noteworthy that not all the disappointing results were in the Type II and Type III injuries as there were three cases of undisplaced fracture where stiffness resulted in a fair result.

Table 7.5 Results at post-treatment review of basal fractures of the terminal phalanx

Fracture type	Outcome of treatment	
	Excellent and good	Fair and poor
I	4	3
II	2	1
III	17	6
Total	23	10

Undisplaced fractures

Type I were those undisplaced fractures of the articular surface of the terminal phalanx not associated with any subluxation or dislocation of the terminal interphalangeal joint. A good prognosis can usually be anticipated though loss of motion at the joint may put the result into the fair or poor category, especially if there has been crushing of the soft tissues or an open wound. Initial treatment requires no more than simple splintage with a plastic mallet splint. As soon as the finger is comfortable and can be moved without pain, early protected motion should be allowed.

Comminuted fractures

Type II fractures were those associated with comminution of the articular surface; often the head of the middle phalanx had driven into the base of the terminal phalanx as the result of a blow or fall on the end of the finger. Others were the result of industrial trauma and were accompanied by untidy skin wounds, laceration of the extensor tendon, and damage to the joint capsule. There is nothing to be gained in these cases by attempts to reduce or fix the fracture by either open or closed methods; early protected movement offers the best chance of a mobile joint. If the joint destruction is severe and is accompanied by an open wound, as seen in industrial crushing injuries, then primary arthrodesis should be considered.

Dorsal marginal

The most controversial fracture in this group is the Type III fracture of the dorsal margin of the terminal phalanx associated with subluxation of the terminal interphalangeal joint. These are often caused by a forceful blow on the fingertip in sport, for example in cricket, baseball or hockey. They have been confused with mallet fractures and in some reports are classified together with those injuries. The true mallet fracture, however, is a small bony fragment associated with rupture of the insertion of the extensor tendon. These Type III fractures are frequently accompanied by subluxation or dislocation of the terminal interphalangeal joint.

Hamas, Horrell and Pierret (1978), in a discussion of the treatment of mallet finger due to intra-articular fracture of the distal phalanx, distinguish three types of structural injury which could cause the mallet deformity Type I, a true tendon rupture, Type II, avulsion of the extensor tendon with a bony fragment less than one-third of the articular surface, and Type III, an intra-articular fracture involving more than one-third of the articular surface. They regard these as troublesome fractures and state that, where there is displacement of a significant part of the surface, accurate open

reduction must be performed to prevent joint stiffness due to secondary arthritis. They recommend fixation of the articular fragment by two Kirschner wires, with the passage of a further wire across the joint to maintain reduction of the subluxation. The wires are maintained for 6–8 weeks. They reported 11 cases with a mean flexion at review of $71°$ and negligible extension lag. Doyle (1982), in discussing mallet finger, identifies two distinct types associated with bony injury: one in which there is a small bony fragment and another in which there is a major bone fragment greater than one third of the articular surface. In the first type, the outcome does not seem to differ from a closed mallet finger without bony injury and the management should be the same. A distinction is made between the second type and a mallet injury and again there is a plea for open reduction and internal fixation after the method described above. A warning is given that the procedure is technically demanding. The K-wires should be inserted with a small power driver and if, as sometimes happens, the fracture becomes comminuted during passage of the wire, a stainless steel wire suture may be passed around the fragments.

The claim that fractures of the terminal phalanx associated with joint subluxation require open reduction and internal fixation seems to be based on theoretical concepts rather than case experience. Whilst it may seem logical to insist on accurate reduction, experience shows that this is, in fact, unnecessary. Wehbé and Schneider (1984) have reported the only substantial series of mallet fractures. They analysed 44 fractures from a total of 160 mallet fingers. These cases were classified into three types, Type I with no subluxation, Type II with subluxation and Type III with physeal injury. Each was then subdivided into group A affecting less than one third of the articular surface, group B one third to two thirds of the articular surface and group C greater than two thirds of the articular surface; 48% were athletic injuries. They were able to follow up 21 cases over a period of six months to eight years; six had been treated by surgery and 15 by simple splintage. Six of these had minor aching at work of which three had been splinted and three had been treated by operation. Three out of the 21 had minor limitation of function and 17 had a minor bump. All but one

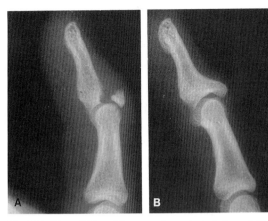

Fig. 7.4 Type III basal fracture of terminal phalanx: (A) dorsal marginal with volar subluxation. (B) Remodelling after two years. Good function

showed bone remodelling, reconstitution of the articular surface, and preservation of joint space. Near normal movement was seen in the great majority. They concluded that surgery was difficult and unreliable, had no advantages, increased morbidity and that the only complication from conservative treatment was a minor cosmetic blemish, namely the bump.

The experience in this review closely follows that of Wehbé and Schneider (1984). Of the 23 cases followed up 17 did well and showed the same remodelling, lack of pain and preservation of joint space noted by the American authors. Of those who fell into the fair or poor category the reason was restriction of motion rather than pain or disability. Figure 7.4 illustrates the remarkable remodelling two years following this injury in a 20-year-old man with a significantly displaced fracture–subluxation which was treated by simple splintage.

Fracture–subluxation of the distal interphalangeal joint is a much more benign injury than its counterpart at the proximal interphalangeal joint. It seldom leads to pain, stiffness or post-traumatic arthritis. Instead, the joint seems to have a remarkable capacity for remodelling. Only the residual dorsal bump remains and some insignificant loss of motion. Although open reduction and internal fixation is frequently advocated to restore congruity of the joint and to reduce subluxation, there is no doubt that the operation is technically demanding. The fragment is small and easily

fragmented. Unless the operator is skilled in the handling of small bone fragments, the procedure could only too easily result in a stiff painful finger. Since long-term reviews indicate the benign prognosis of this injury, there should be a move towards a more conservative approach. Treatment should therefore be confined to simple support with a plastic mallet splint for three weeks followed by active motion. The patient should be warned that a bump will be present but reassured that motion and function will not be significantly impaired. Local discomfort is always a feature of injuries at the terminal interphalangeal joint but settles within six months.

Volar marginal fractures

The reverse injury is unusual and seldom reported; it resembles the more common fracture-dislocation with volar marginal fracture seen at the proximal interphalangeal joint. Whilst it seems logical to reduce the fracture to restore congruity to the joint, this injury seems to behave in the same benign fashion as the dorsal marginal fracture. Figure 7.5 shows a volar fracture with a subluxation of the terminal interphalangeal joint presenting six weeks after injury with minimal symptoms and a

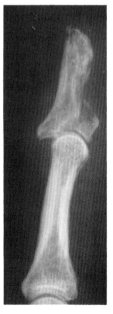

Fig. 7.5 Type III basal fracture of terminal phalanx: volar marginal with dorsal subluxation. Minimal disability at six weeks

range of movement from 0 to 60°. This limited experience may not be universal and where there is clear evidence of instability then treatment should be along similar lines to that used for the comparable lesion at the proximal interphalangeal joint. Figure 7.6 shows a volar marginal fracture with subluxation of the terminal interphalangeal joint. Reduction was easily achieved by flexion but subluxation recurred as soon as extension was allowed. Management of the injury by extension-block splinting, which will be described in relation to the proximal interphalangeal joint, is the procedure of choice. Only if there is a very large fragment with gross instability should open reduction and internal fixation be considered. The volar marginal fracture has been seen in association with a dislocation of the terminal interphalangeal joint (Fig. 7.7). In this instance the fragment is small and after stable reduction of the dislocation can be ignored.

Condylar fractures

These have been divided into the three types illustrated in Figure 7.3. Table 7.4 shows that of the 21 fractures involving the terminal interphalangeal joint, one was undisplaced, ten were unicondylar and ten were bicondylar or comminuted. The number of comminuted fractures reflects the ease with which the terminal digit is trapped or crushed in industrial machinery or domestic accidents. These comminuted fractures are often associated with soft tissue damage to the

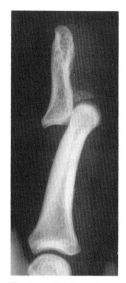
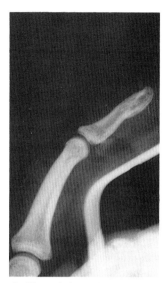

Fig. 7.7 Dislocation of terminal interphalangeal joint with volar marginal fracture. Stable after reduction and therefore treated by simple volar splint

tendons, ligaments or capsule of the joint and may be complicated by an open wound.

The results of 16 fractures followed up at review (Table 7.6) emphasise the poor prognosis in the comminuted fractures, particularly where there is major disruption of the joint surface or serious soft tissue damage.

Table 7.6 Results at post-treatment review of condylar fractures of the middle phalanx

Fracture type	Outcome of treatment	
	Excellent and good	Fair and poor
I	0	1
II	4	2
III	2	7
Total	6	10

Undisplaced fractures

The only apparently undisplaced fracture in this group was that of a child who caught her cardigan in a door and suffered a unicondylar fracture. Within 10 days the fracture had displaced to become a Type II injury with an obvious 25° angulation (Fig. 7.8). This case illustrates the instability of this fracture and the need to fix internally any condylar fracture which shows even the slightest tendency to shift. It is uncertain whether displacement can be prevented by splint-

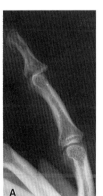
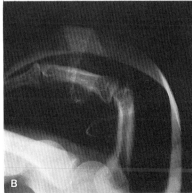

Fig. 7.6 Type III volar fracture subluxation (A) managed on extension-block splint (B)

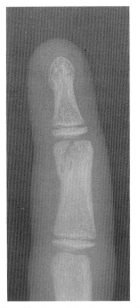
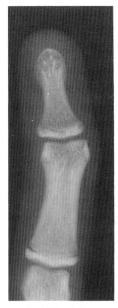

Fig. 7.8 Type II unicondylar fracture of middle phalanx. Initial displacement minimal progressing to angulatory deformity

ing the fracture before deformity occurs, but it is safer to intervene rather than to delay.

Unicondylar fractures

The displaced unicondylar fracture (Type II) is unstable and will certainly result in deformity of the finger, incongruity of the articular surface, and secondary arthrosis. It has none of the benign features of the basal fracture at this level. All authors are agreed that stabilization by internal fixation is required; the fragment cannot be reduced or held by closed techniques. The management of this fracture is discussed in relation to the proximal interphalangeal joint since the problems are similar at the two joints.

Comminuted fractures

Of the nine fractures at this level which were reviewed, seven were open, all the result of industrial crush injuries, one involving a grindstone. Fractures were of the bicondylar Y shape, comminuted, and in one case associated with bone loss; these seven open fractures all had a poor prognosis and the joint became totally ankylosed in four cases.

The extent of the bony injury does not lend itself to accurate open reduction and the additional complication of soft tissue damage to joint, tendon, and ligament makes stiffness inevitable. Where the prognosis is hopeless, it is preferable at the outset to aim for a stable primary fusion in optimum position by arthrodesis (Fig. 7.9). In less severe closed injuries, where there is no soft tissue damage, an attempt may be made to fix a bicondylar fracture by a cross K-wire between the two fragments and a second wire into the shaft, or by interfragmentary wire loops. The fragments are small and fragile, their blood supply is precarious, and the collateral ligaments impede access. If these difficulties can be overcome, then occasionally the joint may be restored to good function. In more comminuted fractures, where there is no soft tissue damage and where ankylosis is not anticipated, early protected movement rather than splintage offers the best chance of a mobile joint.

Avulsion fractures

In this category are included those bony fragments associated with ruptures of the long extensor or flexor tendons, or with ligamentous injuries. The latter will be discussed in relation to proximal interphalangeal joint injuries.

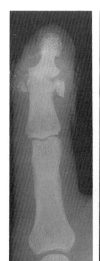
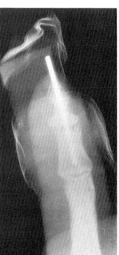
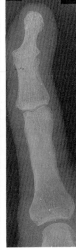

Fig. 7.9 Type III bicondylar fracture middle phalanx. Severe open crush injury. Primary arthrodesis

Extensor tendon injury

The small bony fragments which may accompany mallet finger should not be confused with intra-articular fractures of the terminal phalanx and it is misleading to classify these injuries together. Mallet injury with a bony fragment behaves in exactly the same way as a pure tendon rupture and requires similar treatment.

Flexor tendon injury

Avulsion of the flexor digitorum profundus may be associated with a large bony fragment detached from the terminal phalanx and including part of the articular surface. The bony fragment may become trapped in the distal (A4) pulley and prevent retraction of the tendon. The fragment should be replaced by internal fixation which offers an excellent prospect of restoring tendon function.

INJURIES OF THE PROXIMAL INTERPHALANGEAL JOINT

Basal fractures

The same three types were identified as at the terminal interphalangeal joint (*see* Fig. 7.2). Table 7.7 shows the results seen in this group at review.

Table 7.7 Results at post-treatment review of basal fractures of the middle phalanx

Fracture type	Outcome of treatment	
	Excellent and good	Fair and poor
I	3	0
II	2	1
III	4	3
Total	9	4

Undisplaced fractures

Type I injuries at this joint are uncommon. They are usually caused by a blow on the fingertip in ball games or by a fall on the extended finger. Since they are stable injuries they should be managed by early protected motion, either by taping the finger to its neighbour or by using a Bedford tubigrip support. Rigid splinting has no purpose and may increase the possibility of stiffness in a traumatized joint.

Comminuted fractures

Type II injuries are also uncommon. The distal joint is more vulnerable to crushing and comminution than the proximal interphalangeal joint. Where comminution precludes reduction, either by closed or open means, there is nothing to be gained by splinting. The best prospect of a mobile joint is early protected motion, supporting the injured digit to its neighbour.

Volar marginal fractures and fracture-subluxations

Type III marginal fractures with displacement are frequently associated with subluxation or dislocation of the proximal interphalangeal joint. This is one of the most challenging injuries to the digital skeleton and has attracted considerable attention. They are not common and few authors have reported more than a handful of cases. Like basal fractures of the terminal phalanx, sports accidents predominate and a blow on the end of the finger by a fast-moving hard ball is the commonest single cause of injury. Eaton and Dray (1982) discussed the mechanism of dislocation of the proximal interphalangeal joint. Where this occurs without an associated fracture, reduction is stable because at least one of the collateral ligaments is intact and will maintain stability once reduction is achieved. When the volar lip fragment is small, there may be sufficient of the collateral ligament attached to the middle phalanx to render the joint stable on reduction and to prevent resubluxation. However, where the marginal fragment encompasses a major part of the joint surface, the collateral ligaments will be attached to the volar fragment so that stable reduction is impossible. The joint will relocate on flexion but dislocate as soon as it is extended again.

The management of this injury must take into account this mechanism of stability. In fractures involving small bony fragments, the joint may well not be subluxed at presentation or there may be a dislocation easily reduced and stable in extension. Such injuries pose no problem and may be treated by simple support to a neighbouring digit with early protected motion.

The more usual case is the unstable fracture–dislocation. These can be reduced by flexion of the proximal interphalangeal joint but a position of acute flexion must be held, either by rigid splinting or transarticular K-wire, for at least three weeks. Even at this time the joint may resublux when it is extended and a further period of flexion may be required. The outcome of such treatment will almost certainly be either a joint stiff in flexion or a chronic subluxation with irregularity of the joint surface (Fig. 7.10).

Failure to treat the fracture adequately will, in most instances, result in a stiff painful joint. Whilst remodelling may take place (Fig. 7.11) this is a rare occurrence in contrast to the more benign behaviour of fracture–subluxations at the terminal joint. The disability arising from stiffness at the proximal joint is certainly a more serious handicap than loss of motion at the distal joint. Healing of the fracture

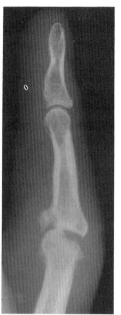
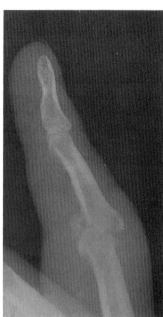

Fig. 7.12   Type III fracture–dislocation. Inadequate primary treatment. Middle phalanx snaps in and out of condylar defect

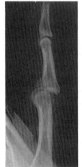
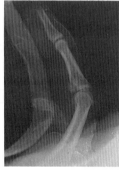
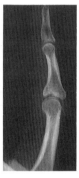

Fig. 7.10   Type III volar marginal fracture of middle phalanx with subluxation of proximal interphalangeal joint. Reduction obtained by flexion on splint. At six months the joint is stiff, the surface is irregular and subluxation has recurred

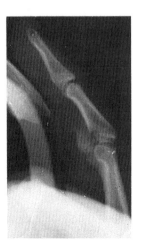
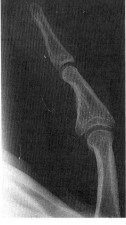

Fig. 7.11   Type III fracture–dislocation. Inadequate reduction, but surprising degree of remodelling at 5 years

in a displaced position may result in a significant step in the articular surface of the middle phalanx. Figure 7.12 shows the late result of an untreated fracture–dislocation in which there is such a step and where a secondary defect in the condyle of the proximal phalanx has developed. The finger snapped as the middle phalanx locked into this condylar depression.

Dynamic fixation. Many different types of treatment have been proposed for this problem fracture. They fall into three groups. The first is some form of *dynamic fixation.* Robertson, Cawley and Faris (1946) reported an ingenious system of three-plane traction through Kirschner wires and claimed good results in seven cases. Subsequently, Agee (1978) described a 'force-couple splint': a complex system of K-wires and rubber bands which maintain reduction without open operation. Only two cases were reported, however. Eaton and Dray (1982) report these methods as difficult for the average orthopaedic surgeon to use.

Open reduction and internal fixation. Second, and favoured by most authors, is a direct approach to the injury by open reduction and internal fixation. The small volar fragment is fixed to the middle phalanx either by fine Kirschner wires or by a wire suture passing from the dorsum of the finger through the phalanx into the fragment and back again to be tied over a button. Lister (1978), the great proponent of intraosseous wiring, reported 24 fractures involving the proximal interphalangeal joint treated by wire sutures, although some of these were condylar and avulsion injuries. If the volar fragment is very small, the wire may be taken around rather than through the fragment. Wilson and Rowland (1966) reported 14 cases, half of which had been struck on the extended finger by a ball. They thought that the mechanism of injury was longitudinal compression and hyperextension and in early cases used open reduction and internal fixation. McCue et al (1970) described 21 patients with fracture–dislocation of the proximal phalangeal joint, but only six were early cases. Kirschner wires were used to fix the volar lip and supplemented by a transarticular wire for three weeks. Eaton and Dray (1982) advocated a similar method, especially for large fragments. The intra-articular wire was removed at two weeks and they used extension-block splinting thereafter to mobilize the joint. Where the volar fracture was comminuted and unsuitable for fixation, they recommend volar plate arthroplasty. This involves removal of the bony fragments and suture of the advanced volar plate into the resultant defect in the middle phalanx.

Extension-block splinting. This is a third method to consider, described by McElfresh, Dobyns and O'Brien (1972). Out of a total of 196 fractures involving the base of the middle phalanx, they found 132 to be stable and 64 associated with subluxation or dislocation. They reported 17 cases treated by extension-block splinting of which 12 achieved full extension while the mean flexion range in the group was 90–105°. The technique (Fig. 7.13) demands close outpatient supervision. A forearm plaster cast is applied to which is attached a dorsal malleable splint holding the finger flexed at the proximal interphalangeal joint. The degree of flexion required is 10–15° more than that necessary to achieve a stable reduction of the dislocation. The finger is left free to flex at the proximal and distal interphalangeal joints but cannot extend. At weekly intervals the degree of flexion is relaxed by adjusting the splint and check radiographs are taken to ensure that reduction is

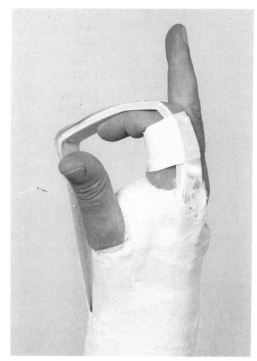

Fig. 7.13 Extension-block splint prevents extension of PIP joint but allows flexion

not lost. Figure 7.14 illustrates a rather comminuted fracture–dislocation treated by this technique with radiographs taken at each stage as the degree of flexion of the splint is reduced. After four weeks the patient should have achieved 90° of flexion but full extension is deliberately delayed for 6–12 weeks. Eaton and Dray (1982), whilst agreeing that the technique is suitable for fracture–dislocations with small interarticular fragments, claim that where larger fragments are involved open reduction and internal fixation is required.

The extension-block splint offers a solution to this challenging fracture which avoids a difficult intra-articular procedure which may itself lead to joint stiffness. Particularly in the case of comminuted or small fragments of less than one-third of the articular surface, open reduction is fraught with difficulty. The fragments may well split when the wire is introduced and sound fixation demands considerable dexterity. Where the fragment is larger, and certainly if 50% or more of the joint is involved, open wiring of the fragment and temporary stabilization of the joint by a transarticular K-wire seems a sound procedure.

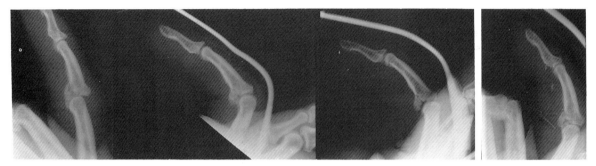

Fig. 7.14 Type III fracture–dislocation of proximal interphalangeal joint managed by extension-block splint. Gradual extension of splint while maintaining reduction

Chronic fracture–dislocation. Despite its obvious severity, it is surprising how often fracture-dislocation of the proximal interphalangeal joint is neglected, inadequately managed or even missed altogether. The interest in this subject, particularly by American authors, reflects the frequency of inadequate treatment and underlines the importance of early recognition of this serious injury. Zemel et al (1981), in a review of the literature, noted three principal techniques for dealing with this problem: the volar plate arthroplasty reviewed by Eaton and Malerich (1980); open reduction, osteotomy and graft as advocated by Wilson and Rowland (1966); and open reduction with intra-articular wiring followed by extension-block splinting recommended by Donaldson and Millender (1978).

Volar plate advancement has the advantage of restoring a smooth articular surface. The small fragment is removed and the volar plate advanced into the defect in the middle phalanx where it is held by a wire suture passed into the defect and through the middle phalanx to be tied over the dorsum. The joint is temporarily transfixed by a Kirschner wire for 2 weeks and then mobilized by extension-block splinting.

A more direct approach, described by Wilson and Rowland (1966), involves correction of the malunion by an opening wedge and graft. The small fragment is fixed by Kirschner wires or a wire loop and the joint is temporarily transfixed in the reduced position by transarticular wire. Zemel et al (1981) reported 14 cases treated by this method with an average improvement in range of motion of 40°.

Donaldson and Millender (1978), adopting a simpler approach, left the fragment undisturbed, reduced the dislocation after soft tissue release, held it at 90° for 11–12 days and then restored motion by using extension-block splinting. Their average range of motion in the four cases described was 86°.

Since these injuries will inevitably lead to pain and stiffness if left in the unreduced subluxated position, an attempt at late reduction by one of these techniques is well worthwhile. Even if the range of motion achieved is not great, the joint will be less likely to become painful or arthritic. Where it is believed that late reduction is not appropriate, by reason of stiffness or secondary arthrosis, then a salvage operation such as arthrodesis or arthroplasty may be considered. Replacement or hinge arthroplasty of the proximal interphalangeal joint has not had the success that has been achieved at the metacarpophalangeal joint and the experience is largely in rheumatoid arthritis. In the present state of development of proximal interphalangeal joint arthroplasty there must be considerable reservation in recommending this procedure in post-traumatic cases, especially in the younger adult.

Dorsal marginal fractures

Fractures of the dorsal lip of the middle phalanx occur much less frequently than the volar fracture. The central strip of the extensor tendon is attached to the small fragment while the volar plate and collateral ligaments will maintain their normal relationships. Volar subluxation of the middle phalanx often accompanies this injury just as it does in the equivalent and more frequent injury at the terminal joint. The aim of treatment is to reduce the subluxation of the joint and to prevent a chronic Boutonnière deformity.

Non-operative management is only appropriate if the fragment is very small and undisplaced. Splinting in extension for four weeks followed by dynamic splinting and exercise is recommended.

Where the fragment is displaced, Weeks (1981) recommends exposure of the fragment and central tendon through a dorsal incision. If the fragment is large it is reduced and held by a K-wire and the joint transfixed by another wire to maintain reduction. When the fracture is comminuted, or the fragment too small for internal fixation, the central slip is sutured directly into the fracture defect and again the joint is transfixed.

Condylar fractures

These fractures were classified into London's (1971) three types (*see* Fig. 7.3). Table 7.8 shows the results obtained in this group at review.

Table 7.8 Results at post-treatment review of condylar fractures of the middle phalanx

Fracture type	Outcome of treatment	
	Excellent and good	Fair and poor
I	9	1
II	2	6
III	0	2
Total	11	9

Undisplaced fractures

Type I injuries should be viewed with considerable caution, for what appears to be a simple undisplaced condylar fracture may, over a period of 7–14 days, develop into a Type II fracture (Fig. 7.15). Whether one can prevent this displacement by external splinting is doubtful and if there is any suspicion of the stability of the fracture, it should be fixed immediately. Careful scrutiny of the X-rays and the use of oblique views may reveal the signs of displacement and instability. Nevertheless, there were 13 Type I fractures treated by simple support to the neighbouring finger and of the 10 followed up 9 were good or excellent.

Unicondylar fractures

Type II fractures are unstable and cannot be reduced by external splinting. If they are allowed to heal in the displaced position, the finger will

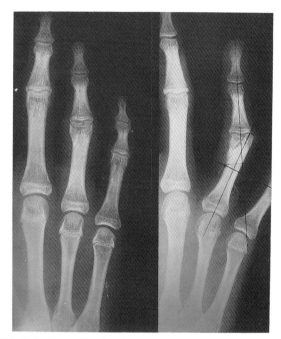

Fig. 7.15 Type II unicondylar fracture of proximal phalanx. Inadequate treatment. Angulatory deformity requiring corrective osteotomy

remain deviated in the lateral plane and may cross over its neighbour. Limitation of motion is likely to accompany this deformity. Of the 19 cases involving the terminal and proximal interphalangeal joints, 14 were followed up and of these there were only six good and excellent results and eight were fair or poor. Of the eight indifferent cases, only three had been treated by open reduction and internal fixation. There is no doubt that improved results can be obtained by accurate fixation of condylar fractures by Kirschner wire (Fig. 7.16) or mini-screw (Fig. 7.17). London (1971) advocated this in his paper and Barton (1984) in his review article on fractures of the phalanges supported this view. The largest series reported has been that of McCue et al (1970). They describe the use of parallel Kirschner wires in the fixation of 32 condylar fractures, dividing the collateral ligament for access. O'Brien (1982) noted the tendency for seemingly undisplaced condylar fractures to become unstable and confirmed the need for internal fixation, for which he recommended Kirschner wires.

Screw fixation provides excellent stability, accurate joint reconstruction and permits unre-

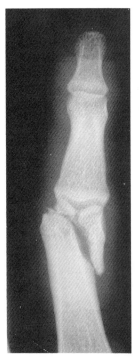
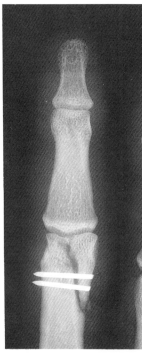
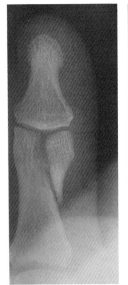
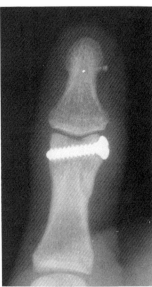

Fig. 7.17 Type II unicondylar fracture of proximal phalanx (A). Open reduction and internal fixation with screw (B)

Fig. 7.16 Type II unicondylar fracture of proximal phalanx (A). Open reduction and internal fixation with two K-wires (B). Good result

stricted early active motion. The method has, of course, been well described by the AO group (Heim & Pfeiffer 1974). Steel (1978), in describing the use of the ASIF small fragment set in hand fractures, warned that care must be exercised not to encroach on the collateral ligament, since the introduction of a screw through its substance may well cause contracture and stiffness. It demands a high degree of skill to obtain accurate, stable fixation without jeopardizing the integrity of the joint and its ligaments. Further miniaturization of the implants and the use of careful technique may obviate these problems and certainly the security of screw fixation permits immediate unprotected movement. Whichever technique is used certain principles are important. The joint surface must be accurately realigned and to do this there must be adequate exposure of the fracture and the joint cavity. At the same time the blood supply of the condylar fragment must be respected, so exposure must not be obtained by extensive dissection prejudicing the vascularity of the fragment. The collateral ligament must either be sectioned and reattached or the fixation implant must pass

through it. Fine K-wires may not cause significant scarring of the ligament, but where screws are employed it is difficult not to encroach on and damage the collateral ligament. Finally, the fragments are small pieces of cancellous bone which are all too easily split by inexpert drilling; the fixation device must be small and be introduced by power tools; the first attempt must, if at all possible, be the last.

Comminuted bicondylar fractures

Type III fractures are either bicondylar or comminuted. Of the 11 cases which could be followed up, nine involved the distal interphalangeal joint and only two the proximal joint. Both had a fair or poor end-result and both of these were open fractures resulting from crushing injuries, and were comminuted and displaced. The terminal joint is more vulnerable than the proximal and is frequently injured in industrial accidents. Whilst it may be possible to stabilize a bicondylar fracture by internal fixation in a similar way to that used for bicondylar fractures of the femur, this is seldom possible because of the comminution and soft tissue damage. O'Brien (1982), whilst recommending this approach, admits its difficulty and the likelihood of diminished motion. For the less severe comminuted fractures early protective movement is advocated.

Avulsion fractures

Small chips of bone, usually located on the volar or lateral aspects of the joint, are indicative of ligamentous injury and should be regarded as sprain fractures.

Hyperextension sprain fractures

The commonest type of sprain fracture is that associated with a hyperextension injury to the proximal interphalangeal joint. This is often the result of sport, horseplay or a fall. The history of a hyperextension strain is usually clear, there is seldom any significant swelling of the joint, movement is preserved and the prognosis is excellent. The bony fragment lies close to the attachment of the volar plate and it is tempting to assume that there has been a partial detachment of that structure. Lee (1963) contrasts the benign outcome of this injury and the frequent loss of motion and persistent swelling which follow dislocation. He is surely correct in assuming that these hyperextension sprain fractures are not the result of subluxation or spontaneously reduced dislocation. Treatment probably does not affect the outcome and should, therefore, be kept simple. Early protected movement by taping the digit to its neighbour is the preference.

Collateral ligament sprain fractures

London (1971) and Barton (1977) rightly stressed the importance of testing for stability when there has been injury to the proximal interphalangeal joint. Where sprain fractures are located near the attachment of the collateral ligaments, displace-

ment of the fracture may well indicate complete ligament rupture and the necessity for operative repair. Large fragments suitable for internal fixation are seldom encountered at the proximal interphalangeal joint and ligament repair should be performed without regard for the bony fragment.

METACARPOPHALANGEAL JOINT

Basal fractures

Three types of basal fracture were again identified (see Fig. 7.2). Table 7.9 shows the results at review in this group of fractures. It will be immediately noted that there is a remarkable contrast between the behaviour of fractures at this joint and that in the distal two joints. The stability of the metacarpophalangeal joint must be a major factor and none of these injuries was accompanied by subluxation or dislocation. Rotational and angulatory strains can be tolerated to a greater degree at this joint than in the more rigid hinge joints, and it is further away than its distal fellows from the vulnerable fingertip. Injuries during football, netball, volleyball, cricket, rugby and hockey were all recorded.

Undisplaced fractures

Type I (undisplaced) fractures had the anticipated good result and their management should be simple. There is no advantage in employing rigid splinting and these stable injuries can start early protected movement as soon as pain allows. Strapping the digit to its neighbour or the use of a Bedford tubigrip permits movement whilst affording some support. These were common fractures but all 13 reviewed were satisfactory.

Comminuted fractures

Seven Type II (comminuted) fractures also did well despite irregularities of the joint surface. Provided there is stability of the joint and early motion can be started, the metacarpophalangeal joint seems to tolerate articular trauma to a remarkable degree. Rigid splinting is positively harmful and achieves no useful purpose. If a fracture is not being held in a reduced position, it

Table 7.9 Results at post-treatment review of basal fractures of the proximal phalanx

Fracture type	Outcome of treatment	
	Excellent and good	Fair and poor
I	13	0
II	7	0
III	6	0
Total	26	0

is futile to splint it. Early protected movement is the treatment of choice. Figure 7.18 shows a comminuted fracture involving a considerable part of the joint surface albeit without any major displacement. After simple splinting, the follow-up radiographs taken after 3 years show a good joint surface and the patient had unrestricted function.

Marginal fractures

The Type III fracture seems appropriate for internal fixation of the displaced articular fragment. Usually the fragments are associated with ligamentous avulsion but seldom is the stability of the joint compromised. The fractures do not behave in any way like their counterparts in the terminal or proximal joints and there is no associated subluxation. This is presumably because the displaced fragment does not take with it both collateral ligaments as at the proximal interphalangeal joint nor is there any extrinsic tendon detachment as at the terminal interphalangeal joint. Lee (1963), in his large series of articular fractures, reported 34 cases of corner fracture of the proximal phalanx. They were not associated with subluxation and

healed with only slight discomfort. Only six cases within this series fell within this category: two were treated by open reduction and internal fixation (Fig. 7.19), and four by simple measures (Fig. 7.20); all did well. Only if there is definite

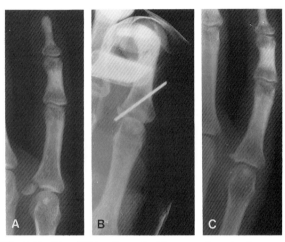

Fig. 7.19 Type III basal marginal fracture of proximal phalanx (A). Open reduction and internal fixation with K-wires (B). Good result at five years (C)

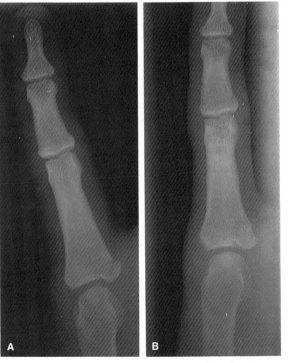

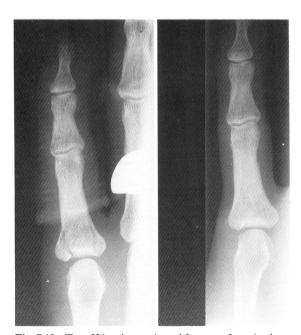

Fig. 7.18 Type II basal comminuted fracture of proximal phalanx. Minimal splinting. Full painless movement at three years

Fig. 7.20 Type III basal marginal fracture of proximal phalanx (A). Minimal treatment. Full painless movement at two years (B)

ligamentous instability, or if a major part of the articular surface is involved, greater than 25%, should internal fixation be applied. Fixation by either Kirschner wire or screw should be sufficiently secure to permit early movement, otherwise restoration of the anatomy may be obtained at the expense of motion.

Avulsion fractures

These are unusual in the fingers where the metacarpophalangeal joints are well protected from injury. The larger fragment has been dealt with above, small fragments can usually be ignored and the ligamentous sprain treated on its merits.

FRACTURES OF THE THUMB

Interphalangeal joint

Basal fractures

These follow the same pattern as that seen in the other digits; all three types of fracture were seen and the causes were not different. Sports injuries (particularly at soccer and rugby football) were common, as were falls on the thumb. The management of basal fractures of the terminal phalanx of the thumb should not differ from that in any other digit. Stiffness of this joint, however, can be tolerated but instability and pain are disabling.

Condylar fractures

The thumb is particularly vulnerable to crushing in industrial accidents and these often involve the condyles of the proximal phalanx. Where there is associated damage to tendon, ligament and joint, and particularly where the fracture is open and comminuted, stiffness is inevitable. In these circumstances primary arthrodesis may be considered. In less severe circumstances early protected movement may result in some retention of joint motion. Displaced unicondylar fractures at this level are suitable for internal fixation either by Kirschner wires or by small screws. Because of the larger size of the thumb, fixation is somewhat easier than in the fingers.

Metacarpophalangeal joint

Basal fractures

Comminuted fractures of the articular surface carry a 'good' prognosis and may be managed, as in the finger, by early protected motion.

Avulsion fractures

Of particular importance in the thumb are those fractures associated with injury to the collateral ligaments. Injury to the ulnar collateral ligament is more common than on the radial side. The mechanism of injury is forced radial deviation and it commonly occurs in falls, particularly on the ski slopes, and in ball games. An avulsion fracture at the base of the proximal phalanx is a common accompaniment of the ligamentous injury and, whilst the fracture may involve quite substantial portions of the articular surface, more often the fragment is small (Stener & Stener 1969).

There is general agreement that, where clinical examination indicates complete rupture of the ulnar collateral ligament, surgical repair is more certain of restoring stability than conservative management. This is supported by the usual finding of the torn ligament lying trapped by the adductor aponeurosis. If a fragment of bone accompanies the ligament avulsion then the displacement of the fragment will indicate the extent of ligamentous separation. Where the fracture fragment lies close to its origin, then it is likely that immobilisation in a plaster cast for four weeks will be adequate treatment; when the fragment is materially displaced then instability of the ligament will usually be found and operative repair should be undertaken. If the fragment is small, that is less than 10–15% of the articular surface, it may be excised and the ligament sutured into the defect with a pull-out wire. When the fragment is large, it should be replaced accurately and held by Kirschner wire or a wire suture (Fig. 7.21), the joint protected in a plaster cast for four weeks and then mobilized cautiously. Some limitation of motion often follows surgery on this joint; this is usually of little functional importance but the patient should be warned that thickening, tenderness, and some discomfort on stressing the joint may persist for several months.

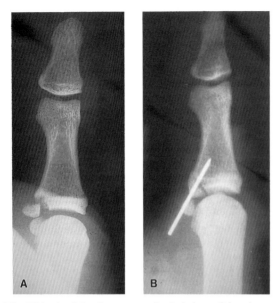

Fig. 7.21 Avulsion fracture proximal phalanx of thumb at attachment of ulnar collateral ligament (A). Fixation by K-wire (B)

Injury to the radial collateral ligament is less common and results from a fall on the thumb with ulnar deviation or adduction. It can be equally disabling if inadequately treated and should be managed in a similar fashion to the ulnar structure, that is by open repair if a complete rupture is demonstrated. Avulsion fractures may also accompany the radial injury (Fig. 7.22) and again may be an indication of the degree of displacement of the ligament. The radial ligament, however, does not become trapped by the aponeurosis. When complete rupture is diagnosed repair should be carried out in a similar fashion to the ulnar side. If there is a small bony fragment avulsed, it may be excised and the ligament sutured to the defect; larger fragments constituting a significant part of the articular surface should be restored accurately by K-wire fixation.

CONCLUSIONS

This is a complex group of fractures ranging from minor cracks in the articular surface to serious fracture–dislocations. No single treatment method is appropriate and it is essential to have a knowledge of the behaviour of each fracture type before choosing the appropriate management. Stable basal fractures without subluxation are suitable for non-operative treatment by early protected movement. Unstable fracture–dislocations, associated with marginal fractures, may demand operative reduction or extension-block splinting. Condylar fractures, if at all unstable, must be accurately reduced and fixed. Comminuted fractures with severe soft tissue damage may require primary arthrodesis or may be salvaged by conservative methods. Avulsion fractures, particularly in the thumb, demand operative reduction when the joint is unstable.

Careful examination to determine instability is as important as radiography in the assessment of these fractures. In most accident units the initial responsibility for these injuries will rest with young, relatively inexperienced doctors. They must be taught how to examine the digits, which radiograph to request, and which fractures will cause problems. Where there is doubt, all fractures involving joints should be referred for a senior

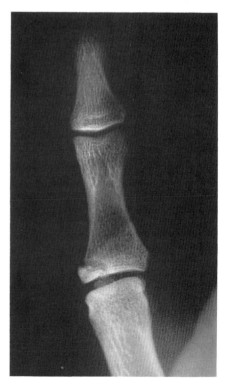

Fig. 7.22 Avulsion fracture proximal phalanx of thumb at attachment of radial collateral ligament

opinion. Failure to institute appropriate management at the outset may result in permanent crippling of the finger joints.

Little has been done in the past to follow up these injuries and there is certainly a need for detailed long-term reviews of articular fractures so that treatment may be based on established experience.

REFERENCES

Agee J M 1978 Unstable fracture dislocations of the proximal interphalangeal joint of the fingers: A preliminary report of a new treatment technique. Journal of Hand Surgery 3: 386–389

Barton N J 1977 Fractures of the phalanges of the hand. The Hand 9: 1–10

Barton N J 1984 Fractures of the hand. Journal of Bone and Joint Surgery 66-B: 159–167

Donaldson W R, Millender L H 1978 Chronic fracture—subluxation of the proximal interphalangeal joint. Journal of Hand Surgery 3: 149–153

Doyle J R 1982 Extensor tendons—acute injuries. In: Green D P (ed) Operative Hand Surgery, Churchill Livingstone, Edinburgh and London, ch 43, p 1460

Eaton R G, Dray G J 1982 Dislocations and ligament injuries in the digit. In: Green D P (ed) Operative Hand Surgery, Churchill Livingstone, Edinburgh and London, ch 16, p 639

Eaton R G, Malerich M M 1980 Volar plate arthroplasty of the proximal interphalangeal joint: A review of ten years' experience. Journal of Hand Surgery 5: 260–268

Hamas R S, Horrell E D, Pierret G P 1978 Treatment of mallet finger due to intra-articular fracture of the distal phalanx. Journal of Hand Surgery 3: 361–363

Heim U, Pfeiffer K M 1974 Small fragment set manual. Springer-Verlag, Berlin

Lee M L H 1963 Intra-articular and peri-articular fractures of the phalanges. Journal of Bone and Joint Surgery 45-B: 103–109

Lister G 1978 Intraosseous wiring of the digital skeleton. Journal of Hand Surgery 3: 427–435

London P S 1971 Sprains and fractures involving the interphalangeal joints. The Hand 3: 155–158

McCue F C, Honner R, Johnson M C, Gieck J H 1970 Athletic injuries of the proximal interphalangeal joint requiring surgical treatment. Journal of Bone and Joint Surgery 52-A: 937–956

McElfresh E C, Dobyns J H, O'Brien E T 1972 Management of fracture-dislocation of the proximal interphalangeal joint by extension-block splinting. Journal of Bone and Joint Surgery 54-A: 1705–1711

O'Brien E T 1982 Fractures of the metacarpals and phalanges. In: Green D P (ed) Operative Hand Surgery, Churchill Livingstone, Edinburgh and London, Ch 15, p 601

Robertson R C, Cawley J J, Faris A M 1946 Treatment of fracture-dislocation of the interphalangeal joints of the hand. Journal of Bone and Joint Surgery 28-A: 68–70

Steel W M 1978 The AO small fragment set in hand fractures. The Hand 10: 246–253

Stener B, Stener I 1969 Shearing fractures associated with rupture of ulnar collateral ligament of metacarpophalangeal joint of thumb. Injury 1: 12–16

Weeks P M 1981 Acute bone and joint injuries of the hand and wrist. A clinical guide to management. C V Mosby Company, St Louis

Wehbé M A, Schneider L H 1984 Mallet fractures. Journal of Bone and Joint Surgery 66-A: 658–669

Wilson J N, Rowland S A 1966 Fracture-dislocation of the proximal interphalangeal joint of the finger. Treatment by open reduction and internal fixation. Journal of Bone and Joint Surgery 48-A: 493–502

Zemel N P, Stark H H, Ashworth C R, Boyes J H 1981 Chronic fracture dislocation of the proximal interphalangeal joint—treatment by osteotomy and bone graft. Journal of Hand Surgery 6: 447–455

P. J. Mulligan

8 Comminuted fractures

The purpose of this chapter is to select comminuted fractures of the phalanges for special consideration. Many of the clinical aspects of phalangeal fractures will have been dealt with already in the other chapters. The methods for treatment will have been described and it is likely that some overlap will occur in this account as there are many basic principles which are common to the less severe injuries as to the severely fragmented bone.

There has been much written regarding the management of fractures of the phalanges, but it is unusual to see special consideration given to comminuted fractures (Barton 1984). This is an opportunity to outline some of the particular features of these injuries. The points of difference between these and the less severe injuries can be seen in the mechanism of injury, the pattern of fractures, the methods of treatment, and the results of rehabilitation. They are commonly regarded as the worst type of fracture occurring in the digits and with the most serious consequences. With regard to the many factors influencing return to function, comminution is a factor in reducing the number who return to full performance (Strickland et al 1982). Over the years, different methods of treatment have evolved whereas only a few years ago (Barton 1979) it was felt that internal fixation was seldom feasible and treatment should be by early movement if this is possible. More recently the newer techniques indicated in that initial report have been extended and we are at last beginning to see some results in comparing different methods of treatment (Diwaker & Stothard 1986).

THE INJURY

Considering various causes of injury, it has been shown that crushing injuries account for almost half of these. One-third may be due to a direct blow and a tenth from a rotational mechanism (Strickland 1982). The severity of the mechanisms will make the pattern of fracture less predictable than in other injuries. Because many result from crush injuries, the force is transmitted to the bone through layers of soft tissues. The injury is in depth and many other structures will have sustained a similar force. There is, therefore, blunt injury to skin, to tendons and sheaths and to ligaments. Vessels and nerves may also be severely traumatized, but it is surprising how frequently they appear to survive. In the most traumatic, the circulation may be severely disturbed and amputation is indicated. In others the composite tissue is badly affected and may be permanently impaired, not just because of stiffness, but because of skin damage and loss of vasomotor control. The crush may have been caused by moving machinery and to the crushing of bone shearing injury to skin and tendons is added. This gives an untidy wound and mutilated digits (Fig. 8.1).

Sometimes only one digit is affected, but frequently more than one finger is damaged. There are many differences when dealing with single and multiple digit injuries, particularly when deciding on management. The recovery of the whole hand depends on a number of factors. The hand will recover quicker from a single digit injury allowing the rest of the hand to return to normal function more easily. The fingers are deformed, the skin is breached and the tendons exposed. The shape and size of the tendon components, together with the position of their attachment to bone, means that flexor tendons are much less commonly involved than extensor apparatus. The cushioning tissues of the volar side protect the ensheathed flexor tendons.

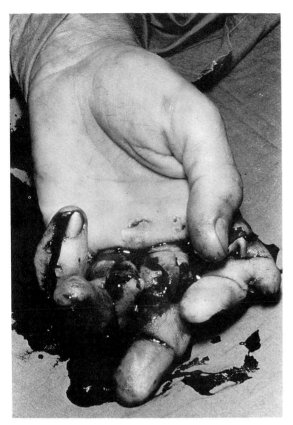

Fig. 8.1 Severely injured hand caught in a milling machine

The extensor mechanism is more frequently exposed and is often torn in the dorsum of the digit by the machinery. When nerves and tendons survive, the digits are still viable and hopefully useful. The appearance of the hand is often of severe destruction with longitudinal wounds. There will be open fractures and deformities of fingers. With a single direct blow or rotational injury, the finger may have retained an almost normal alignment with little wounding, although it may be swollen. Great care must be taken to identify the type of injury and never to under-rate the severity of trauma to the soft tissues.

THE FRACTURES

The assessment of fractures must be with the realisation of the total injury. It is the severe soft tissue damage which will, in the long run, be the limiting factor in achieving the return of function.

It has been shown (James 1962) that the results of fractures of proximal and middle phalanges are clearly related to the degree of soft tissue wounding, including the skin, tendons, vessels and joints. The fracture pattern can confirm the magnitude of the force by the degree of comminution. The reconstruction of the fractured phalanx will, and must, constitute the first step in the repair of the functional soft tissues. Particular note is made if the fractures are into the joints. The bone may be in so many fragments that pieces of bone are avascular or may be missing from the wound site. Frequently the roller-type injury produces a pattern of longitudinal splitting of the phalanges, extending through joints from one phalanx to another (Fig. 8.2). In the direct blow, more transverse or condylar fractures occur. In rotational injury, the fractures are likely to be more spiral or oblique. Spikes may have punctured through the surrounding skin and are frequently contaminated by dirt and debris from the machine. The bones

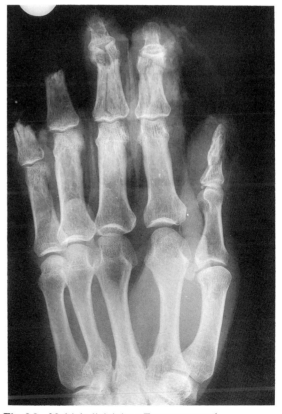

Fig. 8.2 Multiple digit injury. Fractures extend longitudinally through joints

can be completely stripped from the tendon insertions and denuded of periosteum. It is not uncommon for small fragments, especially around the condyles, to have rotated through an arc of $180°$.

During the assessment, radiological examination should be undertaken. This is most helpful in dealing with individual fractures. Sometimes, however, in multiple severe injuries, there are so many fragments and such disturbance of phalanges that the radiograph confirms the severity of the injury but is unhelpful in distinguishing individual fractures. One must concentrate, therefore, on the total effect of the injury with all elements rather than just the bones.

ASSESSMENT OF THE TOTAL INJURY

This part of the management is very important. The anatomical loss and destruction must be related to the functional disturbance. The planned repair will be governed by the return to function which can realistically be achieved. It will be undertaken in the knowledge of which surgical techniques are practical and available. The rehabilitation period and the patient's occupation play a large part in these decisions. The course of treatment should be projected as far forward as the return to work. A provisional outline can be given to the patient, but it is also helpful to the surgeon planning the programme of treatment. This reassures and encourages the patient to participate in recovery from the start. It is also reassuring for the patient to know that there is some hope that use will return to the hand. He may have thought, because of the severity of the injury, that all hope was lost. It is important that the surgeon who will follow through with the treatment is involved with this plan of action. Experience in assessing long-term recovery is required and it is the same experience that will decide on the technique and the instruments which have to be used. This is often more difficult to decide upon than the techniques of the surgery.

Care should be taken not to damage the tissues any further during the assessment. It is worthwhile attempting to get an outline of tissue viability and sensation. Frequently this is difficult to achieve in an anxious patient fresh from injury. The initial examination findings will be confirmed at operation when the reconstruction is undertaken. It is common for patients to admit to sensation being present in severely damaged digits when, in fact, there has been total nerve destruction. This may be an involuntary attempt to preserve tissue. Careful documentation of the injury is always worthwhile. Every feature should be noted and the intact structures should be documented as well as those that have been damaged.

PRINCIPLES OF MANAGEMENT

Many ways of treating these injuries have been described (O'Brien 1982). The spectrum of management ranges from splintage to complex internal or external fixation. In some cases the injury is so severe that careful and judicial amputation is indicated. There is no single treatment. All the different methods must be available and considered. Every technique requires practice and the ability to achieve good results. A guideline might be to seek the earliest return to movement in a functional position with the least pain or further destruction to the tissues.

The fractures must be positioned in the way best to achieve this. Bones must heal and the soft tissues must also be allowed time to heal. If the recovery of the soft tissues can allow movement, then the fractures must also be stable enough to allow this. Some severely comminuted fractures in cancellous bone will stabilize in splintage and allow movement after ten days or so without further displacement. Other less stable fractures will not be so safe to move at this time and should be controlled by fixation. Soft tissues also require a certain time to heal and should be maintained in a position of function during this time. Early mobilization in unstable soft tissue leads to poor healing and deformity. A good example would be in injuries adjacent to the proximal interphalangeal joint where boutonnière deformity frequently follows movement which has been begun too quickly. Thus the nature of the fracture and the soft tissue healing time must be considered when choosing the means of treatment.

The phalanges give attachment to the dynamic components of finger movements. Like an articulated flag pole, they depend on delicate balance to achieve the dextrous movement required; any disturbance of this leads to imbalance of the 'guy ropes' and so contracture and disuse may occur. The 'guy ropes' are the long tendons, the intrinsic muscle insertions and the stabilizing joint capsules. To maintain balance, the phalanges must be correctly aligned and not rotated. The bone should be pulled out to length. Shortening, malalignment and rotation all cause deformity. Soft tissues around the phalanx are closely applied or inserted into them. If these are intact then the position of function can allow the soft tissue envelope to functionally brace the bones in a good position for healing, provided they are pulled out to length. The soft tissue envelope controls the bone position. This is sometimes easier in comminuted fractures than in short oblique or transverse fractures. When there is less comminution, then the effect of muscle pull can be deforming. In most cases the position of immobilization with the metacarpophalangeal joints flexed and the interphalangeal joints extended is the best for recovery. Individual interphalangeal joints should be held in extension by external or internal means if necessary.

During the time of healing, every effort should be made to reduce the swelling. Elevation is standard practice. It is also very helpful to protect the skin. Splintage is often ruled out in skin trauma. There should be no external pressure on the skin. This will be dealt with more fully in the next section. The type of treatment may also be decided upon by the equipment available. The high technology instrumentation in major teaching centres is not always available in many country hospitals or in the Third World. It is important that the *principles* of management are good anywhere, no matter what is the local situation. Even if the means of achieving satisfactory treatment are different, the principles on which this is based are always the same. Many very effective materials can be bought cheaply and, when applied well, will still give excellent results despite their simplicity (Joshi 1979).

METHODS OF TREATMENT

External splintage

There is very little indication for treating unstable fractures by external splintage and the presence of traumatized skin rules this out completely. It can be considered in single-digit injuries, but requires stability of bone and soft tissue, no matter the extent of the fracture. There are many ways of splinting fractured phalanges. Some have been found to be dangerous or at least ineffectual. In years gone by there was great skill in applying plaster of Paris to digits. There are now few who have this skill and to have such a splint applied by someone of little experience must be dangerous. Many of the newer materials could be considered, however, and these are certainly improving.

In stable injuries, only a resting splint should be used. The resting splint should hold the position of the fracture in the soft tissue to prevent muscle pull causing deformities. The external splint should not be used as a means of holding a reduced fracture. The traditional position of holding phalangeal fractures with the metacarpophalangeal joint and interphalangeal joints flexed in the splint is very dangerous. This practice should be discontinued. Malleable metal splints are often used; these can never be adopted as an accurate means of holding a fracture. It is best strengthened by doubling it back on itself with the foam outwards, and again as a resting position with the finger gently strapped in the safe 'position'. It can be very useful if done properly in single digit injuries. The newer plastic and resin materials can also be considered as moulded resting splints, or used as a gutter to hold the proximal interphalangeal joint in extension (Fig. 8.3).

Splinting one digit to another is a common practice in accident departments. In comminuted fractures there is very little application for this, and it should never be used in unstable fractures. It should also be abandoned if an injury extends across a joint with instability to the articulation. There are frequently extensive flexion contractures which are difficult to overcome. Like any other type of external splint it needs very careful and cautious application and arrangements should be made for frequent check visits to the hospital. Adjustments required should be made at an early stage.

Sometimes a single-digit injury is best treated with a well-padded bandage. This will form a restraining splint which can be used until the tissues are almost healed. Thereafter, a more

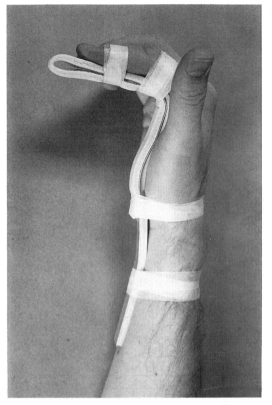

Fig. 8.3   Finger resting in malleable splint achieves position of immobilization—tight strapping is dangerous to injured skin

definitive carefully made splint can be fitted to the finger. This can be extended to a dynamic splint which will allow repair of the tissues (Fig. 8.4).

Although these methods of external splintage are common, their results are poor with comminuted injuries, and they are more likely to be indicated in single-digit injuries. They should only be used when equipment for internal fixation is not readily available.

Internal fixation

Wire fixation

The Kirschner wire is an extremely valuable instrument in dealing with fractures of finger bones. It has become more useful over the last few years because of the improvement in power drills used for insertion. The wires can now be used with much greater accuracy than before. Fragments of a small size can be transfixed without splintering. The rotational force of drilling need no longer tear

nor strip the tissues from the bone. The drill end of the wire is sharper and more efficient. It is imperative to choose good quality drilling wires (*see Appendix*). Many companies providing the power drills will also supply their own efficient wires with them.

There are many different ways of using K-wires in these fractures. They can be used for fracture transfixion or external fixation. They have also been used for pulp traction in the past, but this practice is less often used now, because it is very difficult to maintain accurate traction on digits when pulling through soft tissue. It is much better to consider traction as being an introduction to more rigid external fixation.

The indications for internal fixation of phalangeal fractures have been described by Robins (1961). He suggests that these methods should be used to afford stability after major hand fractures. When the fractures are very comminuted, the shape and size of the fragments must be studied carefully before deciding on treatment. The surgeon has to decide whether internal fixation is feasible or not.

Percutaneous fracture transfixion

This is the most common method of surgical intervention. There is much written about the technique in relation to the tubular anatomy of the phalanges (O'Brien 1982).

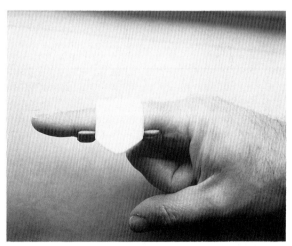

Fig. 8.4   Later a more definitive splint may be used when swelling is less

With practice the bone can be virtually undisturbed and the wires introduced with accuracy. In comminuted fractures the wound will often allow visual reduction of the fractures while the wires are introduced. Sometimes closed reduction also allows accurate percutaneous fixation (Joshi 1976). This can be done under the guidance of an X-ray image intensifier. Perhaps these methods have better application when the fracture is less comminuted, as described in Chapter 5. The wire is of a drill-head type and usually 0.045 inch (1.14 mm) in diameter. In smaller fragments 0.035 inch (0.9 mm) or less may be used. The wire is expected to get two-point fixation on the cortices, but frequently this is not enough and so two wires are needed.

Crossed wires are often advised, but these can distract the fragments apart if introduced from opposite sides of the medulla (Fig. 8.5). This technique has been improved by retrograde introduction of the wires holding the fragments solidly together as they are introduced (Edwards et al 1982). It is frequently worthwhile using one longitudinal wire along which the fracture can be held compressed, while a second oblique wire is inserted to control rotation (Fig. 8.6). It is also possible to introduce them both obliquely or to use two parallel wires through an oblique fracture from the same side. A crossed oblique introduction, both from the same side of the bone, can also be worthwhile. One must feel that the drills penetrating the cortical bone gain security. The wires can be left externally and if not secure they should be turned back on each other before cutting. There seems to be very little problem with infection from these wires. The fractures are held in position and

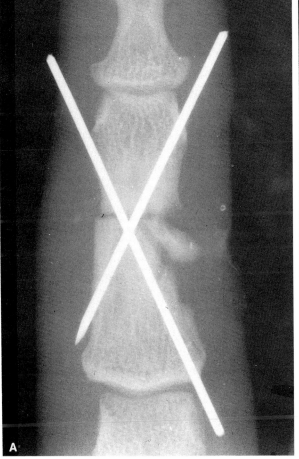

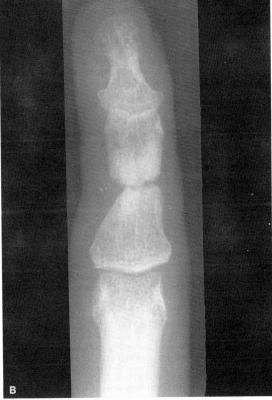

Fig. 8.5 A Oblique wires holding fracture apart.
B Established non-union of fracture

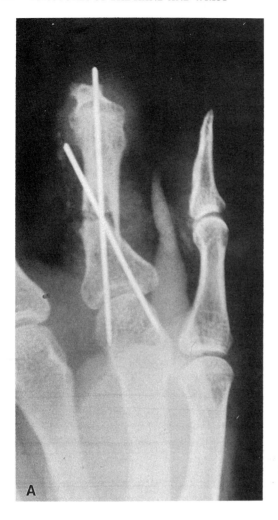

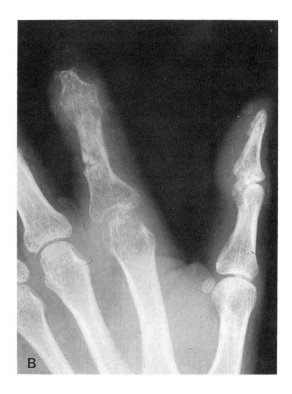

Fig. 8.6 (A) Longitudinal and oblique wires allow more compression. The wire may extend through a flexed metacarpal phalangeal joint. (B) Fracture now united in acceptable alignment

the joints mobilized. The fingers are immobilized for a period of three weeks. Immobilization for longer than this reduces the amount of recovery in the interphalangeal joint (Wright 1968). There are some situations when joint penetration is acceptable. Sometimes the only chance of longitudinal fixation is through a flexed metacarpophalangeal joint or through an extended interphalangeal joint. Many advise against this but again, in practice, it has been found to give very little joint stiffness or infection. If this is the only means of getting stability, then the slight risk is outweighed by the marked benefit from the secure position. Another useful tip is that when introducing the wire through a confined space, for example on the flexor surface, it is often better to drill it right through the other surface and then to withdraw it so that it is flush

with the point of entry. This then means that the wire can later be removed through its exit hole and the difficult point of entry need not be disturbed again.

The additional security of a wire loop in a fracture should be considered (Lister 1978). This has been used in arthrodesis. However there does not appear to be too much application for this in comminuted fractures where a second K-wire would be more helpful. It would be difficult to justify further dissection in order to put in the wire loop. A cerclage wire has the same problems, with the risk of devitalizing the periosteum.

When the digits have been made secure by the chosen means of stabilization, then the fracture should be in a position to allow as much finger movement as possible. It has been shown that properly placed wires do give stability and therefore allow finger movement (Fyfe & Mason 1979). It should be noted that when the wires are removed to allow further mobilization of the joints there will frequently be little evidence of bony union on the radiograph. The time for radiographical union is usually considerably longer than the time for removal of wires. However, it can be as much as 14 weeks in the hard cortical bones of the middle phalanx, and at this level it may be necessary to leave in the wires until there is radiological evidence of union. When the wires are removed it may be worthwhile adopting the benefit of a lively splint.

Wire outriggers

An extension of K-wire principles is to use them not just to transfix the fractures of bone, but to stabilize the whole sections of digit which has been severely traumatized. This is sometimes necessary, particularly in multiple injuries. It is also useful when joints have been severely disrupted. It can be used in a single digit, or a formal external fixator may be better. This technique has been described for phalangeal fractures (Mulligan & Scott 1985). It uses K-wires inserted transversely through digits and maintained at length and rotation by longitudinal external wires. These are fixed to the transverse wires by acrylic cement and form a semi-rigid frame. Several wires can be used in

either direction. The wires can transfix the fractures or be inserted through normal bone as anchorage points. They can also be extended into normal fingers in a search for stability and alignment (Fig. 8.7).

Insertion of the wires is quick and easy and does not require any further tissue disruption; the hand is positioned in the 'position of immobilization'. Interphalangeal joints have frequently been so damaged that there is little hope of recovery. The arrangement of wires holds the fingers in some alignment so that there is recovery of joint movement with a reasonable amount of mobility in many cases. The aim is to allow the severely traumatized tissues to heal while achieving stability and giving the patient a feeling of security. The most frequent result is to recover a hand in a position of coarse grip. This can be strong and painfree and often has a bonus of recovery of interphalangeal joint movement to a greater or lesser extent. With the dressings removed early, the patient begins rehabilitation after a few days of elevation (Fig. 8.8). In severe injury, the confidence is immediate and where there was little hope of anything but amputation, the patient feels surprisingly secure. These fingers are viable and often sensitive, but too traumatized to replant. Many of these patients achieve a quick return to work for such severe multiple injuries to digits (Scott & Mulligan 1980). In single digits, the effect is even quicker.

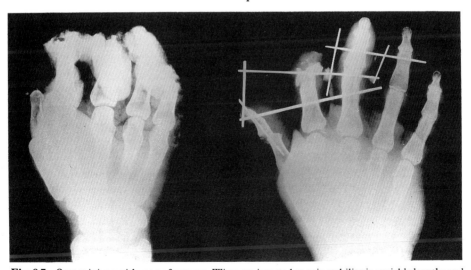

Fig. 8.7 Severe injury with many fractures. Wires are inserted to gain stability in variable lengths and direction

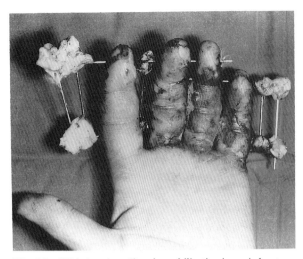

Fig. 8.8 With dressing off, early mobilization is carried out

There are other advantages of this technique. The apparatus is relatively cheap, it is versatile in its application and is probably more so than an external fixator. Compared to external fixators, however, it is not quite as secure in its rigidity. The pins are left in position for 3 to 4 weeks, by which time the patient should have regained

considerable movement. The pins can now be removed and further rehabilitation undertaken (Fig. 8.9).

Formal external fixators

The extension of the principle of external fixators from major long bone fractures to the digits was inevitable. The equipment is much smaller and the pins an improvement on K-wires in that sometimes they are threaded. Although used for the purpose of fixing fractures by Henry Jaquet, external fixation had been used before this for digit lengthening (Matev 1975). It has frequently been used in war injuries (Kesler 1978). The apparatus, therefore, can be used for fracture fixation, distraction or compression. It can fix the fragments in one phalanx, or one to another, or a metacarpal to a phalanx. It is applied longitudinally and is, therefore, more reasonably used in single-digit injuries. In some cases the pins are introduced as transfixion pins with control through both sides of the digit; in other cases a two-plane introduction of the pins is indicated. The fixation should be very

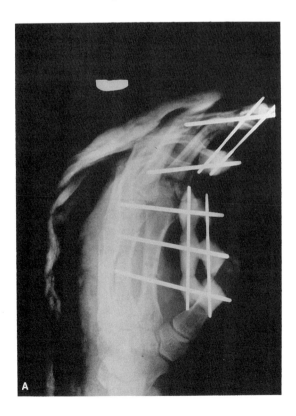

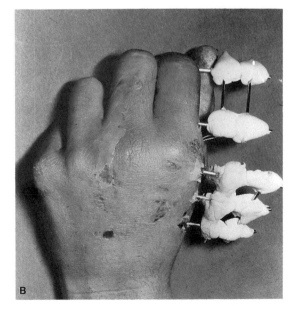

Fig. 8.9 (A) Marked stability in single digit injury with accompanying metacarpal fractures. (B) Early movement achieved

secure and more so than the wires with outriggers. It is, however, not so applicable as the K-wire system to severely comminuted fractures. The design of the restraining jig often limits the adaptability of the apparatus (Fig. 8.10).

The variety of fixators is changing and their use becoming more realistic. Despite their introduction some years ago, there has still been very little written about the results. It is hoped that adjacent joints can be allowed to move freely (Allieu 1985) and they can hold a position to allow further reconstruction or skin grafting to be undertaken. The techniques of introduction are still being developed. They have been used to undertake interphalangeal joint fusion and fracture fixation at the same time (Riggs & Cooney 1983). There are still some complications from this method. There is a rather higher rate of infection than one might expect.

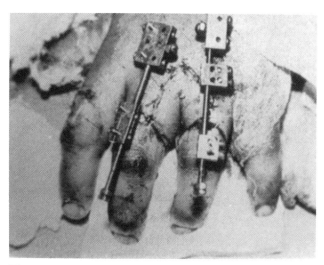

Fig. 8.11 External fixator in multiple digit injury

Riggs and Cooney felt that they could be used for compound, segmental or extremely comminuted fractures of the hand, but only when simple K-wire fixation was not applicable. Their use in multiple digit injuries is infrequently described (Rousso 1985) (Fig. 8.11).

Further details and illustrations of different types of external fixators which can be purchased for use on the phalanges or metacarpals are given in Chapter 13.

Screw and plate fixation

The transfixing screw has been designed to a highly refined point of development. The application of rigid fixation to major long bones has long since been established in smaller fragments. The techniques are clearly described by Heim and Pfeiffer (1982) in their AO Small Fragment Set Manual. When indicated, it can be used with great skill and accuracy. This has been a major contribution to the fixation of fractures of this size. The small fragment set allows screws as small as 1.5 mm diameter to be introduced. Plates are also small and adaptable. The end results of fixation are good if the indications have been properly adhered to. It has the disadvantage that multiple fractures of many bones would require considerable exposure of the soft tissues in order to gain fixation. It should not be allowed to exceed safe tourniquet time. In some multiple injuries Heim states that the surgeon

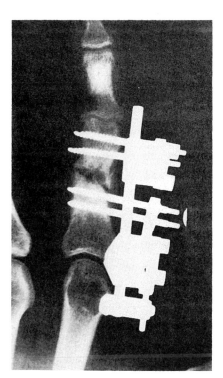

Fig. 8.10 Mini-Hoffman external fixator on phalangeal fracture

should consider whether simple K-wires inserted obliquely, axially, or transversely should be used and combined with cerclage wires (Heim & Pfeiffer 1982). The results obtained using the AO small fragment equipment in hand fractures were considered by Steel in 1978. He concluded there was no place for the set in comminuted fractures of the phalanges. It is very difficult for this type of fixation to achieve the stability of injured soft tissues such as tendons and ligaments where wires can be more helpful. The decision to use these methods should be very carefully considered and they should probably be used in combination with other techniques. The mini screw is best applied to periarticular fractures, where accurate reduction is indicated. Many would also use this technique in non-union of fractures (*see* Chapter 24).

The surgeon undertaking these methods must be specially trained in the technique as it is very easy, when introducing screws, to split fragments (Fig. 8.12). The screw should be introduced with the least exposure. The proximal and middle phalanges may be exposed with least dissection from the posterior or lateral approaches. The extensor apparatus should be carefully replaced and reconstructed at the end of the exposure in order to restore finger balance. Choosing the correct

size of drill and screw is mandatory. Every attempt should be made to avoid splintering of bone, and transfixion with K-wires before insertion of the screw can be helpful. Even when fixed with multiple screws the digits can only mobilize when soft tissues have healed. This is one of the main difficulties as screws do not always achieve soft tissue stability, which may be provided by K-wires if they go across joints or are used with outriggers crossing joints. It may be that they should be used in combination with other techniques.

Despite the criticism of this technique, its application in fractures of the proximal phalanx was compared to other methods by Diwaker and Stothard in 1986, and they found that earlier joint movement was achieved, as was an early return to work. I feel from their report, however, that the method cannot yet be used effectively in multiple comminuted digital fractures but that more will be heard of this in the future (Fig. 8.13).

CONCLUSION

There is no doubt that the management of severe comminuted fractures of the phalanges is still in its developmental stage. The results in the past

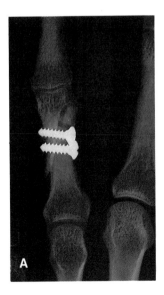

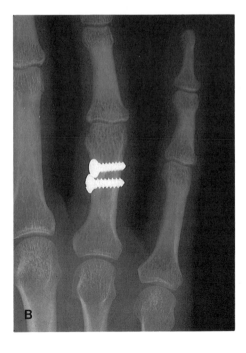

Fig. 8.12 (A) AO screws in fracture, comminuted by insertion. (B) Good radiological result but stiff finger

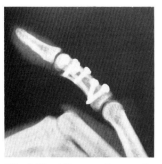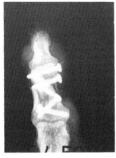

Fig. 8.13 AO screws in severely comminuted fracture of phalanx: stabilizes bone not soft tissue

from open reduction and internal fixation led many to suggest that conservative management was better (Barton 1984). However, techniques for fixation of these fractures have improved, particularly in the last 5 years, and there is some evidence in the literature to suggest that the results are improving with these developments. The fractures are frequently open injuries and fixation is becoming the most common method of treatment of these severe injuries. Many are associated with joint involvement, so joint stiffness is very likely. To avoid this, the treatment must be secure, allow time for tissue healing in the most functional position and achieve an early return to mobility.

In some cases the comminution, though severe, is relatively undisplaced and the soft tissues are stable. Splintage in these cases can be considered and this becomes a functional bracing exercise (*see* Chapter 4) with an early return to movement from a secure position. I make no excuse for repeating the emphasis on soft tissue healing, as it is only by functional recovery of these tissues that a good result can be achieved. Fixation of the bone is designed to allow this to happen.

On many occasions splintage is not possible and so stabilization is achieved by one of these other forms of fixation. The amount of damage to soft tissues decides the prognosis. Strickland et al (1982) showed that the results are worse when there is damage to skin and tendon or when there is tendon involvement. Not surprisingly they also emphasised that the age of the patient had a considerable effect on the prognosis. The security of the fracture allows the position of the soft tissues to heal in order to achieve return to function. The indications for fixation of fractures are now clearer.

The numerous methods have been discussed. K-wire fixation of such fractures is now very common and should be a highly developed and accurate technique. Careful thought should be given to the types of wire and power drill involved. The planning and application of the wires should mean that the fractures are made secure by a relatively harmless technique. There have been great advances in the introduction of these wires.

When the injuries are even more severe and there is dramatic soft tissue involvement, then many digits are severely deformed and unstable. External fixator techniques should now be considered. This can be done by using the K-wire method with outriggers as described. It is cheap, quick and does very little damage. It gives immediate security to the whole hand and rehabilitation starts early. Dressings are removed to allow the patient to see the functioning hand as soon as this is possible. One would expect the patient to return to work within 6 months. The formal external fixator is an extension of this technique. It is more easily restricted to one digit in a longitudinal manner. No one design has yet met with universal approval and there are very few results published of this technique. The design and application will surely get better as time goes by and more will be heard of this type of treatment. The complications seem to be even more significant than for other techniques at present and deserve special consideration.

The use of plates and screws can give good bone fixation, but they should only be used when there is also stability within the soft tissues. Further damage to soft tissue makes this technique less applicable than was first thought. It is best applied to non-comminuted injuries. It should still be used in combination with other methods. Fairly early mobilization of the fracture is shown to give good results if the soft tissues are secure. If not, a period of up to 3 weeks has sometimes to be allowed for soft tissue healing before mobilization is begun.

Finally, there is no one way of treating severely comminuted fractures. The variety of techniques described can be used alone or in combination. The surgeon should be able to adapt each of these and to apply them with variation and skill. The severity and irregularity of such injuries mean it is extremely difficult to assess the results of the techniques involved. The choice of apparatus is important, but no less important is the expertise in rehabilitation which is employed after the surgery. I have been most influenced in selection of techniques by the ability to stabilize the tissues quickly and allow the patient to begin his own rehabilitation at the earliest stage possible. The provision of confidence and security dramatically improves the return to function and employment. The provision of newer surgical techniques which have allowed this has made the biggest improvement in the results we achieve from such injuries. There seem to be fewer of these injuries now than

a few years ago. This is because of changes in industrial practices in many parts of the world, though in under-developed countries and agricultural societies these grotesque injuries are still not uncommon. In such cases, one would advise the rapid and accurate introduction of stabilizing apparatus such as Kirschner wire in a determined effort to allow patients to begin moving quickly. Only when we have a very large number of cases available, and are able under proper experimental conditions to assess these, will we have some idea of the true results of various techniques.

REFERENCES

Allieu Y 1985 External fixation in osteoarticular surgery of the hand. In: Tubiana R (ed) The Hand, Vol. 2, W. B. Saunders Co., Philadelphia, ch 57, p 525

Barton N J 1979 Fractures of the shafts of the phalanges of the hand. The Hand 11:119–133

Barton N J 1984 Fractures of the hand. Journal of Bone and Joint Surgery 66B:155–167

Diwaker H N, Stothard J 1986 The role of internal fixation in closed fractures of the proximal phalanges and metacarpals in adults. Journal of Hand Surgery 11B:103–108

Edwards G S Jr, O'Brien E T, Heckman M M 1982 Retrograde cross-pinning of transverse metacarpal and phalangeal fractures. The Hand 14:141–148

Fyfe I S, Mason S 1979 The mechanical stability of internal fixation of fractured phalanges. The Hand 11, 50–54

Heim U, Pfeiffer K M 1982 Small fragment set manual, 2nd edn. Springer-Verlag, Berlin

James J I P 1962 Fractures of proximal and middle phalanges of the fingers. Acta Orthopaedica Scandinavica 32:401–412

Joshi B B 1976 Percutaneous internal fixation of fractures of the proximal phalanges. The Hand 8:86–92

Joshi B B 1979 Simple and economical splints for the hand. In: Pulvertaft G (ed) The Hand, 3rd edn. Operative Surgery Series, Rob and Smith. Butterworth, London, p. 303

Kessler I 1978 War injuries of the hand with special emphasis on reconstruction of the thumb. In: The war injuries of the upper extremities. Progress in Surgery, Karger Publications, Basel, vol. 16, p 89–100

Lister G 1978 Interosseous wiring of the digital skeleton. Journal of Hand Surgery 3:427–435

Matev I 1975 Gradual elongation of the first metacarpal as a method of thumb reconstruction (Lausanne May 1967), Proceedings, Second Hand Club, The British Society for Surgery of the Hand, London, p 431

Mulligan P J, Scott M M 1985 Multiple compound comminuted phalangeal fractures. In: Tubiana R (ed) The hand, vol. 2, W B Saunders Co., Philadelphia, ch 23, 801–805

O'Brien 1982 Fractures of the metacarpals and phalanges. In: Green David P (ed) Operative hand surgery. Churchill Livingstone, New York, p 582

Riggs G A, Cooney W P 1983 External fixation of complex hand and wrist fractures. Journal of Trauma 23:332–336

Robins R H C 1961 Injuries and infections of the hand. Edward Arnold, London

Rousso M 1985 Multipurpose unilateral external fixator for Hand Surgery. In: Tubiana R (ed) The hand, vol. 2, W B Saunders Co., Philadelphia, ch 58, p 550

Scott M M, Mulligan P J 1980 A method of stabilising severe phalangeal fractures. The Hand 12:44–50

Steel W M 1978 The AO small fragment set in hand fractures. The Hand 10:246–253

Strickland J W, Steichen J B, Kleinman W B, Flynn W 1982 Factors influencing digital performance after phalangeal fractures. In: Strickland J W (ed) Difficult problems in hand surgery, The C. V. Mosby Co, New York

Wright T A 1968 Early mobilisation in fractures of the metacarpals and phalanges. Canadian Journal of Surgery 11:491–498

PART

B

Fractures of the metacarpals

Edward C. McElfresh

9 Metacarpal head fractures

A consistent part of any active hand surgical service is the relatively uncommon intra-articular fracture involving the metacarpal head. Dobyns and Fuqua (1972) found an incidence of 15% in their study of 373 intra-articular fractures involving the hand. McElfresh and Dobyns (1983) have reported on 103 intra-articular metacarpal head fractures and have seen more since writing the paper. Metacarpal head fractures vary from the occult to the markedly comminuted. Males are injured about three times as often as females with a majority of fractures occurring in the second and third decades of life, although fractures may be found in any age group.

The second and fifth metacarpal heads are afflicted more often than the other metacarpal heads. This is probably due to the mobility of the thumb and the protection afforded the long and ring fingers by the bordering index and little fingers respectively. Fractures of the metacarpal head may occur with almost any violent activity in which the metacarpal head either strikes or is struck by another object. They are also seen in crushing and machinery type accidents. Open injuries are seen in about 20% of cases, particularly those involved in machinery accidents and gunshot wounds, but may occasionally be seen with altercations, automobile accidents, and other mechanisms of injury.

HISTORY AND PHYSICAL EXAMINATION

As with any injury involving the upper extremity, an appropriate evaluation needs to be carried out starting with the history and physical examination. It is important to establish the mechanism of injury. This includes the subtleties, if they can be recalled, in order to gain clues as to the type of force involved as well as the direction of the force. One should also ask about the magnitude of the force striking the hand since there is a tendency for more violent forces to cause more comminution in the subsequent fracture.

On physical examination one should first observe the wounds, looking for the evidence of breaks in the integument or an open wound. This is particularly important in those injuries incurred while fighting. Puncture wounds or lacerations over the metacarpal heads should receive meticulous evaluation for osteochondral defects, as well as debridement and general wound toilet, because of the potential complication of an anaerobic or micro-aerophilic bacterial infection developing from intra-oral flora. One must also evaluate the amount of swelling, neurovascular status, musculotendinous function as well as ligamentous stability. This will occasionally require a regional block type of anaesthetic or possibly even general anaesthesia.

RADIOGRAPHICAL EVALUATION

Radiographs are obtained in the usual manner. Routine anterior-posterior and lateral views are taken, as well as oblique views. The oblique views at most institutions are obtained with the hand in a pronated position, but one should also consider taking oblique radiographs in the supinated position if no obvious fracture is seen on the other views and if the clinical evaluation suggests the possibility of a fracture.

Occult fractures, particularly of the osteochondral type, often require specialized views such as a coronal view or a Brewerton view as recommended by Lane (1977). The Brewerton view is obtained by placing the fingers flat on the X-ray plate: the metacarpophalangeal joints are flexed about 65°, and the X-ray beam angled from a point 15° to the ulnar side of a point perpendicularly drawn from the hand. A coronal view is used to look at the dorsal aspect of the metacarpal head. This view is obtained by placing the dorsal aspect of the proximal phalanges on the X-ray plate and flexing the metacarpophalangeal joints maximally. An X-ray beam is then directed towards the metacarpal head along the shafts of the metacarpals.

Specialized techniques such as arthrography, tomography, computerized axial tomography, and radioisotope uptake studies have not been adequately studied in relationship to metacarpal head fractures but may be of value in problem cases, particularly tomography in occult fractures and the use of a pinpoint collimator for radioisotope uptake studies involving areas of avascular necrosis.

CLASSIFICATION

Intra-articular metacarpal head fractures have been classified (McElfresh & Dobyns 1983) by anatomical involvement as seen on the radiographs. There has been a total of ten different groups of fractures noted. These groups are as follows:

1. epiphyseal fractures involving the metacarpal head;
2. collateral ligament avulsion fractures in which the fragment involves the metacarpal head;
3. osteochondral fractures;
4. obliquely directed fractures in a sagittal plane of the metacarpal head, entering the metacarpophalangeal joint;
5. vertically directed fractures in a coronal plane of the metacarpal head;
6. horizontally directed fractures in a transverse plane of the metacarpal head distal to the collateral ligament attachments;
7. comminuted fractures;

8. boxer's type metacarpal neck fractures with an intra-articular split of the metacarpal head;
9. fractures involving loss of substance; and
10. possible occult fractures leading to avascular necrosis of the metacarpal head.

Each group of fractures will be discussed along with mechanisms of injury (when known) possible aetiologies, distinguishing characteristics, complications, and methods of treatment. The author will also state his own approach, including preferred methods of treatment.

Epiphyseal fractures

Other than the Salter-Harris type II fracture (Salter & Harris 1963) of the growth plate and metacarpal neck, the epiphyseal fracture most commonly seen is the Salter–Harris type III fracture extending into the joint space (Fig. 9.1).

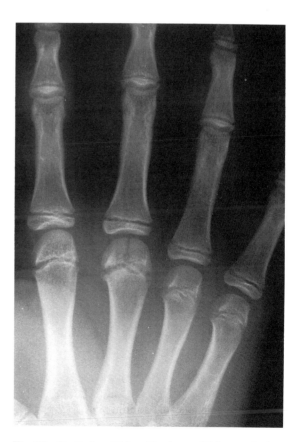

Fig. 9.1 Undisplaced Salter–Harris type III fracture in the third metacarpal head of a 14-year-old boy

These fractures are usually caused by a direct blow over the metacarpal head, those of the second or third metacarpals being most often damaged in this way. The second and third metacarpals are fairly rigid and stable, while the fourth and fifth metacarpals are more mobile and therefore tend to sustain instead a fracture of the metacarpal neck or a Salter–Harris type II fracture. The thumb epiphyseal plate is at the base of the metacarpal and therefore one cannot sustain an epiphyseal fracture of the first metacarpal head. Early adolescence is the age in which this type of fracture is usually seen, although the author has seen radiographs of this fracture in an 8-year-old. Sandzen (1979) has shown a case of a Salter–Harris type V injury of a second metacarpal head from a crush injury with early closure of the epiphyseal plate.

The Salter–Harris type III epiphyseal fracture is usually *not displaced* (*see* Fig. 9.1): these may be treated by 2–3 weeks of splinting to protect it from further injury and then gradual mobilization. As with any epiphyseal fracture, periodical radiographs need to be done prior to completion of skeletal maturity to watch for premature closure of the epiphyseal plate.

If the Salter–Harris type III fracture is *displaced*, it needs to be reduced and held in an anatomical position. The displaced fracture is approached through a dorsal incision, splitting the extensor tendon. The displaced fragment is replaced and held with small Kirschner wires. The wires should be removed in 3–4 weeks. Again, one needs to follow these epiphyseal plates with periodical radiographs until skeletal maturity is reached. The author has seen radiographs of a patient who had a displaced Salter–Harris type III epiphyseal fracture which was moderately displaced, was not reduced, and went on to develop avascular necrosis of the metacarpal head.

Collateral ligament avulsion fractures

Lateral deviation forces in the young child lead to Salter–Harris type II fractures of the base of the proximal phalanx. In a skeletally mature person the same force may cause an injury to the collateral ligament or an avulsion fracture at either end of the collateral ligament. The digit is more susceptible with the metacarpophalangeal joint fully flexed,

due to the shape of the metacarpal head and its axis of rotation making the collateral ligaments taut in full flexion but lax in extension.

Fingers

Any finger may be involved, and either side of the joint in the index and middle fingers, but only the radial collateral ligament attachment has been seen to be avulsed in the ring and little fingers. There may be some protection afforded to these latter two fingers by the index and long fingers against an adduction force. Dobyns and Fuqua (1967) reported a higher percentage of ulnar collateral ligament avulsion fractures than on the radial side. Most collateral ligament avulsion type fractures are closed injuries.

If on examination there appears to be an injury in the collateral ligament complex, radiographs should be obtained prior to markedly stressing the ligament complex. If no fracture is seen, one should consider obtaining a Brewerton view before stressing the joint. If a fracture is identified but is *not displaced*, this is usually treated conservatively with splinting in an intrinsic-plus position for a couple of weeks and then guarded motion started with buddy-taping to the adjacent finger. Longer support periods are used with the radial collateral ligament of the index finger due to the stresses applied with pinching and with the radial collateral ligament of the small finger due to the pull of the abductor digiti minimi muscle. Moberg and Stener (1953) repaired ruptures of the collateral ligament of the small finger. Metacarpal avulsion fragments and collateral ligament injuries, according to Eaton (1971), usually have insufficient displacement to warrant open reduction and fixation and he feels they should be treated conservatively with the possible exceptions of the index and little finger radial collateral ligaments. If there is marked *displacement* (Fig. 9.2), the fractured fragment should be pinned back in place if it is large enough or, if too small, it may be excised and the ligament re-attached by means of a pull-out wire for 4–6 weeks.

This type of fracture can be *associated with dislocation of the MCP joint* which proves irreducible; this is very rare, only two cases having been reported (Flatt 1966, McElfresh & Dobyns 1983).

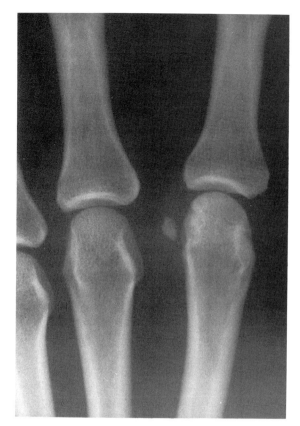

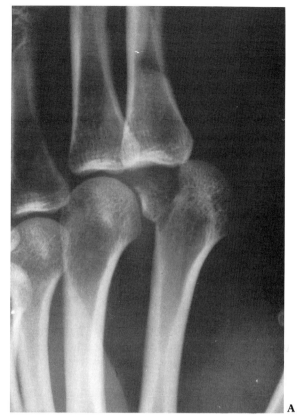

Fig. 9.2 Displaced collateral ligament avulsion fracture of the ulnar side of the second metacarpal head in a 17-year-old girl

They both involved the index finger with a large ulnar fragment of the metacarpal head.

> *Example.* A 25-year-old man injured the left index metacarpophalangeal joint when he was kicked in a karate match. He had an irreducible fracture-dislocation of the metacarpophalangeal joint without neurovascular deficit (Fig. 9.3). The patient was taking prednisone for Crohn's disease. He had an open reduction through a palmar incision and the metacarpal head fragment was stabilized with a Kirschner wire. The wire was removed after two weeks, and the patient then started on active motion.
>
> When seen $3\frac{1}{2}$ years later, the patient had a full range of motion with neither pain nor instability of the index metacarpophalangeal joint. The radiographs showed a defect in the superioulnar aspect of the index metacarpal head which probably represents an area of avascular necrosis.

This type of dislocation may be approached through either a volar or dorsal approach. A volar

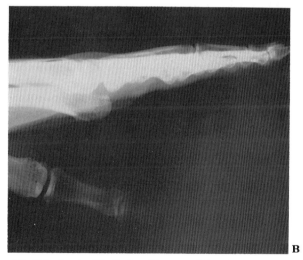

Fig. 9.3 Irreducible displaced fracture-dislocation of the second metacarpal head (A) oblique view. (B) lateral view

approach may be better for viewing the tendon-ligamentous constriction effect on the metacarpal head, but has the disadvantage that the neurovascular bundles are stretched tautly just below the skin surface and susceptible to iatrogenic injury during the surgical approach. The dorsal approach allows adequate reduction of the fracture fragment, and it is usually easier to reduce the dislocation if it is associated with a fracture than if it is an irreducible isolated dislocation. Following reduction, the fragment may be fairly stable when the dislocation is reduced.

Thumb

The first metacarpal head may also suffer a collateral ligament avulsion fracture, but here the fracture is nearly always on the radial side. All large studies of acute ulnar collateral ligament complex injuries report the fracture to be at the base of the proximal phalanx or a tear in the ligament proper (Smith 1977, Lamb et al 1971, Stener 1962, Coonrad & Goldner 1968, Frank & Dobyns 1972, Bowers & Hurst 1977, Smith 1977, Palmer & Louis 1978). Fracture of the metacarpal head on the ulnar side is quite rare, only one instance having been reported by Neviaser et al (1971) in their review of 18 patients.

Undisplaced radial ligament avulsion fractures of the thumb metacarpal head should be immobilized for a period of 6 weeks in a modified thumb spica cast. A well moulded fibreglass thumb spica applied to the hand but leaving the wrist free to move (Fig. 9.4), with adhesive backed sponge padding placed at the wrist level, will allow a great deal more

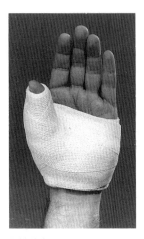
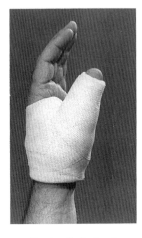

Fig. 9.4 Fibreglass thumb spica cast allowing limited wrist motion. The cast needs to be well moulded to prevent slippage

freedom than the traditional thumb spica and is generally better tolerated by the patient.

Displaced fragments should be replaced through a dorsal approach, paying special attention to the small peripheral branches of the superficial radial nerve. If the fragment is large enough, it should be fixed by Kirschner wires; if it is too small, the fragment may be excised and the ligament complex repaired with a pull-out wire. Another technique that may be used for the ligament repair, instead of the pull-out wire, is to use a 2/0 prolene suture on small straight tendon needles. The suture may be placed through the ligament in a Bunnell fashion and then passed through drill-holes (made with a Kirschner wire) through the metacarpal head and tied to a well-padded button on the opposite side. The thumb is then immobilized for 6 weeks in a modified thumb spica cast. At 6 weeks, the cast is removed and the suture cut on one side. The suture, which is quite smooth, can then be pulled out leaving no foreign body in the ligament. One has to pay special attention to further disruption of the dorsal capsule which, if not meticulously repaired, will allow the proximal phalanx of the thumb to sublux in a volar direction, with eventual development of joint incongruity and its associated problems.

Sequelae

Patients with collateral ligament injuries of the thumb and fingers, whether treated by closed methods or open reduction, generally have pain and swelling with use (particularly stress) for several months after the injury. This may take up to a year to settle down.

Osteochondral fractures

Fingers

Osteochondral fractures may be open or closed and are generally found in patients under the age of 30 years. The mechanism of injury varies markedly but one of the most common mechanisms is when a clenched fist strikes an opponent's mouth in a fist-fight. When the fist strikes the mouth, the dorsal soft tissues are stretched and may split, and the sharp edges of the teeth can cut the soft tissue open. A piece of tooth may break off in the joint or be retained in the metacarpal head; this should be looked for in the X-ray examination. This type of injury frequently leads to a septic arthritis due to the oral flora. These wounds need to be appropriately debrided and often an undetected fracture not seen on X-ray examination will be found due to the tooth impaction.

If there is only an impaction type fracture and any infection or potential infection has been appropriately treated, one should then start early range-of-motion exercises. Any small osteochondral fragments which are displaced into the joint should be surgically excised either primarily or secondarily to prevent further damage to the joint surface.

Thumb

Stener (1964) has described an osteochondral fracture of the first metacarpal head which occurs following disruption of the ulnar collateral liga-

ment mechanism when the joint dislocates and the proximal phalanx shears off a fragment from the metacarpal head. If this is seen during a repair for disruption of the collateral ligament complex, it should be surgically excised.

Oblique sagittal fractures

Oblique sagittally directed fractures of the metacarpal head, which extend into the joint surface, are one of the most common types of fracture of the metacarpal heads. They are usually closed injuries but may be open. The fractures usually affect either the second or fifth metacarpal heads. In the fractures of the second metacarpal head, the distal condylar fragment is routinely on the ulnar side while those of the fifth metacarpal head are on the radial side (Fig. 9.5).

This is considered primarily a shearing type of injury. The reason it is seen with a distal ulnar

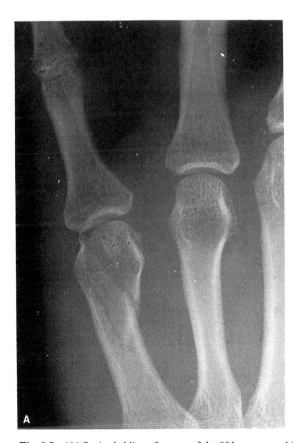 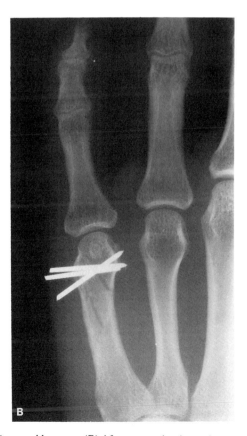

Fig. 9.5 (A) Sagittal oblique fracture of the fifth metacarpal in a 26-year-old woman. (B) After open reduction and internal fixation

condylar fragment in the second metacarpal head and a distal radial condylar fragment in the fifth metacarpal head is felt to be the protection against adduction afforded to the index and small fingers by the long and ring fingers, thus leading to the shearing mechanism.

Any displacement at the joint surface leading to joint incongruity needs to be corrected. If left untreated, these fragments will settle proximally and lead to a block of flexion of the joint due to the protruding spike of metacarpal. Reduction and fixation can occasionally be done percutaneously with multiple Kirschner wires, under regional or general anaesthesia, but usually require an open reduction through a dorsal extensor tendon-splitting approach. The Kirschner wires are left in place for about four weeks.

Example. A 26-year-old woman was struck on the end of her left little finger by a softball. She sustained the closed intra-articular vertical oblique fracture of the fifth metacarpal head shown in Figure 9.5A. This was treated by open reduction and internal fixation with three 0.045 inch (1.1 mm) Kirschner wires (Fig. 9.5B). She was placed in an ulnar gutter splint for 3 weeks, after which the pins were removed, and the patient started on motion with buddy-taping to the adjacent finger. By six weeks the patient flexed the finger from $0°$ to $75°$ and was quite comfortable. At two years she had a full range of motion without pain.

Kirschner wire fixation is normally adequate, but these fractures can also be fixed with a small screw. After splinting for approximately three weeks, the joint is mobilized.

If the fragment has been allowed to settle and has healed with a protruding spike from the remaining end of the metacarpal (Fig. 9.6A), this may need to be excised surgically to allow resumption of full flexion. This may be done several months later if indicated (Fig. 9.6B).

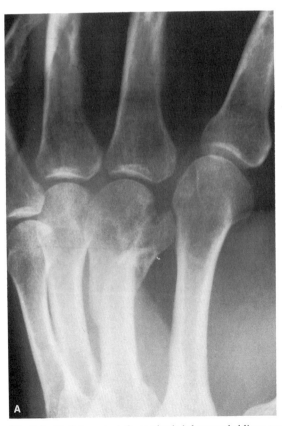 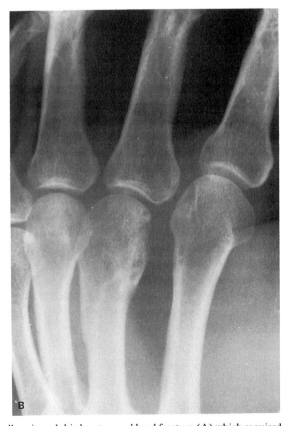

Fig. 9.6   Radial exostosis from a healed shortened oblique vertically oriented third metacarpal head fracture (A) which required excision of the protruding exostosis to obtain full flexion (B)

Vertical (coronal) fractures

Vertically directed* fractures (that is to say, in a coronal plane) of the metacarpal head are uncommon. They may be either dorsal or volar. The *dorsal* injuries are often associated with open extensor tendon injuries and, as with any open fracture, the potential for infection exists. These injuries are due to a shear mechanism from either a direct blow dorsally or a force directed through the proximal phalanx volarly.

Example. An 18-year-old male was involved in an automobile accident in which he injured his left hand. Radiographs showed a fragment in the fourth metacarpophalangeal joint (Fig. 9.7A). There was no evidence of any other fracture and it could not be determined where the fragment had come from until a coronal view was obtained which showed a defect from the dorsal aspect of the metacarpal head (Fig. 9.7B). The fragment was excised since it was not involved in the active range of motion of the joint. The hand was immobilized with an ulnar gutter splint for 4 weeks. The patient regained a full range of motion without pain in another six weeks.

* Assuming the patient to be in the anatomical position, with the metacarpals vertical.

If the dorsal fragment is small and not involved with the plane of active motion, it may be excised but if it is a large fragment it should be replaced with small Kirschner wires and held for approximately 4 weeks before removing the wires and starting active motion.

There has been only one reported case (Mc-Elfresh & Dobyns 1983) of a *volar* fragment. A full description of this case has not previously been published and will be given now.

Example. A 20-year-old man was involved in an accident when his automobile left the road and struck a telephone pole. He injured his right fourth metacarpal head and the radiographs revealed a horizontally directed fracture of the metacarpal head with the volar fragment displaced proximally (Fig. 9.8A). The patient had an open reduction (Fig. 9.8B & C) and internal fixation with two 0.035 inch (0.9 mm), Kirschner wires (Fig. 9.8D). He was splinted for four weeks and then started on early motion. By four months he lacked 5° extension and flexed to 90° but complained of some stiffness. Radiographs showed what appeared to be early avascular necrosis of the metacarpal head (Fig. 9.8E).

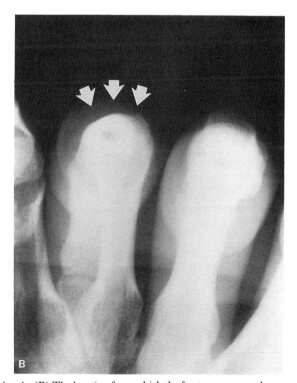

Fig. 9.7 (A) Dorsal horizontal shear fracture in an 18-year-old male. (B) The location from which the fracture came can be seen on the coronal radiograph view

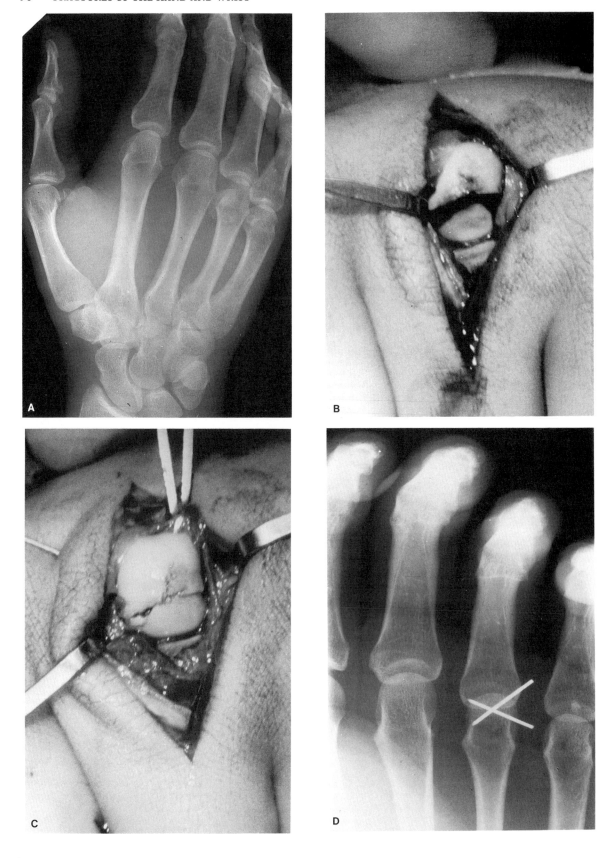

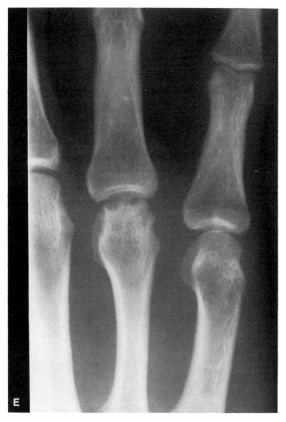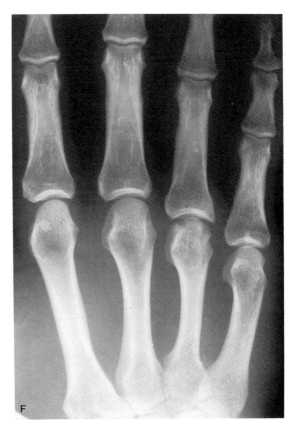

Fig. 9.8   A 20-year-old man with a volar vertically directed fracture of the fourth metacarpal head (A) requiring open reduction (B) and internal fixation (C & D). By 4 months evidence of avascular necrosis was present (E) which showed some remodelling but definite incongruities at $2\frac{1}{2}$ years (F)

After six months the patient had a full range of motion of the metacarpophalangeal joint. One-and-a-half years later, he had only mild aching and a full range of motion. Radiographs showed what appeared to be gradual filling in of the areas of avascular necrosis. At $2\frac{1}{2}$ years the patient noted mild discomfort with heavy use. He still had a full range of motion and the appearance on radiographs showed some remodelling but definite metacarpal head incongruities (Fig. 9.8F).

For cases such as this it is felt that despite the possibility of developing avascular necrosis, open reduction and internal fixation with Kirschner wires should be performed in an attempt to get a congruous joint surface.

Horizontal (transverse) fractures

Horizontally directed* fractures in a transverse plane, distal to the attachments of the collateral ligaments, are unusual and in general have a poor prognosis. These are due to shear force from a direct blow to the metacarpal head. The fracture may impact and be relatively stable which has a good prognosis for satisfactory healing. Displaced fractures often rotate and can rotate almost to 180° because of the absence of capsular attachments (Fig. 9.9). The displaced rotated fractures will usually unite but later show some evidence of avascular necrosis. This causes generalized aching of the joint with use and a decreased active and passive range of motion.

These fractures should be reduced, if displaced, by means of a dorsal extensor tendon-splitting incision and fixed using multiple Kirschner wires. When introducing the wires, one should try to avoid as much of the joint surface as possible but

* Again, this is with the patient in the anatomical position, the metacarpals being vertical.

still obtain compression and stability. Often early passive motion is possible, but the Kirschner wires need to remain in place for 4–6 weeks.

Comminuted fractures

Comminuted fractures of the metacarpal heads comprise one of the most frequent subgroups of intra-articular metacarpal head fractures encountered in a clinical practice. In general, these fractures occur after more violent injuries and are often associated with injuries of the adjacent metacarpals and phalanges. There may be marked soft-tissue damage, including open wounds. Any treatment must also take these other problems into consideration.

The treatment of comminuted intra-articular metacarpal head fractures will depend upon the integrity of the articular surfaces and the amount of displacement. *Undisplaced* fractures with fairly

good integrity of the joint surfaces (Fig. 9.10) are best treated by brief immobilization, followed by active motion avoiding undue stress upon the involved joint. Fractures with large *displaced* articular fragments should be reduced and held with small Kirschner wires, though this is very difficult technically as there may be additional tears of the articular cartilage. The fragments should be pieced together and motion started as soon as fracture stability allows.

Example. A 21-year-old man was seen for a comminuted intra-articular metacarpal head fracture of the left second metacarpal which was sustained when he was struck by a policeman's night-stick at a rock concert (Fig. 9.11A). Six days after the injury, the patient had an open reduction and internal fixation with multiple Kirschner wires done under axillary block anaesthesia (Fig. 9.11B).

The patient was held in a radial gutter plaster splint for three weeks and then started on active motion. The wires were removed at five weeks after operation.

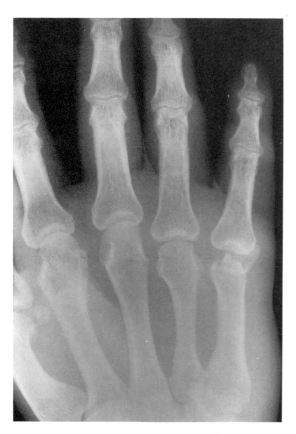

Fig. 9.9 A 45-year-old man with a horizontally transverse fracture of the fifth metacarpal head

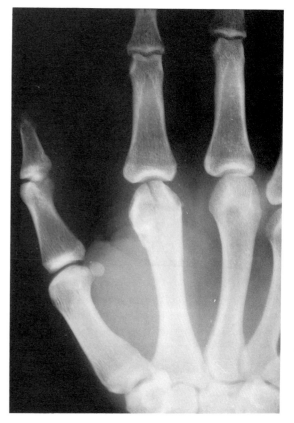

Fig. 9.10 Undisplaced comminuted metacarpal head fracture treated with early protected active motion

By six weeks his motion was from $0°$ to $70°$. One year later, he had $0°$ to $95°$ motion. Two years later he had a full range of motion. He had no pain except for minimal aching in extremely cold weather although there were some arthritic changes on radiographs (Fig. 9.11C).

The fracture which shows marked comminution and displacement that cannot be technically pieced together should be briefly immobilized and then started on active motion, avoiding undue stress upon the joint. In general these fractures are difficult to treat and do not do well. If there is also a fracture of the proximal phalanx or a very comminuted shortened metacarpal head fracture, skeletal traction (Fig. 9.12) is an option for 2–3 weeks before starting on a gentle active motion programme. The skeletal traction can be placed through a metal cylindrical tube created by passing an 18 gauge needle through the proximal phalanx

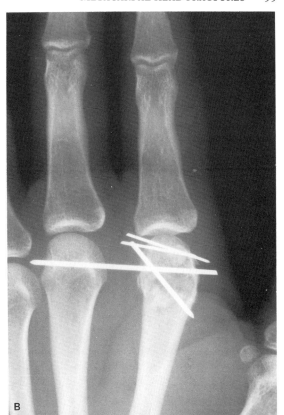

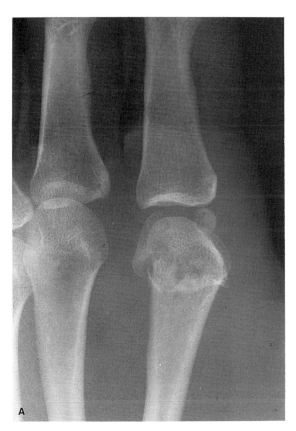

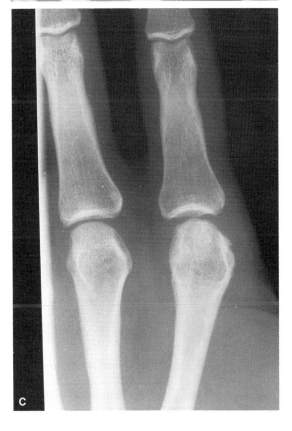

Fig. 9.11 Comminuted fracture of the second metacarpal head (A) treated by open reduction and internal fixation (B). Two years later, there was some incongruity on radiograph (C) but patient was doing well

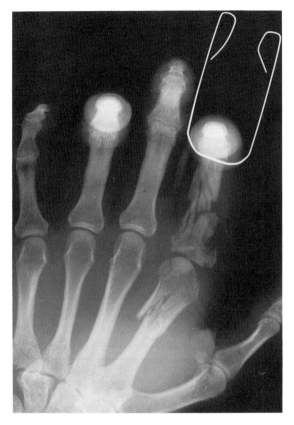

Fig. 9.12 Comminuted second metacarpal head fracture held for two weeks by skeletal traction before initiating active range-of-motion exercises

distally. The needle should be scored at both sides of the finger before breaking the needle to avoid crimping of the ends. The traction wire is then passed through the tube to avoid irritation created by the traction wire.

It is usually impossible to use screw fixation in comminuted metacarpal head fractures due to the size of the fragments and one must rely on Kirschner wires, cerclage wires or a combination of the two techniques. Suggestions have been made in the literature that there might be a place for performing a primary arthrodesis (Heim 1974) or arthroplasty (Beasley 1981) in the severely comminuted type of fractures.

Boxer's fracture into joint

Patients may sustain an undisplaced longitudinal split extending into the metacarpal head from the metacarpal neck fracture commonly referred to as a boxer's fracture. The patient will usually give a history of having been involved in a fist-fight in which he felt the initial fracture occur but kept on striking his opponent. These are usually closed injuries.

Example. A 21-year-old male was involved in a fight and injured his right fourth metacarpal head. He noted that he felt something break but kept hitting the other individual. When seen two days later he was markedly swollen and flexed only from 30° to 55°. Radiographs showed a fracture of the fourth metacarpal neck with 25° angulation and an intra-articular split of the metacarpal head that was undisplaced (Fig. 9.13). He was started on early motion with buddy taping to the adjacent finger. At three weeks he had started to show callus formation and had motion of 15° to 85°.

When there is no displacement, the fracture is treated as any other boxer's fracture. Usually, as in the example described, a conservative approach with early range of motion exercises is the preferred technique. If there is displacement of the longitudinal split (not the metacarpal neck fracture), open reduction with fixation by multiple Kirschner wires, or possibly a small screw, would be warranted.

Fractures with loss of substance of the metacarpal head

Machinery-induced or crushing injuries of the hands can cause loss of bony substance of the metacarpal head. These are open injuries with severe soft tissue damage and therefore the potential of superimposed infection. It is not uncommon to see reflex sympathetic dystrophy after such injury: it may affect the whole upper extremity or be localized to one area or digit.

Treatment of bone loss requires an individualized approach trying to achieve as congruous a joint as possible. Methods used include osteocartilaginous grafts from adjacent non-viable joints, filling with proplast, cartilage resurfacing, and other techniques which are discussed below in the section on reconstructive surgery.

Example. A 20-year-old male college student's left hand became entangled in a table saw. He severed the extensor tendons and sustained multiple fractures, including one with loss of substance of the second

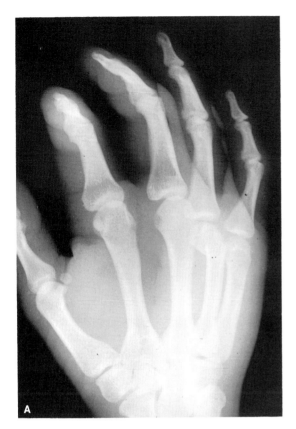
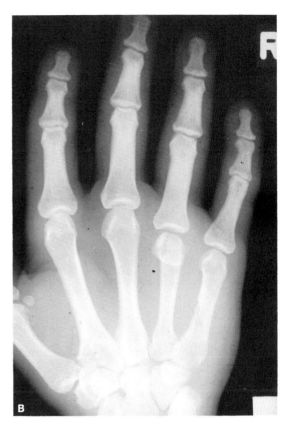

Fig. 9.13 Boxer's fracture with an intra-articular split of the metacarpal head. The oblique view (A) shows the head fracture. The anteroposterior view (B) shows the split in the head extending into the MCP joint

metacarpal head (Fig. 9.14A). A bone graft was cut obliquely from the amputated distal end of the proximal phalanx of the middle finger and fitted into the defect in the index metacarpal head (Fig. 9.14B). The patient was started on early range-of-motion exercises after the wounds healed. By six weeks, the graft had incorporated and the patient's motion at the second metacarpophalangeal joint was $0°$ to $45°$ (Fig. 9.14C). This motion has not changed appreciably over the ensuing five years.

Avascular necrosis of the metacarpal head

A rare defect in the metacarpal head is the development of avascular necrosis following trauma in which no obvious fracture was seen. There have been 17 cases reported in the literature, a majority involving the second and third metacarpal heads (Table 9.1).

The reports have all been of cases involving only one metacarpal (Dieterich 1932, Friedl 1934,

Grosskettler 1935, Schinz et al 1952, Seyss 1961, Franke 1962, and Carstam and Danielsson 1966), with the exception of that of Bopp (1938) which involved both the second and third metacarpal heads. The ages of the patients ranged from 14 to 51 years, most of the patients being fairly young. All the cases reported in the English literature were 14 or 15-year-old boys who had sustained injuries of the metacarpophalangeal joints without evidence of fracture of the metacarpal heads on X-ray examination. Retrospectively, the radiographs all showed widening of the metacarpophalangeal joint spaces. At 6–12 months following the initial injury, the patients were re-evaluated because of persistent

Table 9.1 Reported cases of avascular necrosis of metacarpal heads associated with trauma but with no obvious fracture

	I	II	Digit III	IV	V
Number of cases	0	5	7	3	2

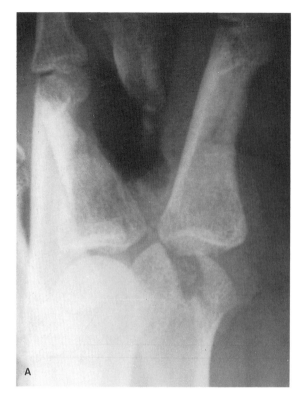

A

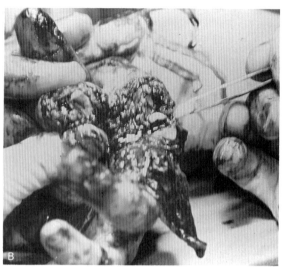

B

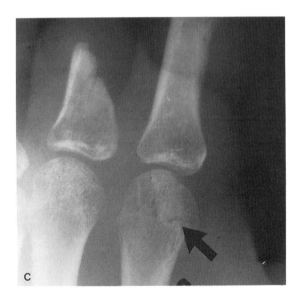

C

Fig. 9.14 A 20-year-old man's unskilful use of a table skill saw resulted in loss of part of the second metacarpal head (A). An osteochondral graft was taken from the head of the proximal phalanx of the amputated middle finger. The graft (B), held in forceps alongside the damaged metacarpal head, is placed in the defect on the index metacarpal. The graft incorporated and healed satisfactorily (C)

aching and discomfort with use of the metacarpophalangeal joint. Radiographs revealed avascular necrosis of the metacarpal joint surfaces which have gradually remodelled but have continued to show only partial recovery with marked irregularities. Aching particularly with strenuous usage has persisted. The radiographs are similar to the late residua of the avascular necrosis seen with the transverse metacarpal head fracture and certain other metacarpal head fractures, suggesting the possibility of an occult fracture.

Example. A 14-year-old boy was playing baseball when he was struck over the right second metacarpophalangeal joint. He developed pain and swelling, but still had a full range of motion. He was seen three days after the injury when radiographs revealed no fracture but in retrospect showed joint space widening (Fig. 9.15A). He was splinted for two weeks because of the pain.

Nine months later the patient returned because of discomfort with use. He flexed from $0°$ to $60°$, and had a palpable defect in the metacarpal head. Radiographs showed evidence of avascular necrosis of the second metacarpal head (Fig. 9.15B).

He was re-examined 8 years after the injury. He then flexed from $25°$ to $60°$, and noted aching with use and crepitus if he tried to hyperextend the joint. Radiographs showed some remodelling but definite subchondral sclerosis with spurring at the margins of the joint (Fig. 9.15C).

The exact aetiology of the avascular necrosis has not yet been demonstrated. Whether or not this is due to an occult fracture or due to a traumatic

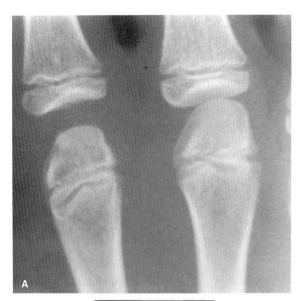

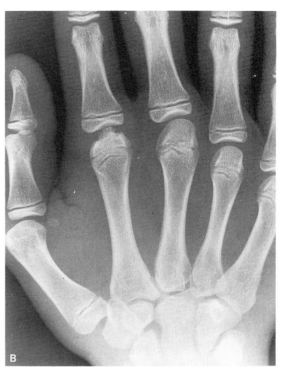

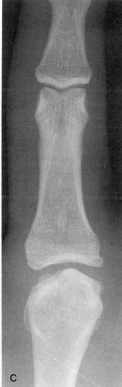

Fig. 9.15 A 14-year-old boy injured his right second metacarpophalangeal joint. Although no fracture was seen on the radiograph, note the widened joint space (A). At 9 months radiographs showed evidence of avascular necrosis (B). By 8 years some remodelling had taken place but there was definite evidence of degenerative arthritis (C)

effusion is unknown, although it is probably the latter. As previously noted, all the radiographs show widening of the joint space; a recent case presented with similar findings and was aspirated of 3 ml of gross blood; when re-evaluated at six months he showed no subsequent changes on radiograph. The metacarpal epiphyses are supplied by radiate epiphyseal arteries which surround the whole circumference of the metacarpal with the distal metacarpal epiphysis being intra-capsular. There are no vessels crossing the physis, but there is a rich anastomosis between the periosteal vessel on the shaft and epiphysis. The physes of the metacarpals fuse at approximately 15 or 16 years in the male and a year earlier in the female. There appears to be a critical period of time when the growth plate fuses but there is still not adequate blood supply across the physis. An injury causing marked joint effusion could then occlude the epiphyseal and periosteal vessels by a tamponade effect leading to decreased epiphyseal vascularity. Avascular necrosis would then result with its associated cartilage collapse. This is somewhat analogous to the femoral head in Legg-Calvé-Perthes disease. It is, therefore, felt that a traumatic effusion of a metacarpophalangeal joint in a young teenager should be aspirated and kept under review with follow-up X-ray examination.

LATER RECONSTRUCTIVE SURGERY

There have been numerous surgical procedures described in the literature for the intra-articular metacarpal head fracture that does not heal in the proper position. These fractures result in joint destruction or arthritic changes. The stiff joint can sometimes benefit from a *capsulotomy* (Fowler 1947, Peacock 1956). Another possibility is to perform an *arthrodesis* of the joint if there is adequate bone stock and no evidence of sepsis. (Peacock 1956, Heim 1974). *Amputations* can be performed either with or without metacarpal transfer, depending somewhat on the deformity and the digit involved (Hyroop 1949, Graham et al 1947, Peacock 1956). Peacock (1956) has even suggested *recession of the proximal phalanx* into the palm.

Arthroplasty

Arthroplasties have a place in the armamentarium of the hand surgeon dealing with the failed intra-articular metacarpal head fracture. Soft tissue interposition arthroplasties have been done utilizing fat (Hamilton 1919, Forrester 1936, Fowler 1947), fascia and tunica vaginalis (Wilmoth 1936). Hemi-arthroplasties used include Burman's (1940) description of a vitallium cap arthroplasty for a shrapnel injury and Isadore Kessler's (1974) use of a silicone implant to replace the metacarpal head.

The most acceptable method of arthroplasty performed at the present time is the flexible silastic arthroplasty of Swanson's design (Swanson 1968, Beckenbaugh et al 1976, Smith and Peimer 1977). A variety of other prostheses are available, including both those that are made of flexible inert materials which act primarily as an interposition (Neibauer and Landry 1971, Beckenbaugh et al 1976) and those that are cemented in place with methyl methacrylate (Linscheid and Dobyns 1979).

Kessler et al (1980) have used a porous implant material, Proplast, to fill defects of articular surfaces penetrating through the subchondral bone in New Zealand rabbits. Twelve weeks later the hyaline cartilage covering the surface appeared normal and bone had grown into the implant. This has been used at least twice by F. Kessler (1982) in clinical situations which exhibited defects in the metacarpal head.

Osteochondral grafts

Osteochondral grafts could be used in a few selected instances, particularly if there was an isolated area

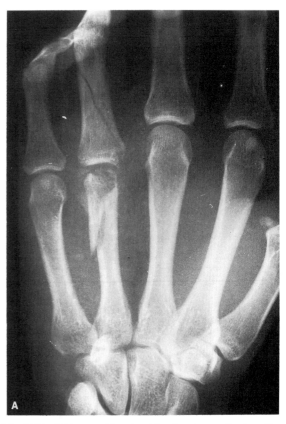

Fig. 9.16 A 20-year-old male schizophrenic sustained a self-inflicted 45 calibre gunshot wound which passed through the left fourth metacarpal head (A). At three weeks he had a metatarsal transfer. The pins were left in place for three months (B). At $1\frac{1}{2}$ years after injury he had a full range of motion without pain but definite evidence of avascular necrosis of the transferred metatarsal head, particularly on the sides (C)

of avascular necrosis present. These grafts survive quite well and show less degenerative changes and failure than half-joint grafts (Kettelkamp et al 1970) although the half-joint grafts are more successful experimentally than whole joint transfers (Entin et al 1962, Erdely 1963a).

Part of a metatarsal bone, usually the fourth or fifth, may be transferred to replace lost bone, as described by Graham and Riordan (1948) (Fig. 9.16A & B). An alternative would be to use an autogenous iliac crest graft with a transferred metatarsal head (Kettelkamp & Ramsey 1971). Most metatarsal transfers eventually show some degree of avascular necrosis of the head (Fig. 9.16C). Whole-joint transfers have been carried out utilizing metatarsophalangeal joints or metacarpophalangeal joints and proximal interphalangeal joints from adjacent damaged digits (Graham 1954, Erdely 1963b, Entin et al 1968). The use of microvascular techniques has spawned renewed

interest in the whole-joint transfer (Tsai et al 1981).

Experimental studies have shown that non-articular cartilage will survive transplantation over long periods of time, as demonstrated by supravital straining and other techniques (Peer 1951, Davis 1956). Entin's experiments (1962) using transplanted articular cartilage showed the cartilage appeared to degenerate more rapidly when subjected to abnormal mechanical stress.

Engkvist and Olesen (1979) used rib and ear perichondrium to cover cartilage defects in animal models. On the basis of this work, Engkvist and Johannson (1980) have performed resurfacing arthroplasty on eight metacarpopalangeal joints in seven patients. Three of the defects were due to intra-articular metacarpal fractures. All three got rid of their pain and had increased motion 12–22 months later. Upton et al (1980) have also reported on perichondral arthroplasties in finger joints.

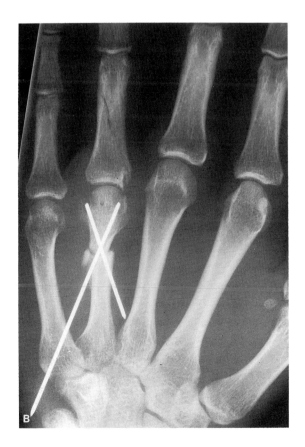

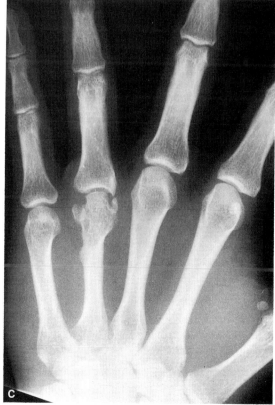

REFERENCES

Beasley R W 1981 Hand injuries. W B Saunders Company, Philadelphia, p 215–216

Beckenbaugh R D, Dobyns J H, Linscheid R L, Bryan R S 1976 Review and analysis of silicone-rubber metacarpophalangeal implants. Journal of Bone and Joint Surgery 58A:483–487

Bopp J 1938 Aseptische epiphysennekrose am os metacarpale II und III. Röntgenpraxis 10:764–765

Bowers W H, Hurst L C 1977 Gamekeeper's thumb. Evaluation by arthography and stress roentgenography. Journal of Bone and Joint Surgery 59A:519–524

Burman M S 1940 Vitallium cap arthroplasty of metacarpophalangeal and interphalangeal joints of the fingers. Bulletin of Hospital for Joint Diseases 1:79–89

Carstam N, Danielsson L G 1966 Aseptic necrosis of the head of the fifth metacarpal. Acta Orthopaedica Scandinavica 37:297–300

Coonrad R W, Goldner J L 1968 A study of the pathological findings and treatment in soft-tissue injury of the thumb metacarpophalangeal joint. Journal of Bone and Joint Surgery 50A:439–451

Davis W B 1956 Absorption of autogenous cartilage grafts in man. British Journal of Plastic Surgery 9:177–185

Dieterich H 1932 Die subchondrale herderkrankung am metacarpale III. Archiv für Klinische Chirugie 171:555–567

Dobyns J H, Fuqua W R 1967 Articular fractures of the hand. Journal of Bone and Joint Surgery 49:1236

Eaton R G 1971 Joint injuries of the hand. Charles C Thomas, Springfield, Illinois, p 47–50

Engkvist O, Johannson S H 1980 Perichondral arthroplasty. Scandinavian Journal of Plastic and Reconstructive Surgery 14:71–87

Engkvist O, Olesen L 1979 Reconstruction of articular cartilage with free autologous perichondral grafts. Scandinavian Journal of Plastic and Reconstructive Surgery 13:269–274

Entin M A, Alger J R, Baird R M 1962 Experimental and clinical transplantation of autogenous whole joints. Journal of Bone and Joint Surgery 44:1518–1536

Entin M A, Daniel G, Kahn D 1969 Transplantation of autogenous half-joints. Archives of Surgery 96:359–368

Erdely R 1963a Experimental autotransplantation of small joints. Plastic and Reconstructive Surgery 31:129–139

Erdely R 1963b Reconstruction of ankylosed finger joints by means of transplantation of joints from the foot. Plastic and Reconstructive Surgery 31:140–150

Flatt A F 1966 Fracture-dislocation of an index metacarpophalangeal joint and an ulnar deviating force in the flexor tendons. Journal of Bone and Joint Surgery 48:100–104

Forrester C R G 1936 Author's method for repair of ankylosed joint of hand. American Journal of Surgery 33:101–103

Fowler S B 1947 Mobilization of metacarpophalangeal joints arthroplasty and capsulotomy. Journal of Bone and Joint Surgery 29:193–202

Frank W E, Dobyns J H 1972 Surgical pathology of collateral ligamentous injuries of the thumb. Clinical Orthopaedics 83:102–114

Franke D 1962 Epiphysäre knochennekrose am metacarpale IV dieterichsche erkankung. Monatsschrift für Unfallheilkunde 65:197–199

Friedl E 1934 Morbus Kohler metacarpi IV. Röntgenpraxis 6:133

Graham W C 1954 Transplantation of joints to replace diseased or damaged articulations in the hands. American Journal of Surgery 88:136–141

Graham W C, Brown J B, Cannon B, Riordan D C 1947 Transposition of fingers in severe injuries of the hand. Journal of Bone and Joint Surgery 29:998–1004

Graham W C, Riordan D C 1948 Reconstruction of a metacarpophalangeal joint with a metatarsal transplant. Journal of Bone and Joint Surgery 30A:848–853

Grosskettler F 1935 Köhlersche erkankung am 2 und 3 metakarpale. Röntgenpraxis 7:606–607

Hamilton G 1919 Arthroplasty of the thumb and finger joints. Texas State Journal of Medicine 14:353–355

Heim U, Pfeiffer 1974 Small fragment set manual. Technique recommended by the ASIF group. Springer-Verlag, New York, p 146

Hyroop G L 1949 Transfer of a metacarpal with or without its digit for improving function of the crippled hand. Plastic and Reconstructive Surgery 17:45–58

Kessler F B, Homsy C A, Berkeley M E, Anderson M S, Prewitt J M 1980 Obliteration of traumatically induced articular surface defects using a porous implant. Journal of Hand Surgery 5:328–347

Kessler I 1974 A new silicone implant for replacement of destroyed metacarpal heads. The Hand 6:308–310

Kettelkamp D B, Kirsch P, Anteman R 1970 Autogenous whole-joint replacement (the effect of the capsule) Clinical Orthopaedics 69:271–278

Kettelkamp D B, Ramsey P 1971 Experimental and clinical autogenous distal metacarpal reconstruction. Clinical Orthopaedics 74:129–237

Lamb D W, Abernethy P J, Fragiadakis E 1971 Injuries of the metacarpophalangeal joint of the thumb. The Hand 3:164–168

Lane C S 1977 Detecting occult fractures of the metacarpal head: the Brewerton view. Journal of Hand Surgery 2:131–133

Linscheid R L, Dobyns J H 1979 Total joint arthroplasty in the hand. Mayo Clinic Proceedings 54:516–526

McElfresh E C, Dobyns J H 1983 Intra-articular metacarpal head fractures. Journal of Hand Surgery 8:383–393

Moberg E, Stener B 1953 Injuries to the ligaments of the thumb and fingers. Acta Orthopaedica Scandinavica 106–186

Neibauer J J, Landry R M 1971 Dacron-silicone prosthesis for the metacarpophalangeal and interphalangeal joints. The Hand 3:55–61

Neviaser R J, Wilson J N, Lievano A 1971 Rupture of the ulnar collateral ligament of the thumb (gamekeeper's thumb). Journal of Bone and Joint Surgery 53A:1357–1364

Palmer A K, Louis D S 1978 Assessing ulnar instability of the metacarpophalangeal joint of the thumb. Journal of Hand Surgery 3:542–546

Peacock E E 1956 Reconstructive surgery of hands with injured central metacarpophalangeal joints. Journal of Bone and Joint Surgery 38A:291–302

Peer L A 1951 The fate of autogenous human bone grafts. British Journal of Plastic Surgery 2:233–243

Salter R B, Harris W R 1963 Injuries involving the epiphyseal plate. Journal of Bone and Joint Surgery 45A:587–622

Sandzen S C 1979 Atlas of wrist and hand fractures. P S G Publishing Company, Littleton, Massachusetts, p 363

Schinz H R, Baersch W E, Friedle, Uehlinger E 1952 In: Carstam N, Danielsson L G 1966 Aseptic necrosis of the head of the fifth metacarpal. Acta Orthopaedica Scandinavica 37:297–300

Seyss R 1961 Dieterichshe erkankung des metacarpale Fortschritte aug dem Gebiete der Röentgenstrahlen 95:279–281

Smith R J 1977 Post-traumatic instability of the metacarpophalangeal joint of the thumb. Journal of Bone and Joint Surgery 59:14–21

Smith R J, Peimer C A 1977 Injuries to the metacarpal bones and joints. Advances in Surgery 11:341–374

Stener B 1962 Displacement of the ruptured ulnar collateral ligament of the metacarpophalangeal joint of the thumb. Journal of Bone and Joint Surgery 44B:869–879

Stener B 1964 Skeletal injuries associated with rupture of the ulnar collateral ligament of the metacarpophalangeal joint of the thumb. Journal of Bone and Joint Surgery 46B:361

Swanson A B 1968 Silicone rubber implants for replacement of arthritic or destroyed joints in the hand. Surgical Clinics of North America 48:1113–1127

Tsai T M, Jupiter J B, Kutz J E, Kleinert H E 1981 Vascularized autogenous whole joint transfer in the hand. Journal of Hand Surgery 6:288

Upton J, John S A, Glowacki J 1980 Neocartilage derived from perichondrium: what is it? Orthopaedic Transactions 4:12

Wilmoth C L 1936 Tunica vaginalis in arthroplasty of small joints. Journal of Bone and Joint Surgery 18:165–168

10 Fractures of the neck and shaft of the metacarpals

Fractures of the head of the metacarpal, involving the articular surface, and fractures of the bases of the metacarpals are uncommon in comparison to fractures of the neck and shaft of these bones which are amongst the most frequent of all fractures. Various studies (James & Wright 1966, Wright 1968, Lamb et al 1973) have confirmed that fracture of the neck of the fifth metacarpal is the most common single fracture in the hand.

Fractures of the neck of the metacarpal are commonly caused by a longitudinal axial compression force applied to the knuckles. They have a characteristic displacement which is one of volar angulation at the fracture site (Fig. 10.1): that is to say, angulation which is concave arteriorly.

Fractures of the shaft are most common in the central metacarpals and most are due to one of two differing mechanisms.

1. Rotational violence, which very often results from a fall on the hand or to a finger being forcibly rotated. This commonly results in a spiral type of fracture obliquely across the mid-shaft of the bone (Fig. 10.2).
2. Direct violence to the hand itself which is more likely to be followed by a transverse fracture of the shaft (Fig. 10.3).

When a fracture of a metacarpal is confirmed by radiograph the question which must be asked is, 'Is it stable or unstable?' Stable fractures are usually undisplaced or displaced very little (Fig. 10.4) and unlikely to displace further. Early movement is encouraged. However, if the fracture is considered unstable, and this is more likely in multiple metacarpal fractures, then immobilization for three weeks either by external support or internal fixation is required.

Fractures of the neck of the first metacarpal are rare but fractures at the base of the shaft of the first metacarpal are not uncommon and are managed in a different way to fractures of the shafts of the other metacarpals.

FRACTURES OF THE NECK OF THE SECOND TO FIFTH METACARPALS

These fractures are seldom greatly displaced. They are commonly impacted and show characteristic volar angulation (Fig. 10.5).

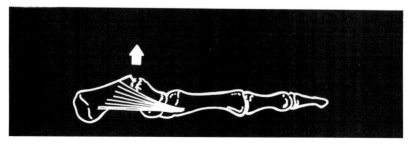

Fig. 10.1 Illustrates the characteristic volar angulation that occurs in fractures of the metacarpal neck

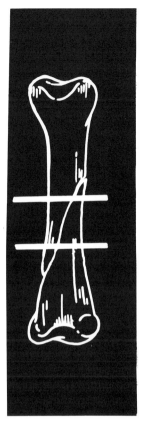

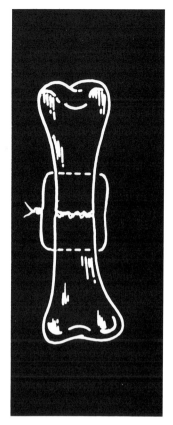

Fig. 10.2   Typical spiral fracture of a metacarpal shaft, showing a method of fixation by transverse Kirschner wires which can be introduced percutaneously. If the fracture has to be opened, screws can be used instead

Fig. 10.3   Typical transverse fracture of a metacarpal shaft, showing a method of fixation by intraosseous wiring

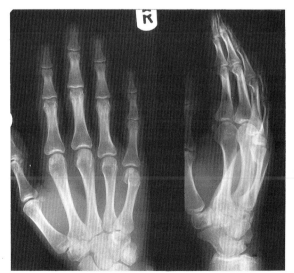

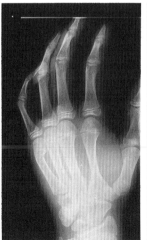

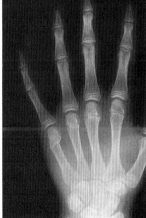

Fig. 10.4   Fracture of the neck of fifth metacarpal with minimal displacement, considered stable and not requiring reduction

Fig. 10.5   Fracture of the fifth metacarpal neck with a degree of volar angulation which was considered acceptable

Minor degrees of angulation (up to about 30°) can often be accepted and no attempt made to correct the deformity. This applies particularly to the little finger. Volar angulation of the metacarpal head of the second, third and fourth metacarpals may produce a tender lump in the palm of the hand which impairs gripping due to discomfort.

Each fracture should be managed on its own merits. If the angulation on radiography seems to be less than 30°, there is seldom any need to try and improve this position in the little finger and only in the other fingers if the head seems unduly prominent and tender. Eaton and Burton (1982) accept angulation up to 40° in fractures of the fourth and fifth metacarpal without requiring correction.

The assessment of the degree of angulation may often be difficult and good quality radiographs are required. It is advisable in any patient who has pain, swelling and tenderness over the head and neck of the metacarpal to suspect a fracture of the neck. The clinical observer has to be suspicious of the mechanism of the injury, which is commonly caused by a punching blow; patients often deny such an incident and think up many ingenious stories to account for their injury. This is particularly important where there is any open wound over the dorsum of the knuckle. Many young doctors have regretted accepting the description by the patient as to the cause of the incident which is nearly always due to an assailant's tooth and has a very high incidence of infection and possible septic arthritis and osteomyelitis.

When the examining doctor feels that a fracture of the neck of the metacarpal is likely, it is wise to ask for radiographs in three planes; postero-anterior (PA), straight lateral and oblique. The oblique radiograph will often show the fracture clearly and the presence of volar angulation (Fig. 10.6). The straight lateral, although there is supraimposition of the other metacarpals, shows the true angle of volar angulation (Fig. 10.7).

Lowdon (1985) studied 12 normal subjects without fractures to determine the normal neck-shaft angle. In an oblique view the normal angle is 25°. On a lateral view the normal neck-shaft angle of the fifth metacarpal is 16.5°. The oblique view thus increases the neck-shaft angle in the normal hand by about 8.5°.

He then studied a series of 73 patients with fractures of the fifth metacarpal neck. In this series none of the oblique radiographs showed a neck-shaft angle greater than 40°; that is, there were none with an angulation greater than 15° more than the normal.

He also assessed the efficacy of manipulation and immobilization on volar plaster slab and found that, if any correction was achieved by manipulation, it was lost in the subsequent management in the volar slab.

Stable fractures

The author feels that an angulation of up to 30° can be readily accepted in the fifth metacarpal neck fracture and will leave no cosmetic blemish or functional impairment. O'Brien (1982) considers that considerable residual angulation can be accepted in fractures of the neck of the fourth and

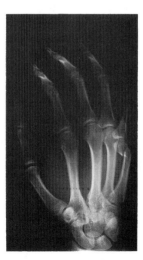

Fig. 10.6   Fracture of the fifth metacarpal neck with clear evidence of the volar angulation on the oblique view

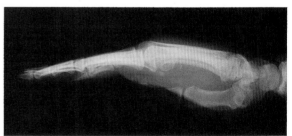

Fig. 10.7   Lateral view of the fracture shown in Figure 10.6 shows the true degree of angulation

fifth metacarpals, as the angulation can be compensated by the mobility of the carpometacarpal joints. Hunter and Cowen (1970) believe that an angulation of up to $70°$ can be accepted in the fifth metacarpal neck fracture. Holst-Neilsen (1976) is prepared to accept a similar degree of angulation in fractures of the neck of all metacarpal bones but Posner (1977) does not consider that any angulation over $15°$ should be accepted in fractures of the neck of the second and third metacarpals because of the lack of compensation at the carpometacarpal joint.

As with all fractures of the hand it is the initial management, often by a junior and inexperienced doctor, that will determine the eventual outcome.

In the great majority of cases in which volar angulation at the fracture is demonstrated, the displacement can be ignored (Furlong 1957, Lamb 1981). The patient should be told that there is a break in the bone with slight angulation but that experience has shown that this displacement is of no functional significance and is unlikely to result in any cosmetic blemish. The fracture displacement is usually stable and active movement should be encouraged from the start. The patient is warned that this will be initially painful but that it is the quickest way to regain function and that the pain will usually be away in a few days. By early active movement, the oedema and swelling is usually dissipated quickly and full flexion regained. An extensor lag of 15 or $20°$ at the metacarpophalangeal joint is common for some weeks after the injury. Pain and tenderness over the fracture site may persist for about three weeks, but as soon as this has settled, patients can usually resume work, even heavy work. The slight extensor lag has usually corrected by 6–8 weeks after injury. Local swelling at the site of the healing fracture may persist, but it is rare for this not to disappear completely and there is usually a most excellent functional and cosmetic result (Fig. 10.8) from conservative management of these fractures (Lamb 1981, James & Wright 1966, Wright 1968).

There has been a tendency in the past for these fractures to be over-treated (Eaton & Burton 1982, Eichenhotz & Rizzo 1961). Some surgeons (O'Brien 1982) use a protective plaster until the pain and swelling has settled. The plaster must be moulded very carefully round the volar aspect of the metacarpal head to push it back into normal position, but not to restrict flexion of the metacarpophalangeal joint. Eaton and Burton recommend that the fracture should be immobilized in a gauntlet cast with the wrist $20°$ dorsiflexed and the metacarpophalangeal joints in $50–60°$ flexion, leaving the interphalangeal joints free. If the plaster is carefully applied it can be effective, but is open to great abuse by those who are ignorant or careless about the proper application of plasters in this area. We have seen too many plasters applied by inexperienced junior staff which obstruct metacarpophalangeal flexion.

Even more reprehensible is the prolongation of any plaster or bandage to immobilize the finger with the proximal interphalangeal joint held in flexion. This usually results in a stiff metacarpophalangeal joint with an extension contracture and a stiff proximal interphalangeal joint with a flexion contracture. The author has seen many examples of this as a result of careless application of plaster or bandage and, even after only three weeks of such immobilization, it may be impossible to correct the contractures. This method of treatment should be avoided if it is a simple fracture with little displacement.

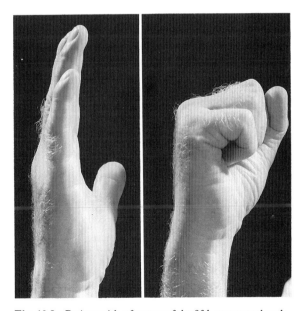

Fig. 10.8 Patient with a fracture of the fifth metacarpal neck with minor angulation was treated by active movement from the beginning. This shows the range of movement two weeks after the fracture

Unstable fractures

If it is considered that the displacement is too great to be accepted, then manipulation should be carried out by pushing the metacarpal head back into normal position. This can be done either by direct pressure backwards on the metacarpal head in the palm (Furlong 1957) or using the flexed proximal phalangeal base to lever the head back into the corrected position (Barton 1982). In the author's opinion, the reduction of the metacarpal head is most readily maintained by percutaneous fixation of a Kirschner wire passed transversely through the metacarpal head into the adjacent one (Furlong 1957, Lamb et al 1973, Bosworth 1937). If it is the fifth metacarpal, it is readily fixed to the fourth, and if it is the second it is fixed to the third. If it is a central metacarpal, it requires the K-wire to be passed across adjacent intact metacarpals while the metacarpal head is held reduced in the corrected position. The wire is inserted with a power drill and usually a 0.035 inch (0.9 mm) calibre wire is satisfactory. It should be introduced proximal to the metacarpal attachment of the collateral ligament as impaling this ligament may restrict active flexion. The aim of this manoeuvre is to correct deformity, maintain the position by firm skeletal fixation and convert the fracture into a stable fracture which can then be treated by early active movement. The whole emphasis on treatment of fractures of the metacarpals, as of other fractures of the hand, is to regain a full range of movement as quickly as possible (Burkhalter 1983).

In the view of the author, there is no place for the use of screws, plates or other methods of internal fixation in these simple fractures of the neck of the metacarpal.

FRACTURES OF THE SECOND TO FIFTH METACARPAL SHAFTS

These fractures are common and are usually either long oblique or spiral fractures produced by torque, or transverse fractures across the middle of the bone usually caused by axial compression or a direct perpendicular force. Isolated fractures of the metacarpal shaft are likely to be stable and their displacement is usually minimal, due to the connection with adjacent intact metacarpals by the interosseii.

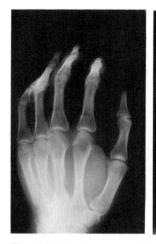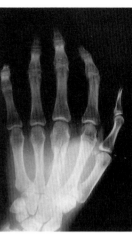

Fig. 10.9   Despite gross swelling of the hand following these fractures sustained in a motor accident, full movement was regained 3 weeks after the injury

Stable fractures

Figure 10.9 shows fractures of the third and fourth metacarpal shafts sustained by a young male nurse in a motor-cycle accident. There was gross swelling of the hand. The fractures were immobilized in a 'boxing-glove' bandage* in the safe position, with the metacarpophalangeal joints flexed and the proximal interphalangeal joints straight, until the swelling had subsided in 10 days. He returned to work three weeks after injury with full movement of his hand and all swelling reduced.

The patient whose radiographs form Figure 10.10 sustained fractures of the second and third metacarpal shafts which were undisplaced and considered stable. Treatment was by early active movement. The fractures healed in three weeks and full mobility was regained.

Another example is provided by a young woman who sustained a comminuted fracture of the shaft of the third metacarpal (Fig. 10.11), treated by early active movement without immobilization. Four weeks after injury, she had a full range of movement in the hand without pain or swelling and the fracture was consolidated.

However, two characteristic deformities may occur in these shaft fractures and their development should be watched for. In the long oblique or spiral fracture it is seldom that there is any

* *See* Chapter 3, page 28–29.

angulatory deformity, but there may be a rotary deformity and shortening may develop as the fracture heals.

Rotary deformity

It is important to watch for development of a rotary deformity. This is unlikely to be detrimental to function in extension but as the fingers flex any minor rotary deformity will be magnified so that the digit obstructs flexion of adjacent digits (Fig. 10.12).

The correct rotation of each digit in extension is determined by relating it to the plane of the nail of the adjacent digits. In flexion, all digits should flex towards the tuberosity of the scaphoid. Any deviation from this may indicate some rotation deformity at the fracture site. Treatment should

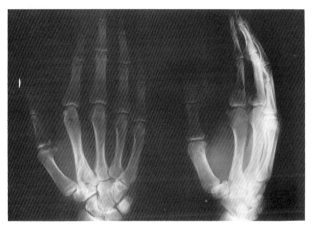

Fig. 10.10 Fractures were considered stable and full movement was quickly restored

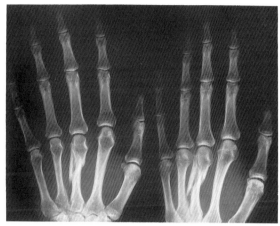

Fig. 10.11 Comminuted fracture consolidated quickly and full movement was regained within four weeks of injury. Active movement was instituted from the start

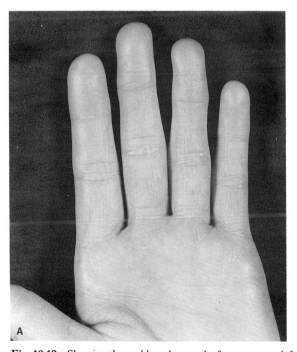

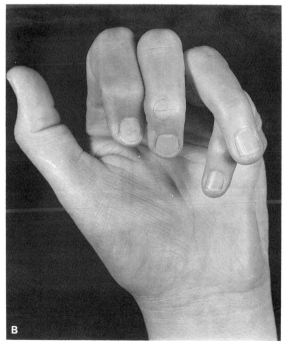

Fig. 10.12 Showing the problem that results from a rotary deformity at the fracture site

aim to prevent the development of rotational deformities (Sutro 1954) as these are difficult to correct once the fracture has healed.

Shortening of the shaft

With a long oblique fracture, insidious shortening of the shaft may occur as the fracture 'settles' while it is healing (Fig. 10.13). This has to be watched for carefully as it will lead to recession of the metacarpal head and an unsightly outline of the metacarpal heads, particularly of the central two metacarpals. The cosmetic disfigurement may be a reason for complaint by the patient, especially in a woman. This is seldom a problem with fractures of the metacarpal shaft of index or little fingers.

Unstable fractures

If rotary deformity or recession seems to be developing, then the fracture is considered to be unstable and should be stabilized either by external fixation or by internal fixation. Brown (1973) recommends the use of a K-wire if shortening of more than 3–4 mm has developed. We seldom use plaster for external fixation, preferring to depend upon a well-fitted and moulded metal splint protected with plastic foam. This splint is applied along the volar surface with the metacarpophalangeal joint fully flexed and the digit of the affected ray immobilized with the proximal interphalangeal joint almost straight (*see* Fig. 3.8). In this way any

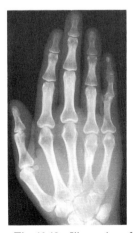
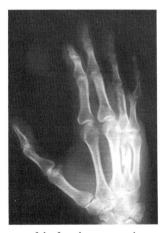

Fig. 10.13 Illustrating a fracture of the fourth metacarpal shaft where a long oblique fracture has 'settled' and produced some shortening

rotary deformity can be corrected and also any tendency to shortening. If a commercial splint is used for this purpose the metal is rather soft and the splint may deform. It is recommended that the edges of the splint be turned with a pair of pliers which will stiffen it sufficiently to maintain the position on application. It is important in its application that the splint should be measured accurately for length and should be bent proximal to the flexion crease for the metacarpophalangeal joints (i.e. the transverse palmar creases) so as not to impede full flexion of that joint. The splint is taped in position and reinforced with a bandage. It is seldom necessary to extend the splint across the wrist but this can be done if it is considered advisable, in which case the wrist is held in slight dorsiflexion. If the splint has not been stabilized to prevent it bending easily, then the wrist must be immobilized as wrist movement will soon straighten the splint at the metacarpophalangeal joint.

Closed reduction and immobilization by a plaster 'gutter' applied either to the ulnar or radial side of the hand is preferred by O'Brien (1982) for the majority of metacarpal fractures and many surgeons also recommend plaster fixation (Barton 1982, Green & Rowland 1975).

Figure 10.14A shows what was considered an unstable fracture of the fourth metacarpal shaft. An attempt was made to reduce this and immobilize it in a plaster. Unsatisfactory control of the fracture was provided (Fig. 10.14B).

Eaton and Burton (1982) recommend for most metacarpal fractures a plaster cast including the metacarpophalangeal joint in flexion and maintained for 4–5 weeks.

In the author's view, any splint or plaster should not be maintained for more than three weeks. It cannot be emphasized too greatly that there is no justification in the management of fractures of the hand to wait for signs of radiological union of the fracture. Clinical union is all that is required and it is seldom in practice that the hand needs to be immobilized for more than three weeks. Wright (1968) found that 68% of patients with fractures of the metacarpals immobilized for more than three weeks had significant loss of function.

An alternative method of management for unstable fractures, particularly when multiple or

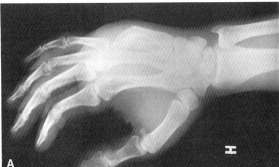

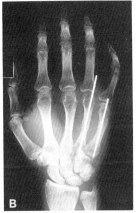

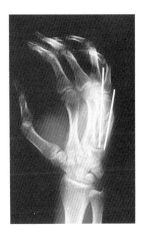

Fig. 10.15 Patient with severe angulation of transverse fractures of fourth and fifth metacarpal shafts (A) had manipulative reduction and plaster fixation. The displacement recurred and the fractures were stabilized by the introduction of longitudinal Kirschner wires (B). The Kirschner wires were left in for several weeks preventing metacarpophalangeal joint movement. Following removal of the Kirschner wires the restoration of flexion of the joints was only achieved after several weeks of physiotherapy

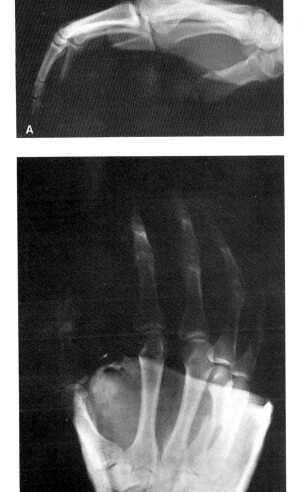

Fig. 10.14 (A) Shows a displaced fourth metacarpal shaft fracture. Despite application of a plaster the displacement persists (B)

associated with open injuries or skin loss, and the one which is preferred by the author, is internal fixation of the fracture by the use of Kirschner wires. Various methods of use of these have been described. Vom Saal (1953) was one of the first to describe intramedullary fixation of metacarpal shaft fractures using a K-wire (Fig. 10.15). Milford (1982) recommends exposure of the fracture

through which a Kirschner wire is passed along the proximal fragment and out of the metacarpal base (with the wrist flexed). The fracture is then reduced and the K-wire passed back along the medullary cavity into the distal fragment. Others (O'Brien 1982) feel that passage of the K-wire along the medullary cavity may not give sufficient fixation and recommend percutaneous fixation inserting the wire into the side of the metacarpal head. While the fracture is held reduced, the wire is advanced across the metacarpal and the fracture line to impinge on the opposite cortex (Fig. 10.16). This is technically not easy to do, but if accurately placed gives good fixation.

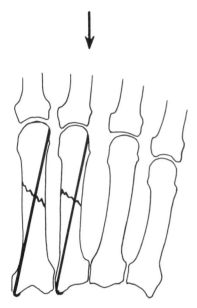
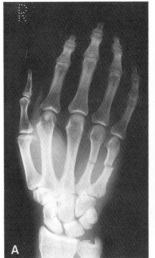
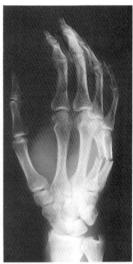

Fig. 10.16 Diagram shows the most satisfactory type of longitudinal insertion of Kirschner wires to control unstable fractures of metacarpal shafts

The author's preferred method in unstable fractures of metacarpal shafts is that of percutaneous Kirschner wire fixation inserted transversely through each fragment, thus stabilizing the fracture to the adjacent intact metacarpals (Lamb et al 1973). It is seldom necessary to expose the fracture site unless there is difficulty in getting reduction: it is extremely rare for there to be any soft tissue interposition in these fractures of metacarpal shafts, but it does occasionally occur. This method of fixation was first described by Bosworth (1937) and recommended by Furlong (1957), Waugh and Ferrazzano (1943) and Berkman and Myles (1943).

It has been found in practice that one wire in the distal fragment and one wire in the proximal fragment is inefficient biomechanically and displacement can recur. It is therefore recommended that two parallel wires should be inserted through the distal fragment and one through the proximal fragment (Fig. 10.17). We have found this method to be extremely satisfactory as it converts an unstable fracture into a stable one and allows early active movement of the fingers. Provided the Kirschner wires are inserted with care in the skeletal plane, there is no danger of damage to important soft-tissue structures. The wires are

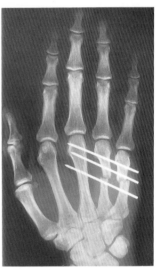
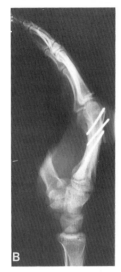

Fig. 10.17 Transverse fractures of the fourth and fifth metacarpal shafts with characteristic angulation (A). Stability was achieved by the percutaneous introduction of transverse Kirschner wires into the third metacarpal from the ulnar side of the hand. Note two wires in the distal fragments and one wire proximally (B). Stability was immediately achieved and full movement was obtained at the time of removal of the Kirschner wires $3\frac{1}{2}$ weeeks after injury

usually inserted from the ulnar side, but occasionally from the radial side for fractures of the second or third metacarpals, and are left protruding slightly from the bone but beneath the skin. The only problem we have encountered with these has been a very few cases of infection. This only occurs if the wires have not been inserted carefully or have been left too prominent and cause irritation to the skin. All infection has settled with removal of the wires and there has been no complication of bone infection.

From the time of insertion of the wires, active movement of the fingers is encouraged and full movement should certainly have been regained well before the time for removal of the K-wires. This usually occurs 3 weeks after insertion.

With the exception of the unstable fractures already specified, it is the author's opinion that internal fixation of single fractures of metacarpal shafts is seldom required unless it is seen that rotary deformity or excessive shortening (Brown 1973) is developing. When managed conservatively by early movement, the function has been excellent. Delayed or non-union is virtually never seen.

In an unstable fracture which cannot be fixed satisfactorily by one of the methods already mentioned, or particularly in multiple fractures, there is a stronger case for open reduction and internal fixation of the fracture. If internal fixation is required for long or short oblique fractures, these are very suitable for fixation with a small screw or screws (Kilbourne & Paul 1958, Ikuta & Tsuge 1974) as illustrated in Figure 10.18. The use of 2 mm or 2.7 mm screws is recommended by the AO group for an oblique fracture of the central metacarpals but in the second or fifth metacarpal or in unstable transverse fractures they rely on the use of a small straight or T-shaped AO plate (Simonetta 1970). Out of 75 metacarpal fractures so treated, eight had infection or developed pseudarthrosis or both—a totally unacceptable incidence. In the author's opinion there is little indication for plate fixation. This inevitably leads to wide stripping of soft tissues from the site of the metacarpal fracture which will cause increased swelling, a greater chance of adherence of tendons to the fracture site, and a greater possibility of infection. O'Brien (1982) believes that screws and plates have no particular advantage over K-wires in the management of metacarpal fractures because they require more extensive stripping of soft tissue for their insertion, and usually require removal. They are occasionally indicated for the rare complication of non-union. An alternative to plate fixation for unstable transverse fractures is the use of intraosseous wiring (*see* Fig. 10.3) (Lister 1978)

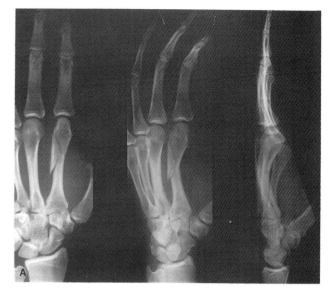

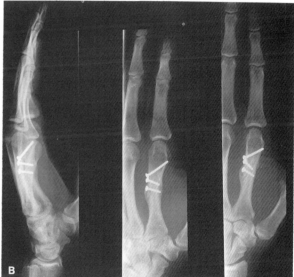

Fig. 10.18   This young man sustained this fracture of the second metacarpal shaft. The fracture was considered unstable and stability achieved by three small screws. Excellent reduction and fixation was obtained, but at the price of infection which took several weeks to clear and restricted flexion of the metacarpophalangeal joint

but, as with plates, its use is seldom needed. Once the unstable fracture has been fixed, by whatever method, the emphasis is again on early active movement. Apart from the Kirschner wires, which should be removed when they have done their job, there is no clear indication or justification for removal of screws, plate or interosseous wiring.

Although the use of traction has been recommended for the management of unstable metacarpal fractures by Swanson (1970), Miller (1965), and also Workman (1964), the author believes that there is never any justification for this.

Provided there is careful wound excision and removal of all devitalized and damaged tissue, infection following wounds of the hand is extremely uncommon. The judicious use of Kirschner wires, interosseous wiring or small screws, as has been described for individual fractures, is not contraindicated in the presence of an open wound.

FRACTURES OF THE FIRST METACARPAL SHAFT

Fractures of the first metacarpal shaft usually occur near to the base (Fig. 10.19) but must be differentiated from the rarer but more unstable fractures of the base known as Bennett's fracture which involve the articular surface and are very unstable. Most fractures of the first metacarpal shaft may be near to the base but do not involve the articular surface. There is often some adduction angulatory deformity but the fractures are usually stable and in most cases the angulatory deformity can be accepted and is unlikely to interfere with the appearance or with function (Green & O'Brien 1972). If it is considered that the deformity is too great to accept, it should be corrected by manipulation and the position maintained by a plaster of the scaphoid type which should immobilize the thumb in a position abducted away from the palm (Fig. 10.20).

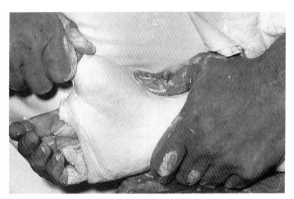

Fig. 10.20 Showing type of plaster recommended for immobilization of fractures of the base of first metacarpal

Immobilization of fractures of the first metacarpal shaft in a plaster in this way is the recommended method of treatment. In the author's opinion it is one of the few occasions in which fractures of metacarpals require plaster immobilization. It is important to ensure that the plaster does not restrict full movement of the other digits. The results of immobilization of these fractures for 3–4 weeks is very good and it is hardly ever necessary to consider open reduction and internal fixation of any kind. Goodwill et al (1969), however, have pointed out that the patient may be off work for about twice as long as the person with an isolated fracture of another metacarpal.

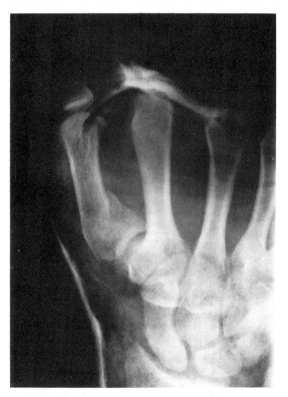

Fig. 10.19 Showing a fracture near the base of the first metacarpal with typical angulation but not involving the joint

REFERENCES

Barton N J 1982 Fractures and joint injuries of the hand. In: Wilson, J N (ed) 'Watson-Jones'—Fractures and joint injuries, 6th edn. Churchill Livingstone, Edinburgh, chap 25

Berkman E F, Myles G J 1943 Internal fixation of metacarpal fractures exclusive of the thumb. Journal of Bone and Joint Surgery 25:816–821

Bosworth D M 1937 Internal splinting of fractures of the fifth metacarpal. Journal of Bone and Joint Surgery 19:826–827

Brown P W 1973 The management of phalangeal and metacarpal fractures. Surgical Clinics of North America 53:1339–1437

Burkhalter W E 1983 Functional treatment of fractures. In: J A Boswick Jr (ed) Current concepts in hand surgery. Lea and Febiger, Philadelphia, chap 21

Eaton R, Burton R 1982 Fractures of the metacarpals. In: David P Green (ed) Operative Hand Surgery, Churchill Livingstone, Edinburgh, chap 11

Eichenholtz S N, Rizzo P C 1961 Fracture of the neck of the fifth metacarpal bone. Is overtreatment justified? Journal of the American Medical Association 178:425–426

Furlong R 1957 Injuries of the Hand. J. A. Churchill (now Churchill Livingstone, Edinburgh)

Goodwill C J, Bridges P K, Gardner D C 1969 The causes and costs of absence from work after injury. Annals of Physical Medicine 10:180–186

Green D P, O'Brien E T 1972 Fractures of the thumb metacarpal. Southern Medical Journal 65:807

Green D P, Rowland S A 1975 Fractures and dislocations in the hand. In: Rockwood C A, Green D P (eds) Fractures, Vol 1, Lippincott, Philadelphia, p 265–343

Heim U F A, Pfeiffer K M 1974 Small fragments set manual. Springer-Verlag, Berlin

Holst-Neilsen F 1976 Sub-capital fractures of the fore-ulnar metacarpal bones. The Hand 8:290–293

Hunter J M, Cowen N J 1970 Fifth metacarpal fractures. Journal of Bone and Joint Surgery 52A:1159–1165

Ikuta Y, Tsuge K 1974 Micro-bolts and micro-screws for fixation of small bones in the hand. The Hand 6:261–265

James J I P, Wright T A 1966 Fractures of metacarpals and proximal and middle phalanges of the fingers. Journal of Bone and Joint Surgery 48B:181–182

Kilbourne B C, Paul E G 1958 The use of small bone screws and the treatment of metacarpal fractures. Journal of Bone and Joint Surgery 40A:375–383

Lamb D W 1981 Fractures of the hand. In: Lamb D W, Kuczynski K (eds) The practice of hand surgery, Blackwell Medical, Oxford

Lamb D W, Abernethy P A, Raine P A M 1973 Unstable fractures of the metacarpals. The Hand 5(1):43–48

Lister G D 1978 Intra-osseous wiring of the digital skeleton. Journal of Hand Surgery 3:427–435

Lowdon I M R 1985 Paper read at Nov meeting of British Society for Surgery of the Hand, London

Milford L 1982 The hand. 2nd edn. C. V. Mosby, St Louis

Miller W R 1965 Fractures of the metacarpals. American Journal of Orthopaedics 7:105–108

Morton H S 1944 Fractures of the wrist and hand. Canadian Medical Association Journal 51:430–434

O'Brien E T 1982 Fractures of metacarpals and phalanges. In: David P Green (ed) Operative Hand Surgery, Churchill Livingstone, Edinburgh, chap 15

Posner M A 1977 Injuries to the hand and wrist in athletes. Orthopaedic Clinics of North America 8:593–618

Simonetta C 1970 The use of AO plates in the hand. The Hand 2:43–45

Smith R J, Peimer C A 1977 Injuries to the Metacarpal Bones and Joints. Advances in Surgery 11:341–374

Sutro C J 1954 Fractures of metacarpal bones. Treatment with emphasis on the prevention of rotational deformities. American Journal of Surgery 81:327–332

Swanson A B 1970 Fractures involving the digits of the hand. Orthopaedic Clinics of North America 1:261–274

Vom Saal F H 1953 Intramedullary fixation in fractures of the hand. Journal of Bone and Joint Surgery 35A:5–16

Waugh R L, Ferrazano G P 1943 Fractures of the metacarpals exclusive of the thumb. A new method of treatment. American Journal of Surgery 59:186–194

Workman C E 1964 Metacarpal fractures. Missouri Medicine 61:68–76

Wright T A 1968 Early mobilisation in fractures of metacarpals and phalanges. Canadian Journal of Surgery 11:491–498

11 Fractures and dislocations at the base of the metacarpals

Junctional areas, which assist in the transmission of energy and in the prepositioning of a terminal device effector agent, are involved in much activity and subject to high stress loading: they are therefore at great risk of injury. The entire junctional area between forearm and hand qualifies in this regard and it is surprising that investigators have been so slow to discern, describe, categorize, quantify and develop techniques of management for the many injuries in the region. The pace of such review is picking up, but mostly in terms of awareness of distal forearm and carpal injuries. The carpometacarpal junctional area continues to attract mostly indifference, except for Bennett's fracture at the base of the thumb. This attitude is not warranted by either the incidence or significance of these problems. As long as 20 years ago, when the more subtle manifestations of injury in this carpometacarpal area were not yet understood or diagnosed, a review of 1425 fractures of the hand and wrist included 120 fractures in the carpometacarpal area (Dobyns et al 1983), an incidence of approximately 1% of all hand-wrist fractures. The spectrum of injury ranges from fairly subtle damage brought on by repetitive, trivial, or occult stresses to injuries resulting from high energy forces and therefore associated with multiple and severe disruption (Gunther 1984): motor-cycle accidents are a well-known source of such injuries.

ANATOMY

The carpometacarpal joints and the metacarpals are the prime determinants of both the transverse and longitudinal arches. They carry out these roles by forming a fixed, firm, and strong central longitudinal arch which supports bilateral, peripheral, transverse arch elements which are sufficiently mobile and flexible to contour the palm and digits to almost any shape of object. These radial and ulnar rays show more versatility and adaptability radially than ulnarward but in both instances can elevate to form an almost flat plane or depress (flex) to form a hollow cup. The critical portions of this junctional region are the carpometacarpal joints with the carpus proximal to the joints subserving the needs of the joints. Detailed anatomical descriptions are given by Eaton (1971), Smith and Peimer (1977) and Gunther (1984).

First carpometacarpal joint

This is the most important joint in positioning of the highly mobile, strong, and constantly active thumb (Gedda 1954). It must, therefore, permit several degrees of motion (Fig. 11.1), yet present a broad platform for transmission of stress. The base of the first metacarpal is convex in the radioulnar (coronal or frontal) plane and concave in the dorsovolar (sagittal) plane. This saddle-shaped configuration matches the dorsovolar convexity and radioulnar concavity of the distal trapezium, which has a larger radius of curvature. This absence of snug articular constraint is augmented by relatively lax ligamentous support, with only one strong connection between metacarpal and trapezium: the thick oblique ligament that extends both anteriorly and posteriorly between deep ulnar tubercles of the first metacarpal and the trapezium. (There is a connection of the same ligament to the

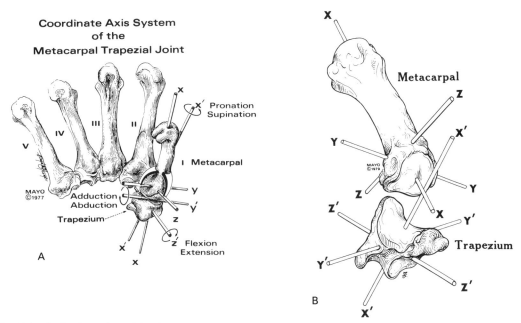

Fig. 11.1 Stylized drawings of the thumb axis and its skeletal associations with the thumb CMC joint closed (A) and opened up (B) dramatize the axes and ranges of the three dimensions of motion available to this loosely constrained, highly responsive joint

base of the index metacarpal.) This construction permits the flexion/extension and abduction/adduction motions of the joint but also means that the joint is relatively unstable, becoming more so with each degree of laxity, attenuation, or damage to the important deep or ulnar oblique ligaments. The short but broad first metacarpal is broadest as it approaches the carpometacarpal joint and is matched by the equally broad, but very short, trapezium proximally. The first metacarpal is strongly anchored to the second metacarpal and the trapezium is strongly anchored by ligaments to the trapezoid on the ulnar side and the scaphoid proximally.

Second carpometacarpal joint

The second metacarpal is usually the longest and is also quite broad as it approaches the carpometacarpal joint. It has both radial and ulnar styloid projections, which grip the trapezoid strongly with the help of firm ligaments. Whereas the first carpometacarpal joint is a discrete joint cavity, the second through the fifth joints are connected to each other and likewise to intermetacarpal joints at each level and also to the midcarpal joint proximally. In keeping with this inter-relationship, the

second metacarpal articulates not only with the small flat trapezoid; its radial styloid articulates with the trapezium and its ulnar styloid articulates with the capitate and the base of the third metacarpal. Extensive tendon insertions for the extensor carpi radialis brevis radially, the extensor carpi radialis longus dorsally and the flexor carpi radialis volarly and radially complement the strong ligamentous connections.

Third carpometacarpal joint

The third metacarpal is also large, with a broad metaphysis at the carpometacarpal area and a proximal surface articulating primarily with the capitate. Radially and dorsally, a styloid process articulates with the second metacarpal and trapezoid. On the ulnar side there are articular facets for the fourth metacarpal. As at the index carpometacarpal joint, the complexity of articulation and the strong ligaments across the joints result in considerable stability and little motion. Also, as at the index, there is a surprisingly deep joint with considerable articular surface in the dorsovolar plane.

The carpal boss (carpe bossu) is a fairly common bony protuberance lying dorsally between trapezoid and capitate proximally, second and third metacarpal bases distally. It may represent osteophyte formation or an accessory ossification centre, the os styloideum. In the latter, it is most often fused to the second or third metacarpal but may occasionally be fused to capitate or trapezoid or even isolated and not fused.

Fourth carpometacarpal joint

Intermetacarpal articulations become even more prominent at the fourth carpometacarpal joint with a ridge in the metaphyseal area, dividing the joint facet into a radial facet, articulating with the capitate and third metacarpal, and an ulnar facet, articulating with the radial half of the hamate and the fifth metacarpal. Approximately 15–20° of flexion/extension and 5° of abduction/adduction are permitted by these articulations.

Fifth carpometacarpal joint

Except for the first metacarpal area, the fifth carpometacarpal junction permits the most motion of these joints. In fact, it simulates to some degree the configuration of the first carpometacarpal joint. The usual metaphyseal flare is present and the metacarpal joint surface articulates with the ulnar half of the hamate and the adjacent fourth metacarpal. The articular surface is saddle-shaped, with convexity in the dorsivolar direction and concavity in the radioulnar direction. This configuration permits 25–40° of flexion/extension and 10–15° abduction/adduction. A small ulnar styloid process gives origin to the abductor digiti minimi muscle. The extensor carpi ulnaris inserts into the dorsal metaphyseal area and the flexor carpi ulnaris inserts, by way of the pisohamate-metacarpal ligament, into the volar metaphysis.

BIOMECHANICS OF THE AREA

Because of their peripheral position, the greater laxity of their carpometacarpal joints, and the increased freedom and mobility of the entire digital ray, the *first and fifth digits* are subject to most risk and most stress, both direct and indirect. Direct blows and axial compression probably account for the majority of carpometacarpal injuries in these two digital rays, but torque and traction injuries are also common. The similarity in anatomy and the similarity in stress application is matched by a similarity in types of injury. The characteristic injury in each location is the fracture–subluxation (Charnley 1961, Ross & Sinclair 1946, Wagner 1950), with the smaller portion of the first metacarpal ulnarward or the fifth metacarpal radially retained in position by its strong ligamentous supports. The major metacarpal fragment ruptures the weaker capsular supports and dislocates proximally in response to the initial stress and to the musculotendinous pull of both extrinsics and intrinsics.

The *second and third carpometacarpal areas* are much more stable and much more protected. Disruption of these areas requires, therefore, a much higher expenditure of energy delivered by either modal stress or direct crush. When the second and third carpometacarpal areas are destabilized, the fourth and fifth CMC (carpometacarpal) joints usually accompany them. On the other hand, the close congruency of the articular surfaces and the relative immobility of index and long finger carpometacarpal joints permit them to be painful with only trivial instability, such as may be incurred by the dorsal compression–volar tension stress of a dorsiflexion injury or the volar compression–dorsal tension stress of a flexion injury. Stress risk dorsally is increased by the strong, repetitive pull of the two radial wrist extensors and the common presence of an accessory ossicle, the os styloideum.

The *fourth carpometacarpal* area lies functionally and anatomically between the rigid elements and the flexible elements. It is perhaps more often involved with injury to the fifth carpometacarpal area but commonly accompanies injury to either of the areas. The frequent subluxation of the major fragment is, however, not as common at the ring finger CMC joint as at the little finger or thumb, and persistent pain with small degrees of incongruency is not as common as in injuries of the CMC joints of the index and long finger.

For further accounts of the biomechanics, see Eaton (1971), Gedda (1954), Gunther (1984) and Smith and Peimer (1977).

INJURIES TO THE FIRST METACARPAL BASE AND CARPOMETACARPAL AREA

In most series, the large majority of fractures (approximately 80%) of the first metacarpal occur at the base of the bone (Gunther, 1984; McNealy & Lichtenstein, 1933; Robinson, 1908).

Classification

There are equal numbers of extra-articular and intra-articular fractures (Macey & Murray 1949). Extra-articular fractures are subdivided into transverse or oblique types, with a special age-related group of epiphyseal fractures (Green & O'Brien 1972). As the oblique fractures approach the capsule, they may even become intra-articular fractures and therefore a variant of the Bennett type of fracture–dislocation.

However the usual Bennett's fracture involves a small fragment, less than one third, of the articular surface of the metacarpal base (Bennett 1882). Nevertheless, there is no consensus concerning use of a name other than Bennett's fracture for any non-comminuted fracture or fracture–dislocation involving the articular base of the first metacarpal whatever the size of the fragment or the amount of dislocation (Ellis 1945, Gedda & Moberg 1953, Goldberg 1951). Double fractures or more comminuted fractures are generally included in the Rolando type classification (McNealy & Lichtenstein 1933). The classical Rolando (1910) fracture involves two articular fracture fragments, one a dorsal articular fragment, another a palmar articular fragment, and a third shaft fragment (Griffiths 1964). Even more extensive comminution is often seen.

Management

Extra-articular fractures

The great majority of extra-articular fractures are reducible by simple traction, counter-traction techniques or by manipulation, provided this is done before healing or surrounding fibrosis have made the fracture relatively immobile (James 1940, Blum 1941, Charnley 1967, Griffiths 1964, Green & O'Brien 1972). Once reduced, most of these extra-articular fractures are stable in a thumb-

spica type of support with the thumb in a neutral resting position (Fig. 11.2). Those that are not stable can generally be handled by percutaneous K-wire fixation techniques, either pinning one fragment to the other or using a technique similar to the Wagner (1950) technique of stabilizing a large metacarpal fragment by pinning it to the trapezium proximally, as described for the Bennett type fractures. The few irreducible fractures are usually due to muscle interposition and respond easily to open reduction and internal fixation. Malunion may occasionally result in such deformity that collapse of the entire thumb may result (Fig. 11.3). Though adequate function may be possible, it is probably better to take down such malunions, reduce them and internally fix the fracture.

Intra-articular fractures

For the intra-articular fractures, where the Bennett's type fracture occurs at about a 4:1 ratio over the Rolando type (Green & O'Brien 1972), an incredible variety of ingenious techniques have been devised (Gedda 1954, Griffiths 1964, Slocum 1973, Wiggins 1954). Because of the inherent instability of the fracture, all external techniques—no matter how ingenious the device—have the potential for creating pressure sores and/or stiffness

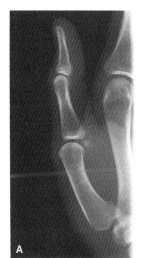
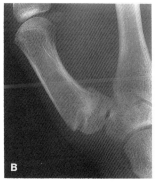

Fig. 11.2 Mildly displaced extra-articular fracture of the first metacarpal at the level of the physis actually displaced slightly more in a thumb spica-cast (A) but nonetheless healed adequately (B)

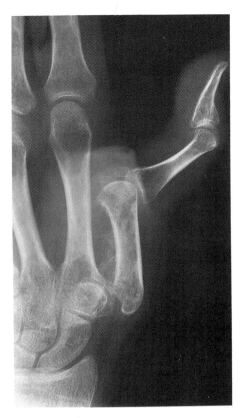

Fig. 11.3 In this patient who had multiple injuries, a fracture of the base of the first metacarpal, which may qualify as a Bennett's, but has more than 90% of the articular surface on the base fragment, was overlooked until malunion developed with a severe dynamic collapse of the thumb articulation chain

(Blum 1941, Charnley 1967, James & Givson 1940). The preferred techniques for those with demonstrable instability are either percutaneous fixation or open reduction and internal fixation (Johnson 1944, Ross & Sinclair 1946, Spangberg & Thoren 1963, Thoren 1956, Wagner 1950). As clearly demonstrated by Salgeback et al (1971) mild residual articular deformity of the base of the first metacarpal is the rule rather than the exception after this injury. Nevertheless, as previously noted, this is a loosely constrained joint and mild degrees of surface irregularity are fairly well tolerated. A very reasonable approach, then, is first to use one's preferred technique of closed reduction and next, if necessary, proceed immediately with one's preferred method of percutaneous fixation (Fig. 11.4). Personally, the Wagner (1950) technique has served me very well, though I have no hesitation

in using two K-wires if one does not seem sufficient or in placing a K-wire across the two fragments if they are large (Green & O'Brien 1972, Salgeback et al 1971). If, for whatever reason, the fixation carried out by this modified Wagner technique does not provide adequate maintenance of reduction, there should be no hesitation about proceeding with open reduction and internal fixation. Whether this is done with K-wires, screws, tension band wiring, threaded bolts, or some other favourite technique is of secondary importance. The minimally comminuted Rolando fractures with large fragments can be handled in exactly similar fashion (Gedda & Moberg 1953).

However, as comminution increases so does the difficulty both of obtaining and maintaining adequate reduction. Traction techniques have been thought desirable in the past for management of excessively comminuted fractures and traction is even more readily available with current techniques employing external fixators. However, it is a rare Rolando-type fracture that will fall into anatomical alignment when excessively comminuted and traction-fixation only is applied. For others, open reduction gives the best possible reassembly of the articular pavement; support of that pavement may require not only internal fixation but restoration of subchondral bone stock by bone graft. Results will deteriorate, regardless of method, as comminution increases.

Adequate access to the thumb CMC joint for most procedures is obtained by a hockey-stick incision, starting dorsally and then curling radially, which gives exposure of both sides of the first extensor compartment tendons. However, in extensively comminuted fractures, the incision can be curved onto the thenar region, the thenar muscles can be reflected distally and the radiovolar aspect of the joint thus made accessible. Curving the incision dorsally and ulnarward across the line of the extensor pollicis longus tendon and into the first web will render the ulnar aspect of the joint accessible too. In this area one must watch for and protect the princeps pollicis branch of the radial artery. In the thenar area, one may encounter the thenar branch of the radial artery. At this broad and irregularly contoured joint, visualization through any porthole should be supplemented by palpation using various types of dental probes.

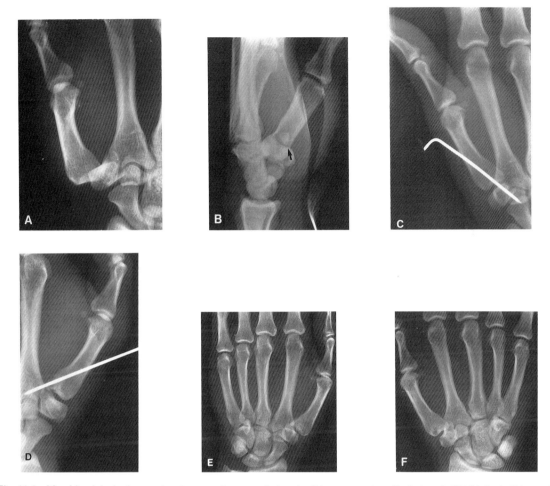

Fig. 11.4 Matching injuries incurred at the same time to each thumb of the same patient. Each thumb CMC joint is dislocated, but one injury is a pure dislocation (A) whereas the other (best seen on a lateral view of the wrist, B) is a Bennett's fracture-dislocation. Each dislocation is shown after closed reduction and percutaneous K-wire fixation—a classic Wagner style pin position on the dislocation side (C); a lucky placement on the other side (D) with the K-wire stabilizing both fragments to each other as well as to the carpus. Five-and-a-half months after injury, both thumb CMCs (dislocation side E; Bennett's side F) were functioning at a near-normal level clinically and radiographs also showed good position and condition

Dislocations of the thumb carpometacarpal joint

Pure dislocations of this joint (Eaton 1971, Eggers 1945, Kestler 1943, Martinez & Omer 1985, Moore et al 1978, Slocum 1973) are rare in normal people, but in loose-jointed individuals (such as those with Marfan's syndrome) are fairly common. For individuals with normal collagen and straightforward trauma, closed reduction and Wagner-type fixation for a period of three weeks, with part-time protection for another three weeks, is quite adequate. For patients with collagen deficiencies or other structural abnormalities, reconstruction

of a capsuloligamentous support system should be considered. Many techniques have been offered (Kestler 1943, Slocum 1973, Martinez & Omer 1985); that recommended by Eaton and Little (1969) is reliable.

Results

Results following extra-articular fractures of the base of the first metacarpal are reliably satisfactory, even in those instances where delays have prevented adequate reduction and a persistent deformity is noted (Robinson 1908, Macey & Murray 1949,

McNealy & Lichtenstein 1933). Results following adequately treated Bennett's fractures or fracture-dislocations are satisfactory in a majority of instances but not in all, and close observation will reveal some residual problem in most (Gedda 1953 & 1954, Salgeback et al 1971). Well-reduced, minimally comminuted, Rolando fractures compare favourably with Bennett's fractures but the more comminuted fractures usually have significant residua of persistent pain, weakness, and sometimes limited motion. These results are in direct proportion to the severity of the original damage and the adequacy of the initial treatment.

INJURIES TO THE CARPOMETACARPAL AREA OF THE INDEX AND LONG FINGERS

Classification

Being less protected, the CMC joint of the index finger is somewhat more prone to injury than that of the long finger, but both are exceedingly stable joints so fractures, dislocations, or fracture–dislocations are all relatively rare (Eaton 1971, Gunther 1984, Smith & Peimer 1977). More common are sprain–impaction syndromes and compression-impaction syndromes (Joseph et al 1981). Sprain-impaction problems are seen after flexion stress injuries resulting in volar impaction and dorsal stretch. A common example occurs when ice-hockey players crash into the wall or fend off an opponent. Compression-impaction is a serious problem in the professional boxer whose repetitive stress to the stable longitudinal arch eventually results in cartilage damage, osteochondral fracture, and a chronically painful arthrosis. High-energy stress may result in fracture anywhere in this carpometacarpal area and there may be a dislocation component, particularly if the stabilizing styloid processes are broken. Simple dislocation without fracture is known to occur but is extremely rare. Axial fracture–dislocations, involving the index and/or long finger rays plus adjacent carpal elements also occur, usually due to the excessive forces of crush or blast.

Management

Treatment of the sprain-impaction syndrome in its early stages is simply that of rest and protection, though this may require support of the entire metacarpal area extending distally beyond the metacarpophalangeal joints. In a chronic form, this is a very difficult problem to control and may eventually require fusion of the three-joint system comprising the index carpometacarpal joint, the intermetacarpal joint between the index and long fingers and long finger carpometacarpal joint (Fig. 11.5).

A similar treatment may be required in the compression-impaction syndrome unless abuse is stopped at an early stage. The rare extra-articular fracture of the base of index or long finger metacarpal is usually stable and often does not require reduction. If unstable, it behaves like the fracture–dislocations and will usually require fixation following reduction. Whether fracture or fracture-dislocation, the destabilized distal fragment will usually align satisfactorily with traction but may remain unstable until internally fixed (usually with percutaneous K-wires even when open reduction is required).

INJURIES TO THE CARPOMETACARPAL AREA OF THE RING AND LITTLE FINGERS

Classification

These injuries are discussed by Hazlet (1968), Hsu and Curtis (1970), Hunter and Cowen (1970), and Shepard and Solomon (1960). Fractures at the base of ring and little finger metacarpals are usually transverse, oblique, or comminuted and often involve the adjacent CMC joint area (Fig. 11.6). Whether they do or not, the instability or dislocation pattern (Dennyson & Stother 1976, Nalebuff 1968, North & Eaton 1980) is much the same with the metacarpals usually displaced dorsally. (However the patient in Figure 11.7 illustrates an exception to the rule.) They may displace *with* the carpometacarpal areas of the index and long fingers, *counter* to the displacement of the other metacarpal bases, *individually* or *together* (Waugh & Yancey 1948). A fairly common fracture-dislocation at the fifth finger carpometacarpal area is analogous to the Bennett's fracture, with a radial articular fragment of the fifth metacarpal base and proximal subluxation of the metacarpal shaft fragment,

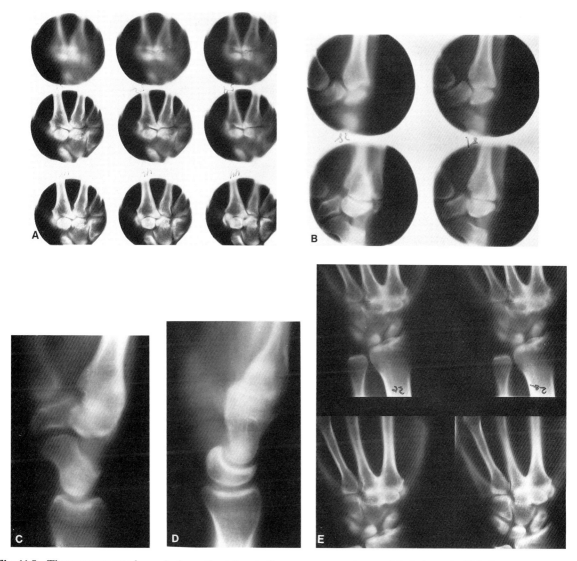

Fig. 11.5 The management of a sprain-impaction injury to the carpometacarpal areas of the index and middle fingers (associated with a carpal boss) is displayed by trispiral tomograms. First are preoperative AP (anteroposterior view) (A) and laterals (B) showing narrowing of the joint space and sclerosis as well as the carpal boss. Postoperative views at one year and four years show various aspects of the successful fusion: C is a lateral tomogram of the fused second CMC joint; D is a lateral view of the fused third CMC joint; and E is AP views that shows the two fused CMC joints plus the fused intermetacarpal joint. Fusion of all three joints is often indicated in this situation

aided by the pull of extensor carpi ulnaris (Fig. 11.8).

Management

These joints are less stable than those of the index and long fingers, and are easier to reduce but more difficult to stabilize. Percutaneous K-wire fixation is usually sufficient to maintain reduction but comminution of the joint surface may be sufficient to indicate open reduction (Hagstrom 1975), primarily for the purpose of reconstructing a better articular pavement (Bora & Didizian 1974). The important range of motion in these two carpometacarpal joints means that every attempt should be made to obtain a congruous joint surface. Fixation, whether percutaneously or after open reduction, should position the joints in some flexion, the

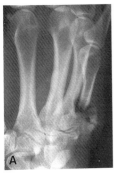 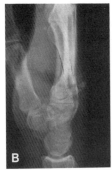 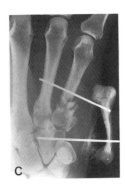 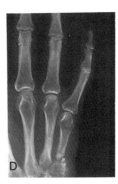 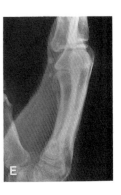

Fig. 11.6 This markedly comminuted, unstable, mostly extra-articular fracture of the fifth metacarpal base and adjacent joint is demonstrated on the oblique (A) and lateral (B) views. Following wound care and repositioning of fragments, position was maintained by a home-made external fixator (C) and views two months later (D & E) show some shortening but good alignment and the beginning of healing

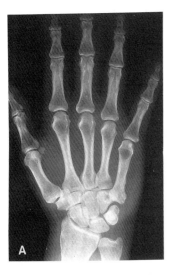 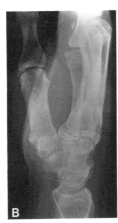

Fig. 11.7 The displacement of most dislocations and fracture–dislocations in this area is dorsal, but there are exceptions to every rule. This palmar dislocation of the fifth metacarpal in a female doctor was diagnosed late and never reduced, because she did not think the disability was great

INJURIES TO MULTIPLE CARPOMETACARPAL AREAS

Classification

Injuries of this type have been reported by Gunther (1984), Hartwig and Louis (1979), Shorbe (1938), Waugh and Yancey (1948) and Whitson (1955). The higher the energy level of the trauma affecting hand–carpal junction, the more likely it is that multiple metacarpal base–carpometacarpal areas are involved (Fig. 11.9). Any pattern may be seen, i.e. dislocation, fractures and fracture–dislocations with displacement most likely to be posterior (dorsal) but also occasionally anterior (palmar) and infrequently divergent (Gunther & Bruno 1985). With the steady increase of high-energy trauma, multiple dislocations are becoming more common and are sometimes associated with bone loss.

Management

They are always unstable and require either closed or open reduction followed by external or internal fixation (Fig. 11.10). If there is bone loss, the fixation of choice is usually distraction–fixation with later reconstruction by simple bone graft or flap with included bone graft (Peimer et al 1981).

COMPLICATIONS OF INJURY TO THE CARPOMETACARPAL AREA OF THE FINGERS

Complications in this region are principally due to the force involved in high energy lesions such as

position in which the palmar arch is formed. Painful arthritis or malunion in this area may be satisfactorily treated by either arthroplasty or fusion, fusion being the simpler procedure. If fusion is chosen, it too should be in a position of slight flexion. The surgical approach for either joint is directly dorsal with the usual care taken to protect branches of the dorsal sensory nerve, the finger extensors in a radial direction, and the ECU tendon in an ulnar direction.

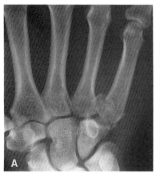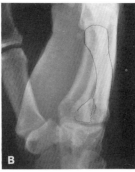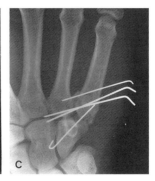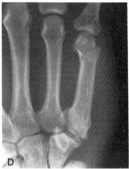

Fig. 11.8 (A & B) An undisplaced fracture of the base of the fourth metacarpal is associated with a comminuted fracture–dislocation at the fifth CMC joint analogous to the Rolando injury of the thumb. (C) shows the AP view after closed reduction and percutaneous fixation. There appeared to be deficient bone stock for complete reduction but a further AP view (D) taken three years later (when he sustained another injury—to the neck of the fifth metacarpal) shows the CMC joint is well preserved

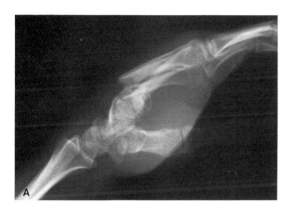

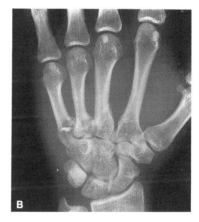

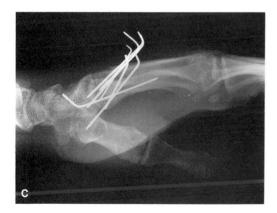

Fig. 11.9 One of the more common multiple fractures of the area is shown on this lateral view (A) of dorsally displaced fractures at the carpometacarpal areas of the ulnar three fingers. With gentle traction, good reduction was possible (B) but was sufficiently unstable that percutaneous K-wire fixation (C) was required

blast, crush, or severe traction–torsion injuries, all of which commonly produce problems in the carpometacarpal area.

Most of the vital anatomical structures in the region are reasonably well removed from these joints, but the extensor tendons and dorsal sensory nerve branches dorsally and the ulnar motor branch and deep palmar arch palmarward are closely related and may be damaged. In most instances, even the palmar structures can be seen satisfactorily through a dorsal approach because of the loss of integrity of the skeletal structures. However, occasionally it is necessary to follow the deep motor branch of the ulnar nerve and related vessels across the palmar aspect of the palm.

It is not uncommon, in the high-energy lesion, for combined metacarpal, carpometacarpal and

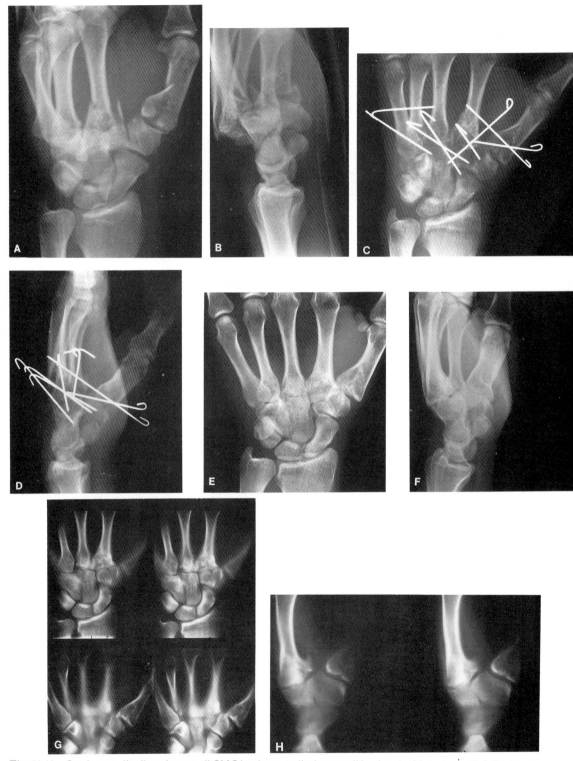

Fig. 11.10   Crush stress distributed across all CMC levels can easily damage all levels as in this instance (A & B) showing a Rolando fracture in the thumb, a palmar fracture–dislocation of the second metacarpal and dorsal fracture–dislocations of the other metacarpals. Open reduction and internal fixation with K-wires gave good alignment (C & D). Radiographs taken 2 years later (E & F) showed surprisingly good reconstitution of the entire carpometacarpal region, even when assessed by tomography (G & H)

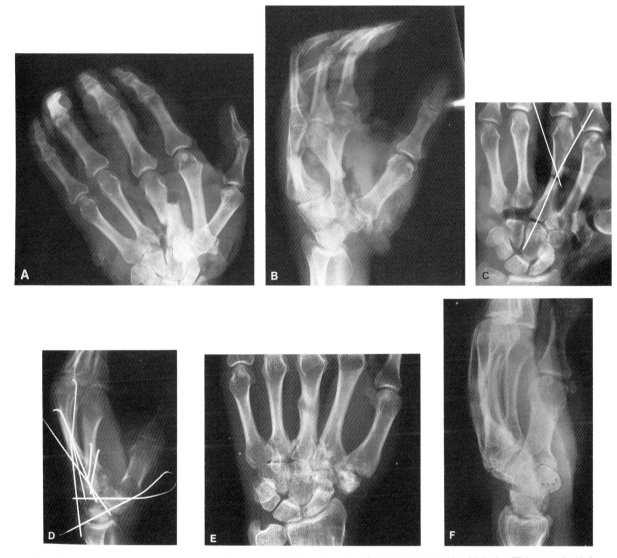

Fig. 11.11 Involvement of various areas of the carpus is fairly common with carpometacarpal level injuries. This example (A & B) shows a fracture–dislocation through the scaphotrapeziotrapezoidal joint, a fracture–dislocation of the index carpometacarpal joint and a displaced fracture of the third metacarpal. Traction and manipulation views (C) show the initial reduction and fixation and also demonstrate damage to the CMC joints of the ring and little fingers as well. Internal fixation was completed (D). Two years later radiographs (E & F) reveal fractures healed and joints ankylosed and stable except for residual subluxation at the scaphotrapezial area

carpal injuries to take place, mostly in a longitudinal destabilization pattern, with one or more digital rays accompanying the supporting carpal elements (Fig. 11.11). While interesting and significant injuries, these do not fall strictly within the parameters of the discussion, so it will merely be mentioned that they do occur and do involve the carpometacarpal area.

Persistent subluxation of the bases of the finger metacarpals does interfere with the dynamic balance of the musculotendinous units to those fingers, usually producing a type of claw deformity with MCP hyperextension and PIP (proximal interphalangeal) flexion. If this is sufficiently severe, even old carpometacarpal subluxations should be reduced.

CONCLUSION

Carpometacarpal area injuries are more frequent and more significant than the literature indicates. The sudden, forceful, repetitive and sometimes awkward force transitions at the forearm–hand junction area result in a multitude of injuries at distal forearm, carpus and carpometacarpal area. The variety, too, is intriguing with sprain-insta-

bility patterns insidiously developing symptoms with minor architectural distortion, whereas major disruptions of the stable arch system may stabilize and become only mildly symptomatic. Identification early and swift, followed by appropriate management is not yet frequent, but can provide successful results for the whole range of carpometacarpal damage.

REFERENCES

Bennett E H 1882 Fractures of the metacarpal bones. Dublin Journal of Medical Science 73:72–73

Blum L 1941 The treatment of Bennett's fracture-dislocation of the first metacarpal bone. Journal of Bone and Joint Surgery 23:578

Bora F W, Didizian N M 1974 The treatment of injuries to the carpometacarpal joint of the little finger. Journal of Bone and Joint Surgery 56A:1459–1463

Charnley J 1961 The closed treatment of common fractures (3rd edn). Livingstone, Edinburgh

Dennyson W G, Stother I G 1976 Carpometacarpal dislocation of the little finger. The Hand 8:161

Dobyns J H, Linscheid R L, Cooney W P III 1983 Fractures and dislocations of the wrist and hand, then and now. Journal of Hand Surgery 8:687–690

Eaton R, Littler J 1969 Ligament reconstruction for the painful thumb carpometacarpal joint. Journal of Bone and Joint Surgery 55A:661–668

Eaton R G 1971 Joint injuries of the hand. Charles C. Thomas, Springfield, Illinois

Eggers G W N 1945 Chronic dislocation of the base of the metacarpal of the thumb. Journal of Bone and Joint Surgery 27:500–501

Ellis V H 1945–1946 A method of treating Bennett's fracture. Proceedings of the Royal Society of Medicine 39:711

Gedda K O 1954 Studies on Bennett's fracture: anatomy, roentgenology, and therapy. Acta Chirurgica Scandinavica (Suppl. 193)

Gedda K O, Moberg E 1953 Open reduction and osteosynthesis of the so-called Bennett's fracture in the carpometacarpal joint of the thumb. Acta Orthopaedica Scandinavica 22:249–257

Goldberg D 1951 Thumb fractures and dislocations: a new method of treatment. American Journal of Surgery 81:227–231

Green D P, O'Brien E T 1972 Fractures of the thumb metacarpal. Southern Medical Journal 65:807–814

Griffiths J C 1964 Fractures at the base of the first metacarpal bone. Journal of Bone and Joint Surgery 46:712–719

Gunther S F 1984 The carpometacarpal joints. Orthopedic Clinics of North America 15:259–277

Gunther S F, Bruno P D 1985 Divergent dislocation of the carpometacarpal joints: a case report. Journal of Hand Surgery 10A:197–201

Hagstrom P 1975 Fracture dislocations in the ulnar carpometacarpal joints. Open reduction and pinning. Scandinavian Journal of Plastic Reconstructive Surgery 9:249

Hartwig R H, Louis D S 1979 Multiple carpometacarpal dislocations: a review of four cases. Journal of Bone and Joint Surgery 61A:906–8

Hazlet J W 1968 Carpometacarpal dislocations other than the thumb: a report of 11 cases. Canadian Journal of Surgery 11:315–23

Hsu J D, Curtis R M 1970 Carpometacarpal dislocations on the ulnar side of the hand. Journal of Bone and Joint Surgery 52A:927–30

Hunter J M, Cowen N J 1970 Fifth metacarpal fractures in a compensation clinic population. Journal of Bone and Joint Surgery 52A:1159–1165

James E S, Givson A 1940 Fracture of the first metacarpal bone. Canadian Medical Association Journal 43:153–155

Johnson E C 1944 Fractures of the base of the thumb: a new method of fixation. Journal of the American Medical Association 126:27

Joseph R B, Linscheid R L, Dobyns J H, Bryan R S 1981 Chronic sprains of the carpometacarpal joints. Journal of Hand Surgery 6:172–180

Kestler O C 1943 Recurrent dislocation of the base of the metacarpal joint repaired by functional tenodesis. Journal of Bone and Joint Surgery 28:626–30

Macey H B, Murray R A 1949 Fractures about the base of the first metacarpal with special reference to Bennett's fracture. Southern Medical Journal 42:931–935

Martinez R, Omer G E Jr 1985 Bilateral subluxation of the base of the thumb secondary to an unusual abductor pollicis longus insertion: a case report. Journal of Hand Surgery 10A:396–399

McNealy R W, Lichtenstein M E 1933 Bennett's fracture and other fractures of the first metacarpal. Surgery, Gynecology and Obstetrics 56:197–210

Moore J R, Webb C A Jr, Thompson R C 1978 A complete dislocation of the thumb metacarpal. Journal of Hand Surgery 3:547–549

Nalebuff E A 1968 Isolated anterior carpometacarpal dislocation of the little finger: classification and case report. Journal of Trauma 8:1119–1123

North E R, Eaton R G 1980 Volar dislocation of the fifth metacarpal. Journal of Bone and Joint Surgery 62A:657–659

Peimer C A, Smith R J, Leffert R D 1981 Distraction-fixation in the primary treatment of metacarpal bone loss. Journal of Hand Surgery 6:111–124

Robinson S 1908 The Bennett fracture of the first metacarpal bone: diagnosis and treatment. Boston Medical and Surgical Journal 153:275–280

Rolando S 1910 Fracture de la base du premier métacarpien.

Et principalement sur une variété non encore décrite. Presse médicale 18:303

Ross J W, Sinclair A B 1946 The treatment of Bennett's fracture with Stader splint. Journal of Canadian Medical Service 3:507–511

Salgeback S, Eiken O, Carstam N, Ohlsson N 1971 A study of Bennett's fracture, special reference to fixation by percutaneous pinning. Scandinavian Journal of Plastic and Reconstructive Surgery 5:142–148

Shepard E, Solomon D J 1960 Carpometacarpal dislocations with particular reference to simultaneous dislocation of the base of the fourth and fifth metacarpals. Journal of Bone and Joint Surgery 42B:771–777

Shorbe H B 1938 Carpometacarpal dislocations: report of a case. Journal of Bone and Joint Surgery 20A:454–457

Slocum D B 1973 Stabilization of the articulation of the greater multangular and the first metacarpal. Journal of Bone and Joint Surgery 55:1655–1666

Smith R J, Peimer C A 1977 Injuries to the metacarpal bones and joints. Advances in Surgery 11:341–374

Spangberg O, Thoren L 1963 Bennett's fracture: a method of treatment with oblique traction. Journal of Bone and Joint Surgery 45B:732–736

Thoren L 1956 A new method of extension treatment in Bennett's fracture. Acta Chirurgica Scandinavica 110:485–493

Wagner C J 1950 Methods of treatment of Bennett's fracture-dislocation. American Journal of Surgery 80:230–231

Waugh R L, Yancey A G 1948 Carpometacarpal dislocations with particular reference to simultaneous dislocation of the base of the fourth and fifth metacarpals. Journal of Bone and Joint Surgery 30A:397–404

Whitson R O 1955 Carpometacarpal dislocation: a case report. Clinical Orthopedics 6:189–195

Wiggins H E, Bundens W D Jr, Park B J 1954 A method of treatment of fracture-dislocations of the first metacarpal bone. Journal of Bone and Joint Surgery 36A:810–819.

PART

C

Special types of hand fractures

Jonathan Noble and Hamish Potts

12 Pathological fractures of the hand

By virtue of its superficial nature and of its function, the hand is most vulnerable to trauma, but fortunately is relatively immune to pathological fractures. Arguments used to explain this, point to the ease with which early swelling may be seen in a superficial structure and pain felt early in so richly innervated an organ. However, this cannot fully account for the very low incidence of pathological fractures in the hand, whether it be from infection, metabolic bone disease, primary or secondary malignancy.

GENERALIZED DISORDERS

Whereas fractures of metacarpals or phalanges may occur due to *bone infection* or *metabolic bone disease* such occurrences are exceedingly rare. When they are encountered, it may be generally said that the management of the fracture will depend almost entirely on the treatment of the metabolic error or the infection. Surgical interference with such fractures has neither been accomplished nor encountered by these authors. It is worth remembering, however, that erosive lesions in the tufts of distal phalanges, which may themselves cause a small fracture, are most likely to be due to a parathyroid adenoma, investigations for which can be initiated by the hand surgeon.

Gout has been described as a rare cause of pathological fracture in the hand (Julliard 1973). Again the fracture is treated on its merits, although the bone quality does not lend itself to osteosynthesis. Julliard also describes a spontaneous avulsion fracture of the dorsum of the base of distal phalanges, such as one encounters in mallet finger

deformities, but in association with *rheumatoid arthritis*.

Fracture of a phalanx of the hand due to *sarcoidosis* has been reported by Landi et al (1983) and by Terranova et al (1985).

Paget's disease sometimes presents with a pathological fracture of a weight-bearing bone. However, fractures in the hand from this condition are extremely unusual—reportably so. Ogilvie-Harris and Formassier (1979) reported two phalangeal pathological fractures and a further case has been reported (Newell 1975) in association with Dupuytren's contracture, a condition which we believe to be commonly associated with Paget's disease. Should so rare a case arise in our practice, we would advise that the fracture be treated upon the merits of its site, deformity and stability. Thus we would treat a Pagetic metacarpal fracture by early mobilization, whereas a phalangeal fracture with rotational deformity we would fix according to the principles set out elsewhere in this book. Paget's disease is a common condition and Grundy and Patton (1969) have estimated that 20% of patients have hand involvement evident on X-ray examination. Against that background it is clear that Paget's disease remains a rare cause of pathological fractures in the hand (Fig 12.1).

LOCALIZED BONE LESIONS

In practice, nearly all pathological fractures of the carpus, metacarpus and phalanges are due to bone cysts, benign or malignant tumours and thus this chapter will concern itself mostly with them. It is important to emphasize that the only tumours

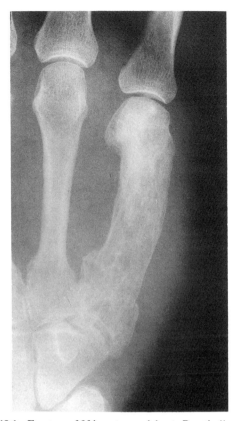

Fig. 12.1 Fracture of fifth metacarpal due to Paget's disease

Table 12.1 Prevalence of bone tumours in the hand

Tumour type	Total	Total in hand	%
Osteoid osteoma	77	5	6.5
Osteoblastoma	364	14	3.8
Osteogenic sarcoma	605	3	0.5
Juxtacortical sarcoma	24	0	0
Solitary osteochondroma	323	16	5.0
Solitary enchondroma	136	48	35.3
Benign chondroblastoma	458	11	2.4
Chondromyxoid fibroma	340	12	3.5
Chondrosarcoma	264	2	0.8
Fibrosarcoma of bone	130	0	0
Giant cell tumour	265	10	3.8
Non-ossifying fibroma	48	0	0
Ewing's sarcoma	167	0	0

which commonly cause a fracture are enchondromata which are said to provide 90% of all bone tumours in the hand. Huvos (1979) has assembled a magnificent collection of bone tumour data from the experience of his own unit and a comprehensive literature survey. We have extracted from that survey the proportion of cases presenting in the hand and this is set out in Table 12.1.

One-third of all enchondromata present in the hand; otherwise only osteochondroma and osteoid osteoma occur in the hand in 5% or more of cases.

Bone tumours causing pathological fracture

Enchondromata apart, a review of the literature reveals that almost any other of the lesions to be outlined, in the hand, would be the subject of no more than a case report or reports, rather than a 'series'. Thus our purpose is merely to highlight those bone lesions which we know have caused, or believe could cause, a pathological fracture. In

common with most other practitioners we can only claim significant personal experience with enchondromata, and those lesions apart (as they seem to have a proclivity to fracture) it would seem in general that pain and/or swelling is more likely to be the initial presentation. One point of great, but very rare, interest is that of *trauma-induced sarcoma.* Dreyfuss et al in 1980 reported a Ewing's sarcoma of the thumb with a fracture line running through it at the exact position of a previous traumatic fracture several years previously. The patient, a mechanic, had been subject to 'repeated trauma' in the interim. The case satisfied Ewing's own criteria (1935) for trauma-induced malignancy and a total of six cases of *Ewing's sarcoma* in the hand were summarized in Dreyfuss's report, in which the well-known appalling prognosis even with radical surgery is re-emphasized.

Aneurysmal bone cyst

This is rare in the hand, although Carroll (1975) has suggested that a number of previously diagnosed giant-cell tumours of bone are aneurysmal bone cysts. In his account he makes no particular mention of fracture, indicating that they have an expanded, bubbly appearance upon X-ray examination and are typically seen in the distal metacarpus and proximal phalanges. This corresponds with Chalmers' (1981a) findings in three cases. Judging from his radiographs, sufficient rapid cystic destruction of the cortex had occurred as to constitute a pathological fracture (Fig 12.2). In this paper the 20–30% postoperative recurrence

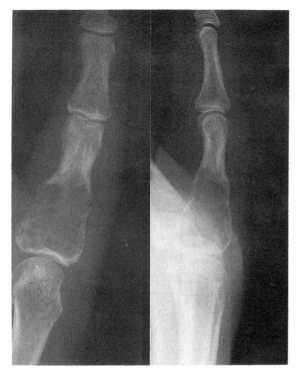

Fig. 12.2 Aneurysmal bone cyst (Mr J Chalmers' case) before and after curettage

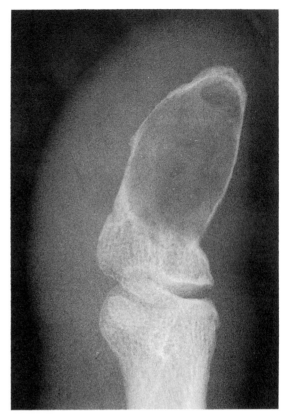

Fig. 12.3 Inclusion epidermoid cyst with pathological fracture, in a man of 58. This is the legacy of a crushing injury of the fingertip when he was 7 years old (Mr N J Barton's case)

after aneurysmal bone cyst is mentioned and the possibility of curettage (as opposed to curettage and bone grafting) being sufficient to secure bone healing was illustrated.

Solitary bone cyst

Solitary bone cyst is described by Carroll (1975) as a fibrocystic disorder which should be distinguished on X-ray examination, like aneurysmal bone cyst sometimes with difficulty, from an enchondroma. The distribution of simple bone cysts is similar to that of aneurysmal ones and in our opinion the distinction may be artificial on purely radiological grounds. Carroll encountered only one pathological fracture in his cases.

Epidermoid (inclusion) cysts

These cysts are common in the subcutaneous tissues, but rarely occur within bone. Being post-traumatic they are most typically seen in the distal phalanx. However, their neat, round, central shape

within a phalanx may make distinction from an enchondroma difficult. Pathological fracture occurs very occasionally (Fig 12.3) and recommended treatment has included curettage or even amputation of a finger tip. If the circumstances were clinically typical of an epidermoid cyst, then in the presence of a fracture we would be very inclined to splint the fracture and thereafter treat the matter expectantly.

Bone cysts in general are found in children and adolescents, whereas enchondromata are generally encountered in young adults. If there is calcification on the radiograph, then this is pathognomonic of an enchondroma and exclusive of any form of cyst.

Benign chondroblastoma

This is a rare tumour, which may also be difficult to distinguish from an enchondroma, although it predominates in teenagers. As it is extremely rare in the hand, almost never fractures (Huvos 1979) and does not undergo sarcomatous transformation it is clearly a rarity whose unlikely existence may be regarded with impunity.

Osteochondromata and osteoid osteomata

These essentially do not cause pathological fractures in the hand. The same would appear to be the case for non-ossifying fibroma as judged by a recent Mayo clinic review (Arata et al 1981).

Giant cell tumour

This constitutes about 5% of all bone tumours and between 1 and 5% of these occur in the hand. The presentation may be any combination of pain, swelling and pathological fracture, typically in the third or fourth decades.

Should a case present with fracture we would recommend curettage (if only to confirm the diagnosis) and bone grafting, with a meticulous long-term clinical and radiological follow-up. Only in recurrent cases, or those in whom the presentation is both late and gross, should radical ray resection/amputation be considered and radiotherapy is notoriously counter-productive with osteoclastomata. It may actually cause a pathological fracture.

Anyway a number of alleged giant cell tumours in the hand may in fact be no more than an aneurysmal bone cyst. This statement exemplifies the 'Catch 22' of bone tumours in the hand. We can only treat and teach authoritatively upon the basis of firm, conclusive diagnoses. Generally they can only be made upon the basis of a biopsy. Such surgical intervention is in fact frequently unnecessary with this group of conditions, particularly if the surgeon is willing to undertake the meticulous follow-up of patients just referred to.

Ganglion

Intraosseous ganglion is another rare curiosity in the hand, although Chalmers (1981b) has illustrated a case arising in the lunate, and causing spontaneous pathological fracture of it. Of the 15 cases of intraosseous ganglion reported by Kam-

bolis et al 1973, four involved the wrist and none caused fracture.

Enchondroma

This is where the story really begins as regards pathological fracture in the hand. Although sizeable series of enchondromata in the hand have been published by Takigawa (1971), Noble and Lamb (1974) and Shellito and Dockerty (1948), there is no uniformity about the findings or the advice offered.

Clinical presentation

Enchondromata of the hand may be part of a more widespread case of Ollier's disease (multiple enchondromatosis). Takigawa (1971), who presented 110 cases of enchondromata in the hand, found that many of his cases were polyostotic, whereas in the other recent large series we found such cases to be in a minority (Noble & Lamb 1974). Two-thirds of our cases presented with a pathological fracture, usually in a young adult; only two of our 40 cases were 50 or more years old and most were under 30 years. This is a higher proportion than that reported by Takigawa, or by Shellito and Dockerty (1948).

The majority of our cases were also phalangeal, usually either side of the PIP joint. Many had been aware of a painless swelling before the fracture occurred. The degree of trauma to cause the fracture varied greatly.

Radiology

These lesions are typically found in the metaphyseal area of the bone. We used a similar classification to that employed by Takigawa. Briefly the lesions may be situated centrally, eccentrically or in the juxta-cortical region of the bone and they may or may not expand the bone width. Calcification is a common feature, particularly in long-standing cases, and it is by this feature that many of the other common benign lesions described may be excluded (Fig 12.4). The bone cortices are frequently very thin, particularly in those presenting with a pathological fracture. Fracture lines, like the basic pathology itself, do not involve joints.

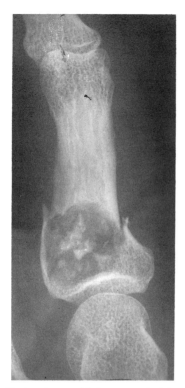

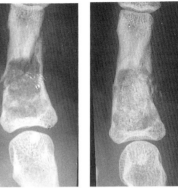
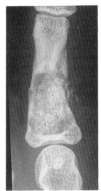
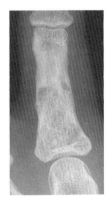

Fig. 12.5   Enchondroma with fracture (A). After bone grafting (B). Healed $2\frac{1}{2}$ years later (C)

Fig. 12.4   Enchondroma with fracture and calcification

Treatment

Of our 40 cases of enchondromata, 25 presented with a fracture. That fracture was treated by the standard and time-honoured method of curettage of the lesion, whose cavity was then packed with autologous bone graft in 13 of those 25 cases (Fig 12.5). It was found that good healing could occur after curettage of the lesion alone (Fig 12.6). We then experienced a case in whom there was a contraindication to surgery, whose fracture was therefore treated conservatively on a Zimmer splint and which healed most satisfactorily (Fig. 12.7). That regime of almost 'studied neglect' was then followed in six cases. At our follow-up study all six cases treated by 'studied neglect' had obtained a good or excellent result, whereas two cases who had undergone curettage and grafting developed problems, which could be attributed to that operation, including one non-union of the fracture.

Since conducting this study during 1973 we have not operated upon an enchondroma of the hand and have treated another six cases of fracture by

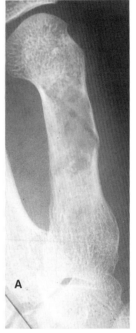
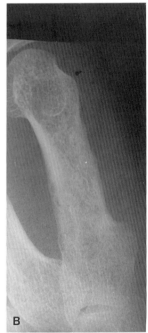

Fig. 12.6   Enchondroma with fracture, curetted (A). Appearances 8 years later (B)

splintage alone. Our follow-up studies in these cases reveal that not only does the fracture heal spontaneously but that there may also be ossification within the enchondroma itself (Fig 12.8).

In Takigawa's series (1971) radical excision or diaphysectomy was described. Unless there is a diagnostic and thus histopathological problem we consider both to be unnecessary in the management of pathological fracture secondary to benign enchondroma. It is interesting that Takigawa men-

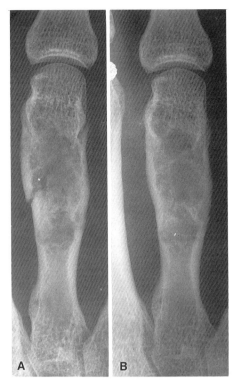

Fig. 12.7 Enchondroma with fracture treated conservatively (A). $2\frac{1}{2}$ years later (B)

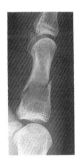
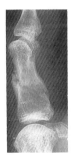
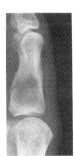
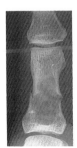
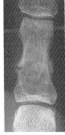
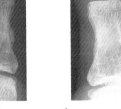

Fig. 12.8 Enchondroma with fracture, treated conservatively, showing ossification 6 months later

tioned a few of his patients who declined surgery and proceeded to heal spontaneously. This coincides with our perplexity at the common textbook advice, which frequently is that the monostotic cases be treated surgically, whereas the polyostotic cases can be left alone with some impunity.

Question of malignancy

The questionable drawback in these cases is that the diagnosis may just be other than benign enchondroma. We can see much good sense therefore in carrying out a biopsy in any case in whom there has been a fracture and with which concern may exist as to the pathological diagnosis. Having opened the lesion to biopsy it, thorough curettage seems the most sensible method. We are however puzzled by a paper which advocates curettage and freeze-dried cancellous bone allograft in all cases of solitary benign enchondroma and states that, because of the possibility of malignant degeneration, all such tumours should be so treated (Jewusiak et al 1971). We would be inclined to the general view that if the surgeon has decided to bone graft then access to the cancellous bone contained within the patient's own olecranon is easy and convenient.

The surgeon, whilst always remaining both sceptical and vigilant, can take a fairly relaxed view for a variety of reasons as follows:

1. Chondrosarcomata in the hand are exceedingly rare and osteosarcomata are even more so.
2. Such malignancy typically occurs in patients over the age of 50, in whom pathological fracture due to enchondromata is very unusual.
3. Usually sarcomata will have their own distinctive radiological appearances.
4. Few sarcomata exhibit calcification, whereas most enchondromata do.
5. These malignant tumours, when they do arise, are slow-growing and generally only give rise to problems locally.
6. Few of these malignant tumours present with pathological fractures. In the series of 19 chondrosarcomata of the hand reported by Roberts and Price (1977), pathological fracture was only mentioned in five patients. It is emphasized that the total number of reported chondrosarcomata (the commonest malignant

hand bone tumour) at the time of Roberts and Price's paper was only 41.

However, we consider the following to be crucial features demanding further investigation, including biopsy: periosteal reaction, patchy destruction of the cortex, absence of calcification, recurrence of previous lesion, and a second increase in size. It is pertinent to note that in one of the very rare cases from the world literature in which malignant transformation of an enchondroma to a chondrosarcoma occurred (Shellito & Dockerty 1948) the patient had experienced five previous curettage operations. This exemplifies the wisdom of judging a case just as much by the clinical features, history and radiological progress, as by the histopathology whose distribution is varied and whose interpretation is always difficult.

As we have previously stated (Noble & Lamb 1974) surgery might profitably be reserved for patients with persistent symptoms, refracture or delayed union.

Ollier's disease

A detailed description of this well-known condition is outside the scope of this chapter. However, in a recent general review of the subject Shapiro (1982) commented that 'lesions of the hand and foot posed relatively few problems'. It is interesting to note that in Shapiro's series all pathological fractures, at all sites, healed with conservative treatment over a normal period of time.

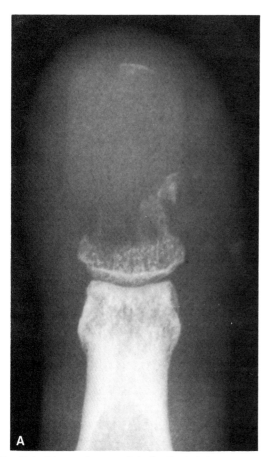 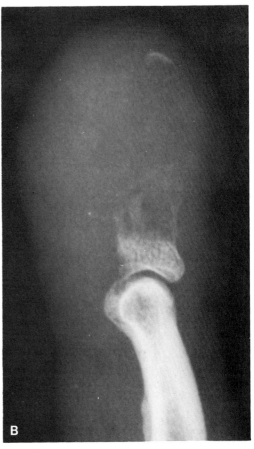

Fig. 12.9 X-rays of metastasis in the distal phalanx from a carcinoma of the kidney in a 53-year-old man (patient of Mr R C Mulholland)

Malignant tumours

Metastatic bone disease

The hand is a most unusual site for metastasis, but it does occur (Fig 12.9) and because it is rare the correct diagnosis may not be made. The subject has been studied by Kerin (1958) and Uriburu et al (1976), who added two cases of their own to the 90 others which they reviewed from the literature, and by Healey et al (1986). These lesions show a preference for the distal phalanges. Lung (42 cases) and breast (15 cases) are the only common primary sites. The presentation of a lung metastasis in the hand is more likely to be as part of a differential diagnosis from an infection than it is to be as a classical pathological fracture. Despite being associated for a number of years with units attracting cases of metastatic bone disease, we have yet to encounter a patient with such a pathological fracture in the hand, requiring surgery. Our approach generally would be as for any other metastatic fracture, with radiotherapy and possible internal fixation foremost in our thoughts. We have heard of such cases which have been best dealt with palliatively by means of amputation.

Osteosarcoma

This is exceptionally rare in the hand. Huvos (1979) states that it is more slowly growing than elsewhere and only locally malignant, with secondary spread unlikely. Thus he advises treatment by radical excision of the ray concerned, rather than by amputation of the hand, which would be the treatment in a case of local recurrence.

This great rarity in the hand is only mentioned here as theoretically it may be a cause of pathological fracture.

Chondrosarcoma

This is the commonest cause of bone malignancy in the hand. However, Roberts and Price (1977) were only able to trace 19 such cases from the Bristol Tumour Registry. They cited another 41 cases from the literature. Whereas fracture is unlikely to be a presentation, it will be noted in about 20% of cases. These patients are likely to be male and middle-aged or elderly and the principles of treatment are similar to those for an osteosarcoma. The 'cure' rate is high and the degree of malignancy is better judged by the clinical behaviour than by histological appearances. Despite isolated reports of chondrosarcomata arising from pre-existing benign enchondromata (Culver et al 1975), those too are cases of great rarity and it is generally agreed that chondrosarcomata in the hand are malignant de novo (Dahlin & Salvador 1974).

CONCLUSIONS

This is a short chapter regarding rare conditions. Generally speaking a pathological fracture in the hand is most likely to be secondary to an enchondroma. The surgeon may treat these conservatively with some impunity, but should always be alert to the possibility of the lesion being otherwise, and in particular being sarcomatous. Investigation need not be sophisticated or protracted. Biopsy, a small procedure, will resolve most diagnostic problems, although it should be appreciated that malignant transformation is as well judged clinically and with radiographs as it is by the histopathology.

REFERENCES

Arata M A, Peterson H A, Dahlin D C 1981 Pathological fractures through non-ossifying fibromas. Journal of Bone and Joint Surgery 63A:980–988

Carroll R E 1975 Tumors of the hand skeleton. In: Flynn J E (ed) Hand Surgery, Williams and Wilkins, Baltimore, pp 676–677

Chalmers J 1981a Aneurysmal bone cysts of the phalanges. A report of three cases. The Hand 13:296–300

Chalmers J 1981b Tumours. In: Lamb D W, Kuczynski K (eds) The practice of hand surgery, Blackwell Scientific Publications, Edinburgh, p. 455

Culver J E, Sweet De and McCue F C 1975 Chondrosarcoma of the hand arising from a pre-existent benign solitary enchondroma. Case report and pathological description. Clinical Orthopaedics 113:128–131.

Dreyfuss U Y, Auslander L, Biakik V, Fishman J 1980 Ewing's sarcoma of the hand following recurrent trauma: a case report. The Hand 12:300–303

Dahlin D C and Salvador A H 1974 Chondrosarcoma of the bones in the hand and feet. Cancer 34:p. 760

Ewing J 1935 Modern attitudes towards traumatic cancer. Archives of Pathology 19:690–728

Grundy M, Patton T J 1969 The hand in Paget's disease. British Journal of Radiology 42:748–752

Healey J, Turnbull A D M, Miedema B, Lane J M 1986 Acrometastases. A study of twenty-nine patients with osseous involvement of the hands and feet. Journal of Bone and Joint Surgery 68A:743–746

Jewusiak E M, Spence K F, Sell K W 1971 Solitary benign enchondromata of the long bones of the hand. Results of curettage and packing with freeze dried cancellous bone allograft. Journal of Bone and Joint Surgery 53A:1587–1591

Julliard A 1973 Les fractures pathologiques des os du main. Acta Orthopaedica Belgica 39:1016–1023

Huvos A G 1979 Bone tumours: diagnosis treatment and prognosis. W B Saunders Company, Philadelphia

Kambolis C, Bullough P G, Jaffe H L 1973 Ganglionic cystic defects in bone. Journal of Bone and Joint Surgery 55A:496–505

Kerin R 1958 Metastatic tumours of the hand. Journal of Bone and Joint Surgery 40A:263–278

Landi A, Brooks D, de Santis G 1983 Sarcoidosis of the hand—report of two cases. Journal of Hand Surgery 9A:197–200

Newell R L 1975 Paget's disease, Dupuytren's contracture and phalangeal fracture. The Hand 7:297–9

Noble J, Lamb D W 1974 Enchondromata of bones of the hand. A review of 40 cases. The Hand 6:275–284

Ogilvie-Harris D J, Formassier V L 1979 Pathological fractures of the hand in Paget's disease. Clinical Orthopaedics 143:168–70

Roberts P H, Price C H G 1977 Chondrosarcoma of the bones of the hand. Journal of Bone and Joint Surgery 59B:213–221

Shapiro F 1982 Ollier's disease. An assessment of angular deformity, shortening and pathological fracture in 21 patients. Journal of Bone and Joint Surgery 64A:95–103

Shellito J G, Dockerty M B 1948 Cartilagenous tumours of the hand. Surgery, Gynaecology and Obstetrics 86:465–472

Takigawa K 1971 Chondroma of the bones of the hand: A review of 110 cases. Journal of Bone and Joint Surgery 53A:1591–1600

Terranova W A, Williams G S, Kuhlman T A, Morgan R F 1985 Acute phalangeal fractures due to undiagnosed sarcoidosis. Journal of Hand Surgery 10A:902–903

Uriburu N F, Norelino F J, Marin J C 1976 Metastases of carcinoma of the larynx and thyroid gland to the phalanges of the hand. Journal of Bone and Joint Surgery 58A:134–136

13

Open fractures and those with soft tissue damage: treatment by external fixation

While the principles of external fixation have become well established in the treatment of severe injuries of the pelvis and lower extremity, their application to injuries of the hand has achieved significant clinical attention only in the last decade. With increasing experience and refinements in the technique and instrumentation, the list of indications for external fixation in the hand continues to grow. At first, the application of external fixation to the hand was hampered by the weight and bulk of the devices and by technical problems in their insertion. Injury to the neurovascular structures and interference by the transfixion pins with the adjacent gliding tendon mechanisms often compromised hand function.

The terminology applied to the different types of external fixator has become rather confused, particularly when 'half-frame' is applied to a device applied to one side of the limb, but 'double-frame' to a device on both sides. In this chapter, the former (see Fig. 13.14) will be described as a single half-pin frame and the latter (see Fig. 13.15) as a transfixion frame. 'Half-pin' means a pin inserted from one side of a bone, usually purchasing on both cortices but not emerging through the skin on the opposite side. Transfixion pins pass through both cortices and the skin on both sides. A half-pin frame applied to each side of the digit or limb may externally resemble a transfixion frame: this is best called a double half-pin frame, and may have the two sets of pins in the same plane or in two different planes.

Transfixion-frame devices became available in 1970 (Matev) for bone lengthening in reconstructive procedures. A variety of transfixion-frame devices later became available for use in trauma

and reconstruction (Mantero et al 1976, Kessler et al 1977; Paneva-Holevitch & Yankov 1980). Initially, such devices were applied to the first ray, whose plane of position with respect to the rest of the hand facilitated through-and-through fixation. Transfixion-frame devices, however, were difficult to apply to the other digits where both the pins and connecting portions of the device tended to interfere with adjacent rays. Because of this, half-pin frame devices were developed which, while less stable than the double frame configurations (Ardrey 1970), offered greater flexibility, particularly for the central rays. Current external fixation devices now offer a variety of pin and connecting rod configurations which make it easier to avoid interference with important gliding tendons and neurovascular structures. The devices have also become smaller, thus avoiding transfixion of adjacent mobile joints.

INDICATIONS FOR EXTERNAL FIXATION IN THE HAND

Most current external fixators can be used in three different ways: for applying compression, for distraction, or simply maintaining neutralization of forces across the intermediate bone or joint segment.

Compression

External fixation devices can be used across joints to apply compression as a means for securing arthrodesis (Micks & Hager 1968, Ferlic et al 1983). Although arthrodesis can in most instances be achieved predictably by internal fixation, external fixation with compression can accelerate

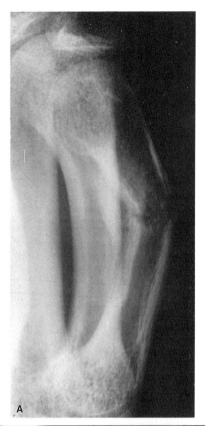

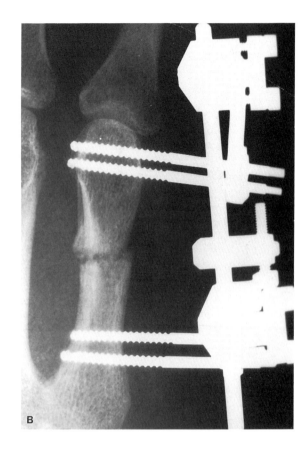

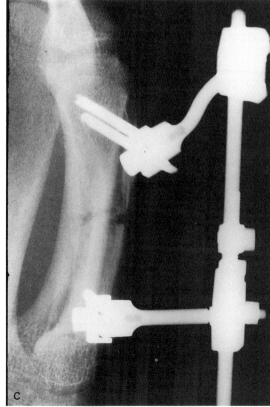

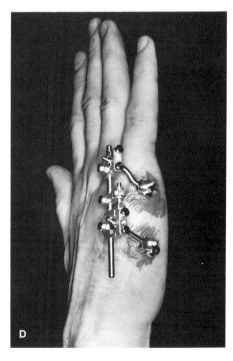

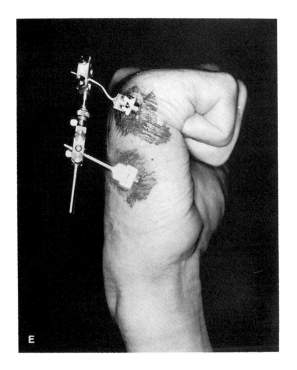

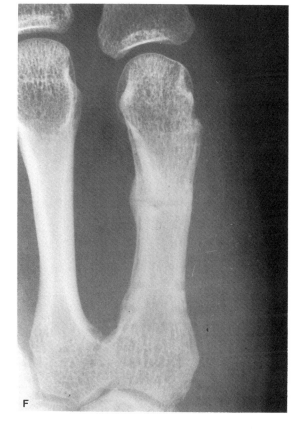

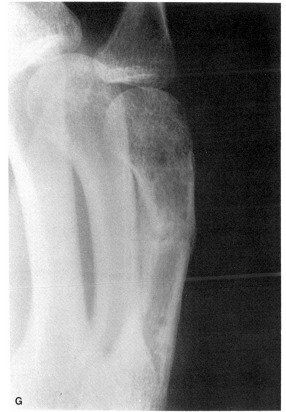

Fig. 13.1   External fixation to provide compression (see text for details)

osseous union and be advantageous in instances where bone stock is deficient and internal fixation more difficult. Similarly, external fixation can be utilized to position and compress correctional osteotomies, minimizing the soft tissue dissection required for internal fixation and avoiding the bulk of an implant. External fixation in such situations can provide sufficient stability to allow adjacent joints to be mobilized by surgery and postoperative therapy. When the osteotomy has united, the device is easily removed.

Example. This 25-year-old man (Fig. 13.1) presented ten weeks after an open fracture of the right fifth metacarpal diaphysis which had resulted in a dorsal angular deformity, an extension contracture of the metacarpophalangeal joint and an extensor lag at the proximal interphalangeal joint (A). (B and C) Extensor tenolysis and dorsal capsulotomy of the metacarpophalangeal joint were performed simultaneously with correctional osteotomy. Reduction was held by a single half-pin frame mini-external fixator which allowed compression across the osteotomy. (D and E) External fixation provided fracture stability while allowing immediate active and passive range-of-motion exercises to preserve the motion obtained at operation. (F and G) The osteotomy healed uneventfully without significant deformity.

Fractures with a stable configuration can be

rendered more stable by compression of the opposing fracture surfaces. Most external fixation devices have the ability to apply compression across the fracture through threaded connecting rods. Compression can also be utilized in treating septic non-unions, after debridement, by applying compression across interposed bone grafts or shortened opposed fracture surfaces (Allieu & Fassio 1974, Asche et al 1979).

Distraction

The most common indication for external fixation of the hand is to provide distraction. This can be achieved by applying longitudinal traction at operation and then tightening the external fixation device to hold the distraction obtained (Morton 1944). Alternatively, traction can be applied progressively through a threaded rod on the device (Allieu 1985, Cooney 1980). This principle, first applied to thumb reconstruction (Fig. 13.2), was introduced in 1967 by Matev and later reported by

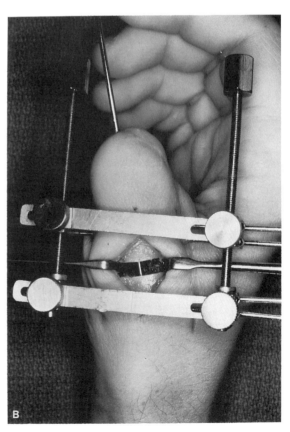

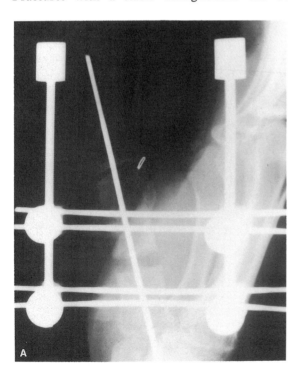

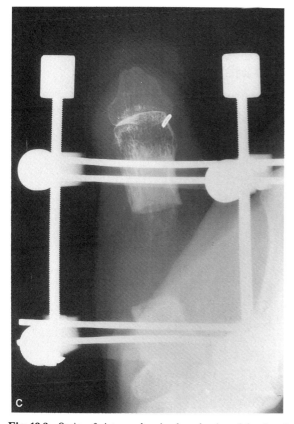
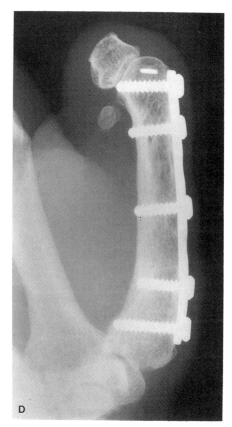

Fig. 13.2   Series of pictures showing lengthening of the thumb metacarpal by distraction and subsequent interpositional bone grafting demonstrating the principle of distraction by external fixation

Kessler et al (1979), Paneva–Holevich and Yankov (1980), and Manktelow and Wainwright (1984).

Extra-articular fractures

External fixation, having been developed for the treatment of congenital anomalies and traumatic amputations, was subsequently applied to injuries of the skeleton of the hand where bone shortening had occurred. Most often this occurs at the metacarpal level as through a gunshot injury, which leads to segmental bone loss and metacarpal shortening. When initially seen, metacarpal length can be maintained by transfixion of the injured metacarpal with Kirschner wires to adjacent metacarpals (Peimer et al 1981). When seen late, such metacarpal shortening usually has to be overcome by gradual distraction prior to interpositional bone grafting (Kessler et al 1979). Similar shortening also occurs in comminuted, segmental

phalangeal defects and requires maintenance of appropriate skeletal length either by internal splints (Fig. 13.3) or external means. External fixation offers greater flexibility in controlling length.

> *Example.* A gunshot wound (Fig. 13.4) of the proximal phalanx (A and B) in this young man was treated with debridement and maintenance of digital length and alignment by external fixation (C and D). Following soft tissue coverage, interpositional bone grafting led to uneventful union (E and F).

Intra-articular fractures

Severely comminuted fractures, particularly with adjacent soft-tissue injury, often surpass our technical ability for internal fixation. Inappropriately applied attempts at internal fixation may further splinter small fragments or strip them of their soft-tissue attachments leading to further loss of reduction. With such comminution, one should

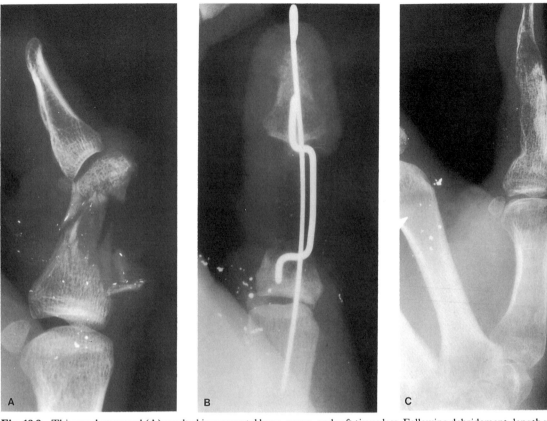

Fig. 13.3 This gunshot wound (A) resulted in segmental bone, nerve, and soft tissue loss. Following debridement, length was maintained by an internal spacer wire (B) allowing flap reconstruction, nerve grafting, and interpositional bone grafting (C)

revert to simpler reduction techniques such as traction.

Vidal et al (1978) coined the term 'capsuloligamentotaxis' which refers to the reduction of articular fragments by traction applied through their capsular and ligamentous attachments. This concept is particularly useful at the wrist (Fernandez et al 1983), but equally applicable to the smaller joints of the hand, most commonly in comminuted fractures of the base of first and fifth metacarpals, and comminuted fracture-dislocations of the proximal interphalangeal joints (Burny et al 1980, Jenkin 1983, Nonnenmacher 1983). In such cases, external fixation is applied through pins placed in bone proximal and distal to the comminuted articular fracture fragments. Mild traction is applied, tightening the ligamentous and capsular attachments of the fragments, and bringing them back into alignment. In the case of fracture-dislocations, the joint can be reduced simultaneously.

When compression has resulted in depressed, comminuted central articular fragments, their lack of soft-tissue attachment prevents reduction by capsular distraction. Open reduction, elevation of depressed articular fragments, and support by cancellous or cortico-cancellous bone grafts is required. This is greatly facilitated by an external fixator which maintains reduction and allows simultaneous freedom of surgical approach. External fixation of the joint is usually required for 3–6 weeks, depending upon the size of the articular fragments and their underlying support. Attendant arthrofibrosis during immobilization is usually prevented by the mild capsular and ligamentous distraction applied which prevents their shortening and facilitates joint mobilization following removal of the external fixation device.

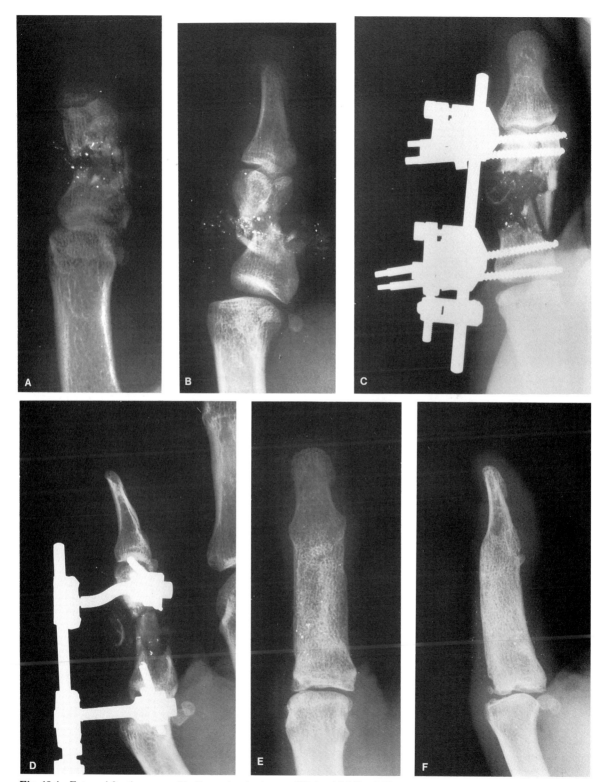

Fig. 13.4   External fixation to provide distraction (courtesy of Richard S Idlers MD)

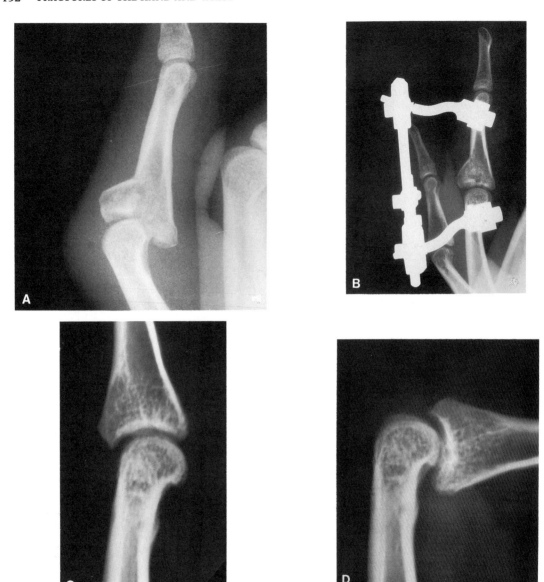

Fig. 13.5 External fixation to provide distraction, augmented by bone graft (see text for details)

Example. This 18-year-old boy (Fig. 13.5) sustained a comminuted fracture–dislocation of the proximal interphalangeal joint (A). Reduction was accomplished through 'ligamentotaxis' achieved through distraction by a half-pin frame mini-external fixator (B). Central depressed portions of the articular surface without capsular attachments were elevated and maintained with autogenous cancellous bone graft. External fixation was discontinued after $4\frac{1}{2}$ weeks, capsular contracture during that time being minimized by distraction of the joint. One and a-half years later, the joint was stable and painless with 95° of active motion (C and D).

In 1975, Volkov and Oganesyan introduced a hinge-distraction concept for treating fractures,

ankyloses, persistent dislocations, and non-unions. An external hinge device is applied across joints, providing stability yet allowing flexion and extension of the joint (Oganesyan 1982). We first used this technique for reconstruction at the elbow (Deland et al 1983) and have subsequently applied the concept to acute and subacute complex fractures and dislocations of the interphalangeal joints in treatment of fractures and dislocations. External fixation in such cases provides distraction of the joint and reduction of dislocation or subluxation while allowing active motion. The most common applications are fracture–dislocations of the proximal interphalangeal joint. In such instances, a

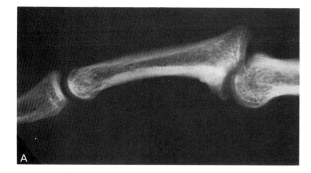
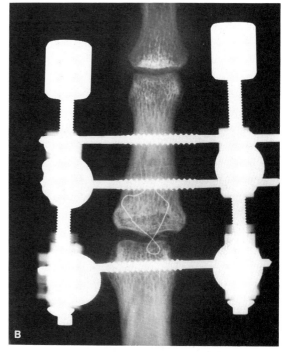
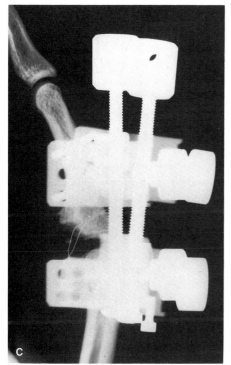
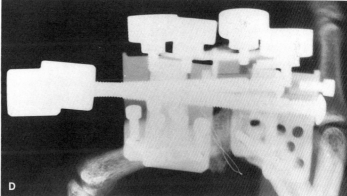

Fig. 13.6 Hinge-distraction fixator (see text for details)

threaded transfixion pin can be placed through the rotational axis in the proximal phalangeal head, perpendicular to the principal plane of flexion and extension. Two additional transfixion pins are placed through the middle phalanx. The external fixation device allows distraction between the proximal pin and the two more distal pins. The middle phalanx can be translated dorsally or volarly to some extent on the most proximal pin with motion through the proximal interphalangeal joint occurring about the proximal pin. By such a method, external fixation will allow immediate reduction of joint dislocation, reduction of comminuted articular fragments by distraction across

the relocated joint, and maintenance of joint motion in the postoperative period. This same technique can be coupled with resection arthroplasty in treatment of post-traumatic ankylosis or arthritis (Oganesyan 1982).

Example. This 30-year-old man (Fig. 13.6) presented nine months after a failed volar plate advancement arthroplasty for a proximal interphalangeal joint fracture–dislocation (A). Open reduction, tenolysis, and revision of the arthroplasty were performed. External fixation maintained the joint reduction obtained (B) yet allowed active and passive motion of the joint postoperatively (C and D).

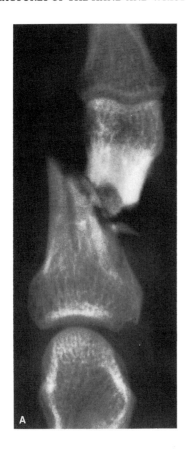

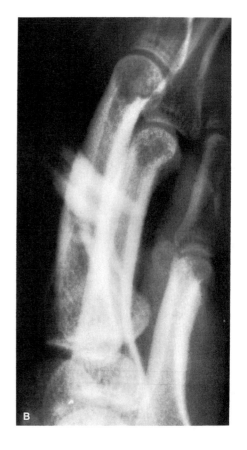

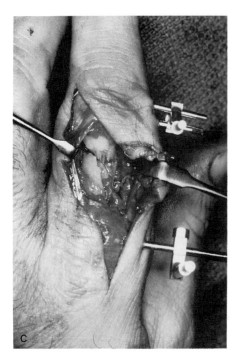

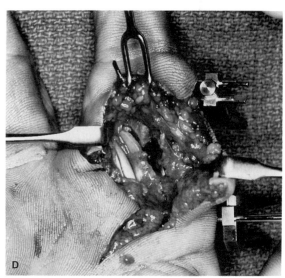

Fig. 13.7   External fixation providing neutralization (see text for details)

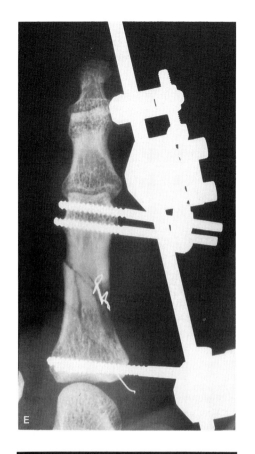

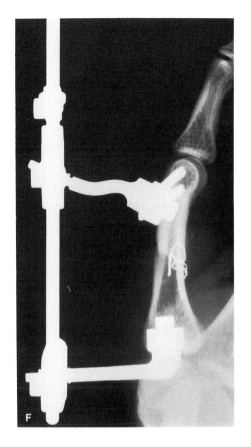

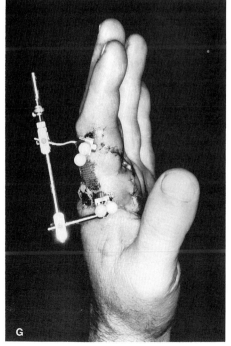

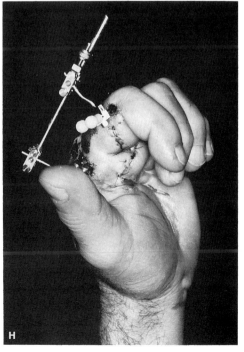

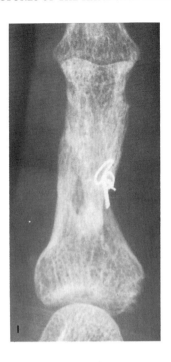

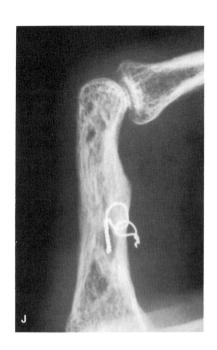

Neutralization

The concept of neutralization is applicable when the fracture pattern is oblique or comminuted, preventing the application of compression. It may also be used to supplement the fixation of difficult fractures where internal fixation is inadequate, for example in unstable comminuted extra-articular fractures with multiple small fragments difficult to fix internally. Usually these fractures are open, with associated skin loss and tendon injury. Because of contamination and skin loss, primary internal fixation is ill-advised since the prognosis depends upon the extent of concomitant soft-tissue trauma which influences subsequent fracture healing (Muller-Farber & Rehn 1983). Dissection which further compromises vascularity of the bone must be avoided. External fixation allows absolute fracture immobilization without further soft-tissue dissection, thus assisting in soft tissue healing as well as fracture vascularization. At the same time, access is provided to the wound for subsequent debridements, bone grafting, and skin coverage. Adjacent joints can be left free for early mobilization.

Example. This 37-year-old man (Fig. 13.7) sustained a through-and-through punch-press injury to the proximal phalanx of his left index finger (A and

B). There was marked soft-tissue stripping and devascularization of the comminuted fracture fragments, with disruption of the dorsal and volar peritendinous structures (C and D). The proximal phalangeal volar cortex was reduced and internally fixed with a wire suture and the second annular pulley reconstructed. Reduction was secured through a Jacquet external fixator applied to the proximal phalanx on either side of the comminuted fracture (E and F). External fixation facilitated open wound management and, as shown here at five days (G and H), allowed early active range-of-motion exercises to prevent tendon adherence. The fracture progressed to uneventful union (I and J).

Neutralization can also be used for temporary immobilization of joints. The slight traction applied across the joint keeps the capsular and ligamentous structures under light tension and assists in later mobilization of the joint.

External fixation is very helpful in positioning the thumb ray and maintaining the first web space. In severe or crushing injuries to the hand and first web space, soft-tissue swelling invariably leads to contraction of the first web secondary to fibrosis of the first dorsal interosseous and adductor pollicis muscles. Spacer wires can be employed to maintain an adequate first web, but usually the web space is already compromised to some degree by immediate soft-tissue swelling and, when this decreases, spacer wires do not allow further distraction. External splints can be used to control the first web space (Kalisman et al 1983) but exert their force more on the proximal phalanx than the metacarpal; in addition, they provide poor control of rotation of the first ray and do not allow access to the wound unless the splint is removed. External fixation is achieved by half-pins placed in the first ray and connected through a rod to similar pins in an adjacent ray. This holds the thumb ray in palmar abduction and pronation more efficiently than can be achieved by external splinting. As soft tissue swelling subsides, further distraction and change in position can be achieved. With severe injuries external fixation must be maintained for a minimum of 6–8 weeks. Premature discontinuance of external fixation will lead to progressive contracture secondary to the underlying fibrosis. During that time, however, motion can be initiated at all joints of the first ray by disconnecting the connecting rods, actively and passively mobilizing the first

ray and, in between exercises, reattaching the connecting rod to maintain the first web space.

Example. This 19-year-old woman (Fig. 13.8) presented with incomplete amputation of the left hand through the first web space, coronally dividing the carpal bones (A). The motor branch of the median nerve had been cut: this was repaired. After fixation of the carpus with K-wires and neurovascular and tendon repairs, the first web space was maintained in palmar abduction and pronation with an AO small external fixator (B and C). The fixation allowed access to the wound for subsequent changes of dressing (D).

After three weeks, active and gentle passive motion of the first ray was possible by intermittent removal of the interconnection bar. Between exercises the first ray was maintained in appropriate position by reinsertion of the connecting bar. External fixation and subsequent reinnervation of the thenar muscles led to full supple preservation of the first web space (E and F).

External fixation for positioning of the first ray is especially helpful during resurfacing tissue proce-

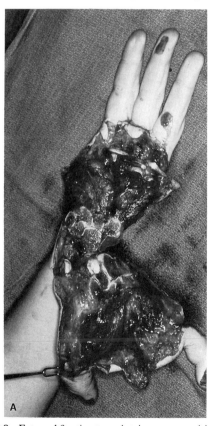
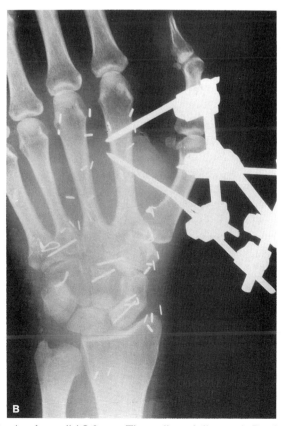

Fig. 13.8 External fixation to maintain correct position of thumb using the small AO fixator. The small metal clips seen in B and C were used to seal and tag arteries and veins. For details of management, see text

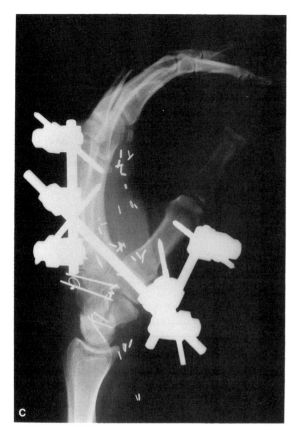

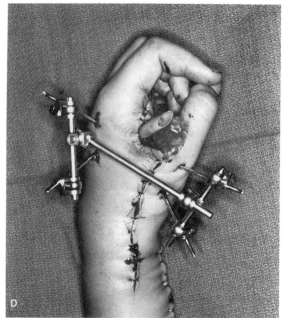

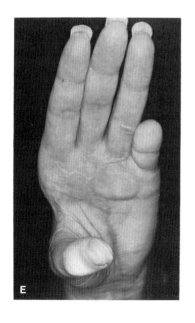

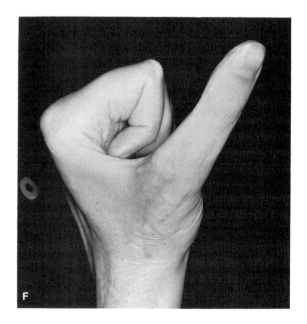

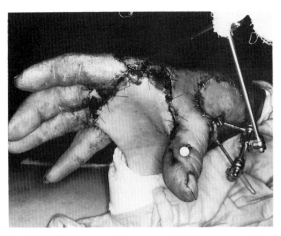

Fig. 13.9 This 56-year-old man sustained a severe crushing injury to his right hand with open fractures of the second through fifth metacarpals, open dislocation of the first metacarpophalangeal joint, and degloving of the palm. Following fracture stabilization, an AO small external fixator was applied with half-pins in the first and second metacarpals to position the first ray. This allowed access to the wound and, in this case, coverage by the attached ilio-inguinal flap. The fixator was also used to elevate and position the hand

dures to the first web space (Fig. 13.9). Wound access is facilitated and position better preserved than by conventional dressings and splints.

SPECIFIC TYPES OF EXTERNAL FIXATION

In our early cases, equipment that was already in common use in maxillofacial surgery, such as that developed by Ginestet (1971), was applied to the hand. Now many fixation devices can be obtained for the wrist, metacarpals, and phalanges. The choice will depend upon the clinical situation as well as the availability of such devices to the surgeon.

K-wires bonded by acrylic resin

Several types of external fixators made from Kirschner wires and acrylic resin have been described. These consist essentially of transverse Kirschner wires on either side of the fracture connected together in various ways. The pins on either side of the fracture can be joined simply by a tube of acrylic resin (Dickson 1975), or by a spanning wire connected to each of the pins with a bolus of cement (Crockett 1974), or through longitudinal wires encased within acrylic resin (Stuchin & Kummer 1984). These techniques should be within the armamentarium of every operating hand surgeon as the materials are universally available and inexpensive. While offering less flexibility than more sophisticated prefabricated systems, the methods perform well (Pritsch et al 1981, Richard et al 1983).

Of the various configurations, the most stable is that utilizing two half-pins proximal to and distal to the fracture, reduction of the fracture assuring proper digital rotation in a position of full flexion, followed by spanning the proximal and distal pins with a longitudinal rod made of wire surrounded by acrylic resin (Fig. 13.10). The stability that can be achieved with such a system has been shown to be greater than that of the mini-Hoffman type external fixator, with 50% more rigidity in anterior bending and 100% more rigidity in mediolateral bending (Stuchin & Kummer 1984).

Lengthening devices

A variety of lengthening devices including the Matev (1970), Kessler (1977), Paneva-Holevich (1980), and Allieu (1985) devices can be utilized for fracture fixation (Fig. 13.11). These devices are particularly applicable when progressive distraction or compression is required. While applicable in many complex fracture situations, they are less versatile than the newer systems such as the Jaquet mini-Hoffman fixator.

Roger Anderson device

Early experience of external fixation in the hand and wrist was achieved with the Roger Anderson device (1944). Smaller models were developed for maxillofacial surgery and are applicable to the hand and wrist. Our clinical usage of the Roger Anderson device* has been supplanted by more specialized designs for the hand.

* Tower Company, Seattle, Washington

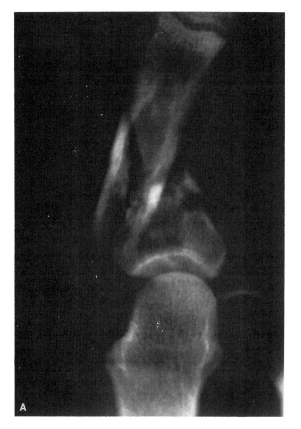

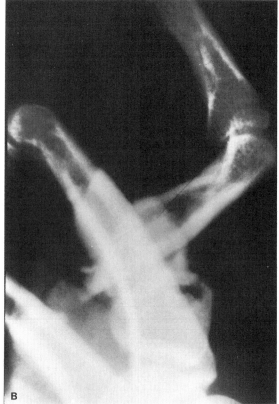

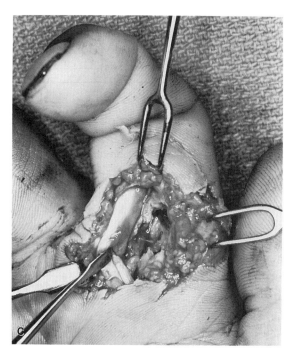

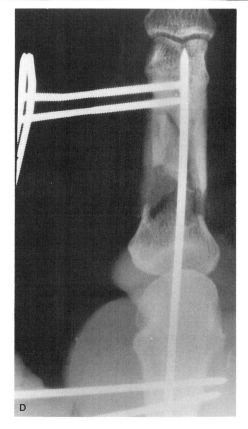

Fig. 13.10 See p. 162 for caption

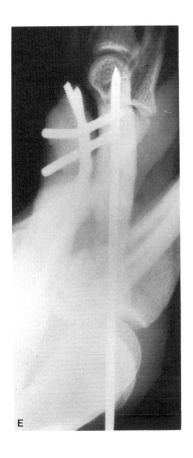

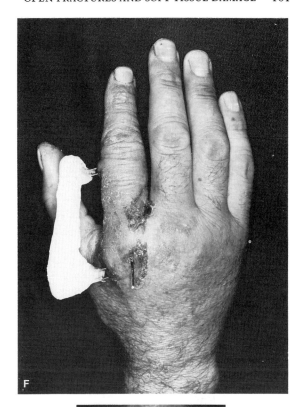

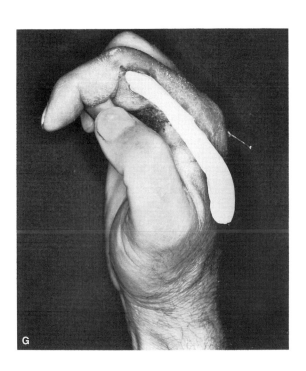

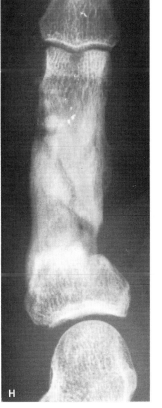

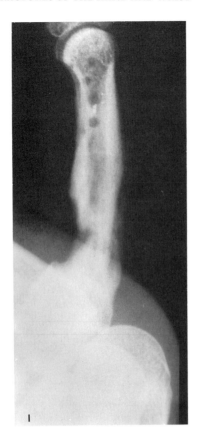

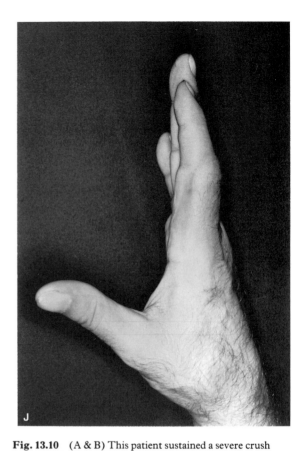

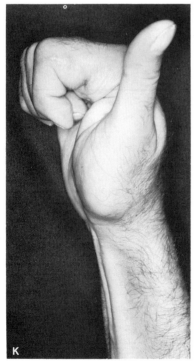

Fig. 13.10 (A & B) This patient sustained a severe crush injury to his right index finger causing an unstable, comminuted extra-articular fracture of the proximal phalanx. (C) There was laceration of the extensor mechanism and volar disruption of the second annular pulley and flexor tendon bed. (D & E) Reduction was obtained by metacarpophalangeal joint flexion and maintained with an internal longitudinal K-wire plus an acrylic external fixator. While the K-wire and acrylic connecting rod were setting up, the digit was held in a position of full flexion to ensure proper rotational alignment. (F & G) External fixation allowed access to the wound and early active motion of the IP joints. (H & I) The bone united uneventfully (J & K) and the final range of movement was quite satisfactory.

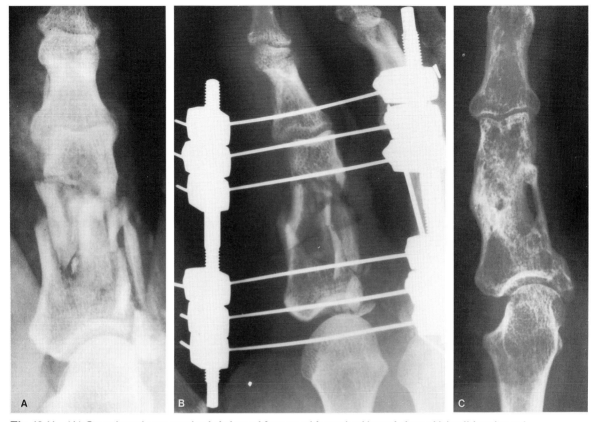

Fig. 13.11 (A) Comminuted open proximal phalangeal fracture with proximal interphalangeal joint dislocation and metacarpophalangeal joint subluxation. (B) Stabilized by external fixation through transfixion wires. Wires through the middle phalanx and metacarpal assisted in initial maintenance of reduction of these two joints. (C) The phalanx united in acceptable position

AO small external fixator

The AO small external fixator is extremely adjustable and is suitable for fixation of complex metacarpal fractures as well as positioning the first ray in major hand injuries to prevent retroposition or supination contractures (*see* Fig. 13.8). The device is too large for application to the phalanges.

The small external fixator set (Fig. 13.12) consists of 2.5 mm threaded half pins which are connected by 4 mm bars attached with clamps which can be fitted both to the pins and the bars. The equipment (shown in Fig. 13.12) is simple and versatile and consists of the following components:

1. threaded half pin 2.5 mm/150 mm
2. clamp 4.0 mm/2.5 mm (connects 4.0 mm bar to 2.5 mm half-pin)
3. clamp 4.0 mm/4.0 mm (connects two 4.0 mm bars or 4.0 mm bar to 4.0 mm Schanz screw)
4. 7.0 mm socket wrench
5. 7.0 mm combination wrench
6. connecting bars 60–200 mm
7. (Schanz screw 4.0 mm/60–100 mm—for fixation of forearm and humeral fixation)

This system is applied by inserting two threaded half-pins on either side of the fracture to be reduced or, in the case of positioning of the first ray, two pins in the first ray and two pins in another stabilizing ray. A 5.0 mm skin incision is made and dissection continued down to and through periosteum. The pins are inserted, with a low speed drill, at 45–60° divergent from each other with each pin purchasing two cortices. A 4.0/2.5 mm connecting clamp is placed on each pin, securing the pin with

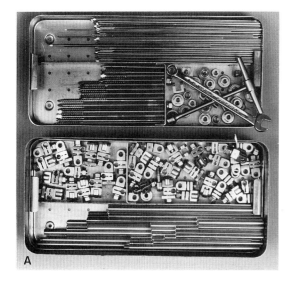
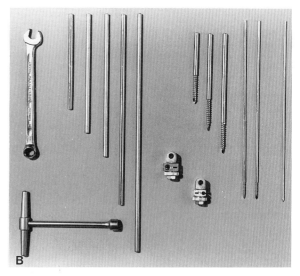
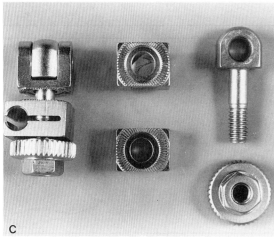
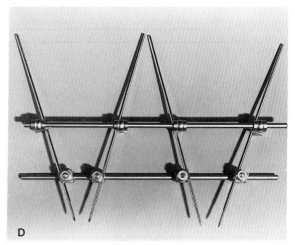

Fig. 13.12 The AO small external fixator. (A) The complete set in its case. (B) Small and large pins, clamps, connecting rods, and spanners. (C) Close-up of interconnecting clamps. (D) Basic frame assembly

the 2.5 mm portion of the clamp and allowing passage of the connecting bar through the 4.0 mm portion of the clamp. The fracture is reduced and the connecting clamps (see Fig. 13.12C) tightened, securing the reduction. If the pins proximal and distal are not in the same plane, a connecting bar is placed between each set of pins and a separate bar used to connect the proximal and distal bars with 4.0/4.0 mm clamps. For positioning of the thumb ray, each set of pins is connected with a short connecting bar. The thumb ray is positioned and the two bars then interconnected with an additional

bar. Figures 13.7 and 13.8 show the AO small external fixator in use.

Jaquet mini-fixator

This mini-fixator was designed and manufactured by Jaquet Orthopédie SA of Geneva for treatment of injuries to the small bones of the hand. It is alternatively described as a mini-Hoffman and is manufactured in the USA by Howmedica. While the additional interconnections and adjustability of the device currently give less stability than K-wire and acrylic resin models, the device provides quite adequate stabilization and currently is the most useful of the external fixators for the metacarpals and phalanges. The system, which is illustrated in Figure 13.13, consists of the following basic components:

1. 2.0 mm diameter half pins, length 33–60 mm, thread length 12–20 mm (Fig. 13.13C)
2. 1.5 mm transfixion pins, length 30–60 mm (Fig. 13.13C)
3. 1.5 mm threaded transfixion pins, length 33–78 mm, central thread length 10–20 mm (Fig. 13.13C)
4. pin holders for 1.5 and 2.0 mm pins: straight, offset, and T-shaped (Fig. 13.13D)
5. connecting clamps (Fig. 13.13E)
   (a) simple swivelling clamp links pin holder to connecting rod and is universally adjustable
   (b) sliding swivelling clamp has a knurled wheel which allows compression or distraction
6. smooth vice for 1.5–2.0 mm pins (Fig. 13.13E)
7. connecting rods—3 mm diameter × 30–300 mm length (Fig. 13.13B)
8. manual pin drivers for 1.5 mm and 2.0 mm pins (Fig. 13.13B)
9. socket wrenches—4.0 mm and 5.5 mm (Fig. 13.13B)
10. spanner wrench—4.0 mm and 5.5 mm (Fig. 13.13B)
11. drill bits—1.5 mm (Fig. 13.13F)
12. point breakers to remove point of threaded transfixion pins (Fig. 13.13B)
13. HM100 drill guide (Fig. 13.13F)

Frame configurations

A variety of frame configurations is possible due to the great flexibility of the device. We have found the configurations described next to be most commonly useful.

The single half-pin frame. This is the most common configuration used on the hand (Fig. 13.14). Two threaded 2.0 mm half-pins are placed on either side of the fracture. A pin-holder is connected to each set of pins. A single swivelling clamp is applied to one pin holder and a sliding swivel clamp to the other. The two clamps are connected by a 3.0 mm connecting-rod of appropriate length. This connecting rod should be positioned dorsally to counteract the predominant flexion deforming forces. The half-frame configuration allows access to local wounds and causes little interference with the adjacent digits.

Transfixion frame configuration. This configuration is particularly useful in lengthening procedures or arthrodesis (Fig. 13.15). It consists of a set of through-and-through transfixion pins on either side of the fracture or joint to be fixed with an offset pin holder applied on either side of each set of transfixion pins. Simple swivelling clamps are applied to two of the pin-holders and adjustable sliding clamps to the other two. Both sets of clamps are then interconnected with the tools of the appropriate length. Through the adjustable swivel clamps on either side, equal compression or distraction across the fracture or arthrodesis site can be achieved.

Triangular configuration. This configuration consists of a pair of transfixion pins on one side of the fracture with a pair of threaded half-pins distal to the fracture. An offset pin holder is applied on either side of the transfixion pins with two pin-holders applied to the pair of distal pins. The proximal and distal pairs of pin-holders are then connected through connecting rods in triangular fashion.

Technique of frame application

Because the swivelling clamps allow 90° of adjustment and there is unlimited rotation of the holders, it is not essential that proximal and distal pairs of pins be placed in proper alignment. The proximal and distal pairs of pins can be inserted independently, fracture reduction or positioning obtained, and the two sets then fixed rigidly to each other through the connecting rods and tightened swivel clamps. Insertion of the pins is carried out through small skin stab incisions. Blunt dissection is carried down to bone. The 2.0 mm half-pins require predrilling with a 1.5 mm drill followed by insertion of the pin with a hand chuck. After placement of the first pin, a drill-guide is placed over this pin and the second pin similarly inserted, parallel to the first. The 1.5 mm transfixion pins are self-

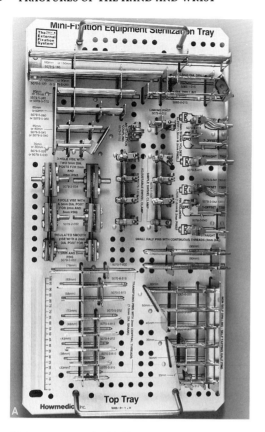

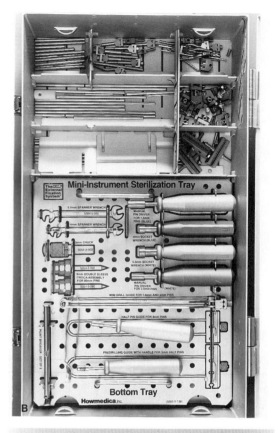

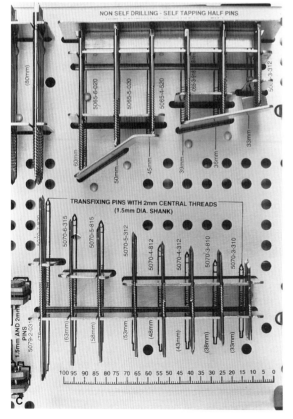

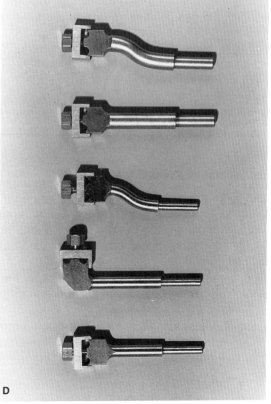

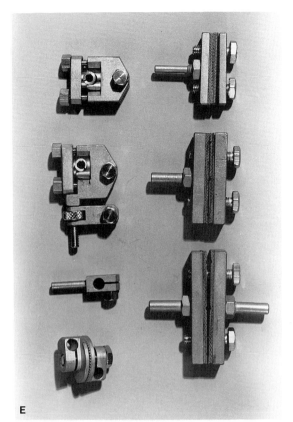

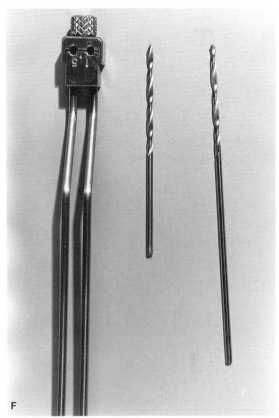

Fig. 13.13   The Jaquet mini-fixator. (A) Top tray. (B) Bottom tray. (C) Close-up of 2 mm half-pins and 1.5 mm transfixion pins. (D) Pin holders. (E) Connecting clamps. (F) Drill guide and drill-bits

drilling and self-tapping. Predrilling is usually not necessary.

In positioning the pins at the metacarpal level, it is important to avoid transfixion and consequent entrapment of the extensor mechanism. This is very easy in the case of thumb, index, and small metacarpals, but requires somewhat greater attention in application to the middle and ring metacarpals. At the phalangeal level, the pins are most commonly placed in a radioulnar direction to avoid interference with the extensor mechanism, but it may be impossible to avoid this along the proximal aspect of the proximal phalanx. In such cases fixation is then placed more proximally in the metacarpal or at the most proximal level of the proximal phalanx where transverse fibres of the extensor mechanism are transfixed, sparing the more oblique components critical to interphalangeal joint motion. Transfixion at this level does not impair metacarpophalangeal motion (see Fig. 13.7H).

COMPLICATIONS

Despite improvement in design and application of external fixators, and the renewed enthusiasm in their use which has generated greater experience, complications continue to occur frequently. Many of the common pitfalls can be avoided if one is aware of the potential problems.

Pin-tract infection

Pin-tract infection has remained the most common problem with external fixation. Transcutaneous pins into bone incite the formation of a membrane between the pin and the surrounding tissues

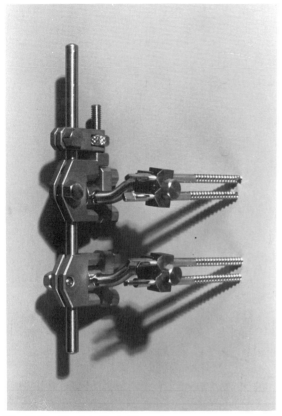

Fig. 13.14   Single half-pin (Jaquet)

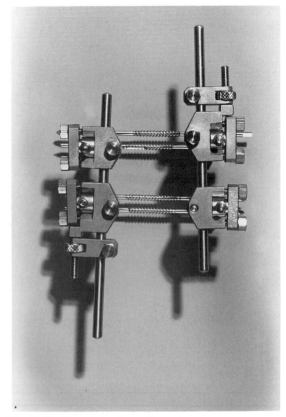

Fig. 13.15   Transfixion frame (Jaquet)

(Browner 1983, Green 1981). Fluid is secreted by this membrane, serving as a potential culture medium for contamination by superficial micro-organisms. As long as free egress of this fluid is maintained, the likelihood of infection is extremely small. When host defence is altered, a hematoma present, or drainage obstructed through crusting at the skin interface, infection can occur. Other local factors such as tissue necrosis or bone necrosis further predispose to infection.

Soft-tissue necrosis can be caused by inadvertent entrapment and wrapping of the surrounding soft-tissues during the process of drilling. To avoid this it is essential to have an adequate incision which allows introduction of a drill-guide/protector to isolate the drill-bit from the surrounding soft tissues.

Tension can occur on the surrounding skin by the transfixion pin. This is particularly true in lengthening procedures. If one anticipates applying distraction it is wise to retract the skin toward the area of fracture, osteotomy, or joint prior to insertion of the pins. After putting the pins in, all soft tissues around them should be released to ensure there is no tension against the pins.

Pin-tracts are more susceptible to infection when the soft tissues above the bone are mobile and thick. At the metacarpal level, pin placement should be through an area of skin as close to the metacarpals as possible (see Fig. 13.1E). Relaxing incisions at the metacarpal level will need to be generous to allow for proximal and distal excursion of the surrounding skin which occurs with digital motion. At the phalangeal level, pins are ideally introduced in the mid-axial line where there is little motion of skin over bone during flexion and extension (see Fig. 13.7G & H). When there is significant swelling or thickness of soft tissue at the pin entrance, relative motion of the skin about the pin can be diminished by wrapping gauze around the pins between the clamps and skin. Pin care should include cleansing of the pin/skin interface with hydrogen peroxide three times a day to remove any crust or debris and ensure a free drainage tract.

Bone necrosis can occur through thermal necrosis. Rouiller & Majno (1953) have shown that osteocytes are damaged by temperatures of over $55°C$. The heat generated during insertion of the pins can be reduced by predrilling a smaller diameter hole before inserting the pin (Matthews & Hirsch 1972). It is essential to avoid the use of high speed drills, blunt drill-bits, and poorly designed pins. Ideally, after predrilling, pins should be put in with a hand chuck.

Bone necrosis can also occur from excessive pressure of the pins on adjacent bone. Such necrosis can be minimized, and the strength of pin fixation maximized, by ensuring the pin passes through the centre of the bone, transfixing the cortices where they are furthest apart. Pins designed for parallel insertion must be accurately inserted using an appropriate drill guide; if they are inserted with some divergence and then forced into parallel slots of a pin-holder, excessive pressure from the pin on adjacent bone occurs and leads to necrosis and loosening.

It is advisable not to back the pins out once they have been inserted as this makes subsequent loosening more likely. It is better to be shy on initial insertion distance, so that any necessary readjustment is by further insertion rather than withdrawal. Fluoroscopy is a helpful guide to pin placement and also the extent of pin insertion.

There is always some unavoidable stress on the pins generated by loads that occur with active and passive motion. Stress by the pins on bone can be minimized by ensuring their parallel insertion, using threaded rather than smooth pins, increasing the diameter of the pin, inserting pins in more than one plane, and increasing the number of pins. Since most hand fractures do not require as lengthy periods of immobilization as in the lower extremity, the race between fracture healing and pin loosening is usually favourable: the external fixation device is removed between 3 and 6 weeks. In cases with significant loss of bone and soft tissue substance, the soft tissue coverage and subsequent bone grafting and internal fixation can be accomplished between 3 and 6 weeks.

Loose pins must be detected early and removed. Leaving them in will lead to additional bone destruction and infection. If removal of a pin jeopardizes the remaining stability, additional pins should be inserted.

Osteomyelitis

True osteomyelitis is rare, but a pin-tract infection with focal osteomyelitis does occur. In our experience, most cases resolve with early pin removal and oral antibiotics. Bony debridement has rarely been required.

Fracture through pin holes

Late pathological fracture through pin holes is rare in the hand due to its limited weight-bearing and protective adjacent joints. Fracture can occur through attempts to insert too large a pin relative to the bone diameter (Fig. 13.16). Pins less than 30% of the diameter of the bone have a stress concentration factor of only 1.6, whereas pin diameters approaching 50% of that of the bone cause a dramatically greater effect (Brooks et al 1970). The pin should therefore be less than 30% of the bone diameter.

Neurovascular injury

Neurovascular injury can occur when pins are inadvertently inserted through a neurovascular bundle, or so close to a neurovascular bundle that the bundle becomes wrapped round a drill-bit or threaded pin. Avoidance of neurovascular structures at the metacarpal level is quite easy. We have not seen neurovascular injuries in the digits, although pins inserted in the mid-axial line are extremely close to the more volar neurovascular bundle. Such damage can be avoided by incision and direct exposure of the bone, allowing tissue retraction for drilling and pin placement. Drill sleeves should be used for both drilling and insertion of pins. In the case of insertion of parallel pins, the second pin has to be introduced through a special parallel drill-guide, of which the present design precludes use of a drill-sleeve.

Distraction and non-union

As with older traction techniques, there is a

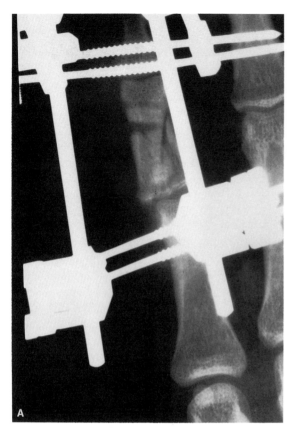 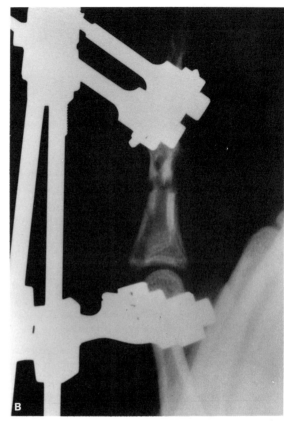

Fig. 13.16 An iatrogenic fracture caused in treatment of comminuted fracture of base of middle phalanx when two distal transfixion pins were placed too close to the fracture. Two attempted pin passages created a hole excessively large for the small diaphyseal diameter of the middle phalanx and fracture resulted. The pins then had to be passed through the distal phalanx instead. Despite some distraction of this iatrogenic fracture, both it and the original fracture at the base of the middle phalanx went on to uneventful union

potential for non-union when fractures are distracted by external fixation.

Reduction must therefore be checked to ensure that distraction is not present. Since the most common applications for external fixation are open fractures with soft tissue and bone loss, early bone grafting is very often required.

Loss of reduction

With any of the adjustable external fixators, there is risk of loss of reduction by loosening of the device. There is a trade-off between flexibility and stability, and from time to time the connections need to be checked and retightened. The stiffness of a given fixator configuration can be increased by increasing the number of pins used, increasing the

distance between pins, increasing the stiffness or diameter size of pins, and shortening the distance from the fracture to the transfixion pins. Regular check radiographs must be taken to make sure that reduction is maintained.

Interference by fixator with adjacent digits

Despite the availability of smaller external fixation devices, it is inevitable that the device to some degree will interfere with motion of the adjacent digits. There is seldom a problem in extension, when divergence of the digits occurs, but in flexion the digits converge and there is limited room for such fixators. The ends of protruding pins should be cut off as short as possible to allow motion of the adjacent digits and their sharp points covered with plastic protectors. The adjacent uninjured digits should also be exercised as well to prevent them from stiffening.

CONCLUSION

The indications for external fixation of the hand are limited. At present the main indications are segmental comminuted fractures (particularly ones with associated soft tissue injury), articular fractures with small comminuted fragments, infected non-unions, and maintaining the position of the first ray in severe injuries otherwise likely to cause retroposition or supination contracture. The greatest advantages are in severe injuries with bone

and soft-tissue loss, where both external splints or cast and internal means of fixation are inadequate. In such cases, external fixation allows access to wounds for subsequent debridement and coverage procedures.

With refinement of external fixation devices, their smaller configurations have allowed the adjacent joints to remain free for active and passive exercises. The adaptability of the latest external fixators allows for progressive reduction by distraction and also permits a second chance to improve reduction. Attention to the technical details of applying the devices will minimize the risk of complications.

Adherence to these precise indications and precautions will provide the hand surgeon with a useful, versatile tool.

REFERENCES

Ardrey J 1970 Le fixateur externe d'Hoffmann couple en cadre. Étude biomécanique dans les fractures de jambes. Thesis, University of Montpellier

Allieu Y, Fassio B 1974 Value of an external fixation device in the treatment of osteoarticular infections of the hand and fingers. Annales de Chirurgie 28:271

Allieu Y 1985 External fixation in osteoarticular surgery of the hand. In: Tubiana R (ed) The Hand, vol II. W. B. Saunders, Philadelphia, p. 525

Anderson R, O'Neil G 1944 Comminuted fractures of the distal end of the radius. Surgery, Gynaecology and Obstetrics 78:434

Asche G, Haas H G, Klemm K 1979 The external mini-fixator: application and indications in hand surgery. In: Brooker A F, Edwards C C (eds) External fixation: the current state of the art. Williams & Wilkins, Baltimore, p. 105

Brooks D B, Burnstein A H, Frankel V H 1970 The biomechanics of torsional fractures. The stress contraction effect of a drill hole. Journal of Bone and Joint Surgery 52A:507

Browner B D 1983 Pitfalls in the management of open fractures with Hoffmann external fixation. Annales Chirurgiae et Gynaecologiae 72:303

Burny F, Moermans J P, Quintin J 1980 Use of minifixator in hand surgery. Acta Orthopaedica Belgica 46:251

Cooney W P 1980 External mini-fixators: clinical applications and techniques. In: Johnston R M (ed) Advances in external fixation. Year Book Publishers, Chicago, p. 155

Crockett D J 1974 Rigid fixation of bones of the hand using K-wires bonded with acrylic resin. The Hand 6:106

Deland J T, Walker P S, Sledge C B, Farberov A 1983 Treatment of posttraumatic elbows with a new hinge-distractor. Orthopaedics 6:732

Dickson R A 1975 Rigid fixation of unstable metacarpal fractures using transverse K-wires bonded with acrylic resin. The Hand 7:284

Ferlic D C, Turner B D, Clayton M L 1983 Compression arthrodesis of the thumb. Journal of Hand Surgery 8:207

Fernandez D L, Jacob R P, Buchler U 1983 External fixation of the wrist. Current indications and techniques. Annales Chirurgiae et Gynaecologiae 72:298

Ginestet G 1971 Le fixateur externe dans le traitement des fractures du maxillaire inférieur. Rev. Odontostomatol 2:455

Green S A 1981 Complications of external skeletal fixation: causes, prevention and treatment. C. C. Thomas, Springfield, Illinois

Jenkin E 1983 The treatment of intraarticular metacarpal and phalangeal fractures with the small external fixation device. Handchirurgie 15:198

Kalisman M, Chesher S P, Lister G D 1983 Adjustable dynamic external splint for control of first web contracture. Plastic and Reconstructive Surgery 71:266

Kessler I, Baruch A, Hecht O 1977 Experience with distraction lengthening of digital rays in congenital anomalies. Journal of Hand Surgery 2:394

Kessler I, Hecht O, Baruch A 1979 Distraction-lengthening of digital rays in the management of the injured hand. Journal of Bone and Joint Surgery 61A:83

Manktelow R T, Wainwright D J 1984 A technique of distraction osteosynthesis in the hand. Journal of Hand Surgery 9A:858

Mantero R, et al 1976 Un apparecchio di Hoffmann modificato per il trattamento delle lesioni della mano. Revue de Chirurgie et Mano 13:134

Matev I B 1970 Thumb reconstruction after amputation at the metacarpophalangeal joint by bone-lengthening. A preliminary report of three cases. Journal of Bone and Joint Surgery 52A:957

Matthews L S, Hirsch C 1972 Temperatures measured in human cortical bone when drilling. Journal of Bone and Joint Surgery 54A:297

Micks J E, Hager D L 1968 A method of accelerating fusion of small joints. Journal of Bone and Joint Surgery 50A: 1269

Morton H S 1944 Fractures of the hand and wrist. Canadian Medical Association Journal 51: 430

Muller-Farber J, Rehn J 1983 Morphologic aspects of bone healing after third-degree open fractures. An experimental study. Arch Orthop Trauma Surg 101: 201

Nonnenmacher J 1983 Osteosynthesis of fractures of the base of the first metacarpal by an external fixator. Annales Chirurgiae des Mains 2: 250

Oganesyan O V 1982 Use of the Volkov-Oganesyan hinge distractor to restore joint function. In: Seligson D, Pope M (eds). Concepts in external fixation. Grune & Stratton, New York, p. 139

Paneva-Holevich E, Yankov E 1980 A distraction method for lengthening of the finger metacarpals: a preliminary report. Journal of Hand Surgery 5: 160

Peimer C A, Smith R J, Leffert R D 1981 Distraction-fixation in the primary treatment of metacarpal bone loss. Journal of Hand Surgery 6: 111

Pritsch M, Engel J, Farin I 1981 Manipulation and external fixation of metacarpal fractures. Journal of Bone and Joint Surgery 63A: 1289

Richard J C, Latouche X, Lemerle J P et al 1983 External fixation in emergency treatment of severe open traumatisms of the hand. An original technique. Annales de Chirurgie 34: 332

Rouiller C, Majno G 1953 Morphologische und chemische untersuchungen und knochen nach hitzecinwir kung. Beitrage zur Pathologie und Anatomie 113: 100

Stuchin S A, Kummer F J 1984 Stiffness of small-bone external fixation methods: an experimental study. Journal of Hand Surgery 9A: 718

Vidal J, Buscayret C, Connes H 1978 Treatment of articular fractures by 'ligamentotaxis' with external fixation. In: Brooker A F, Edwards C C (eds) External fixation: the current state of the art. Williams & Wilkins, Baltimore, p. 75

Volkov M V, Oganesyan O V 1975 Restoration of function in the knee and elbow with a hinge-distractor apparatus. Journal of Bone and Joint Surgery 57A: 591

14

Severe fractures including those with loss of bone

The statement that finger fractures cause as much compensation expense as do fractures of the long bones (Bunnell 1953) was recently supported by the conclusions of a review by Strickland et al (1982), who found that the digital performance following fractures, both simple and comminuted, falls far short of normal functional restoration (Strickland et al 1979). This applies even more to the increasingly large number of severe multistructural hand injuries (Fig. 14.1) which include skeletal disruptions: these are multi-level-, multi-ray-fractures, with substantial loss of bone as well as of soft tissue structures. Since reconstruction of the skeletal load-bearing function is considered to be the prerequisite of further repair of all functionally important soft-tissue structures (Vilain 1971, Pannike 1972 Segmüller 1976, Foucher et al 1977, Meuli et al 1978, Meyer et al 1981), two conclusions follow:

1. In severe hand injuries with damage to soft tissues as well as bone, the restoration of skeletal function (i.e. load-bearing) provides the basis for the planning and performance of simultaneous soft tissue reconstruction, including all vitally and functionally important structures such as arteries, nerves, tendons, etc.
2. Primary skeletal stability must be achieved independently of the nature, the type and extent of skeletal destruction.

There are only a few exceptions to these principles such as neglected or obviously contaminated wounds. Devitalized tissues, however, do not necessarily imply a delay in surgery since reconstruction of the skeleton may be combined with skin coverage by local or distant, pedicle or free flaps (Büchler 1984).

As we approach the close of this century, efforts are being continued to improve techniques of routine closed fracture treatment in the hand and of ordinary internal fixation. But, most importantly, skeletal repair by bone grafts, stabilized by techniques of rigid internal fixation, are also being perfected. Future developments may include internal fixation applied to free combined bone and soft-tissue transfers (Taylor 1973, Taylor 1977). These are fortunately seldom necessary, for the vascular supply to the hand is abundant and revascularization of autologous traditional bone grafts is fast and predictable. Finally, external fixation is most valuable in many intermediate situations when wound contamination or doubtful soft-tissue viability preclude primary definite reconstructive procedure.

METHODS OF FIXATION

Stabilization

Stabilization of fractured bones aims at mechanical control of the fragments following reduction. This may be efficiently achieved in cases where an intact envelope of soft tissue surrounds the bone (Charnley 1967, Brown 1973, Barton 1979, Strickland 1979).

External stabilization

External stabilization (by plaster cast) of fractures in the human hand can cause many problems because of the almost inevitable damage to the

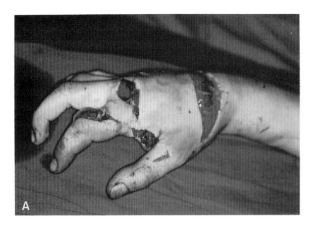

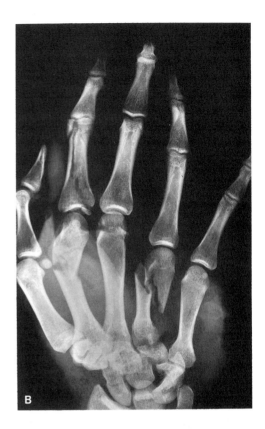

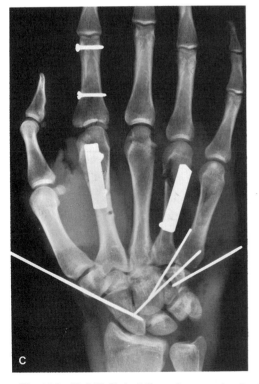

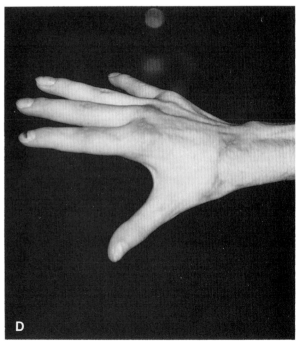

Fig. 14.1   (A & B) Skeletal disruptions at various levels and rays: left hand caught in printing press machine. (C) Primary skeletal stabilization. (D) Final functional result

gliding structures in this sensitive anatomical area. In the fracture pathology of man the incidence of comminuted fractures in the hand is higher than in any other part of the body. Even pressure by the plaster cast may not be tolerated; contused and damaged periarticular tissues mean that complete immobilization, even of short duration, of the involved articulations may result in permanent stiffness. Postoperative care of soft tissue, especially following flap-transfers of any kind, may require priority, and immobilization of fractures may be neglected in favour of primary soft tissue healing.

Kirschner wire techniques

Internal fixation was dominated for decades by percutaneous or buried K-wire techniques and was considered the most gentle method of operative stabilization (Joshi 1976, Chase 1968, Fyfe 1979, Belsole 1980, Jupiter 1985). The limitations of this technique are by now obvious:

1. Exact anatomical reduction and retention of the fragments is not guaranteed except in the most simple of unstable fractures.
2. The stability necessary during the healing period of bone may be lacking and this may limit the patient's ability to mobilize the hand.
3. Lack of stability is such that external splintage is also necessary; the risks inherent in any operative procedure (with or without opening the fracture site) are inevitably combined with the shortcomings of immobilization of the injured ray.
4. In the presence of multifragmentary fractures and even more so of fractures characterized by loss of bone substance, K-wire techniques are inadequate. Exceptionally, K-wires may serve as a temporary spacer while awaiting a second bone graft procedure (Jupiter 1984).

Stable internal fixation

In all fractures not amenable to K-wire fixation, stable internal fixation is preferred. The advantages of stability outweigh the inevitable disadvantages of the additional operative trauma, by allowing soft tissue healing under the most favourable conditions. Stable fixation makes possible the early resumption of function independent of the extent and severity of the skeletal injury (Kilbourne 1958, Vilain 1971, Tubiana 1971, Heim 1973, Crawford 1976, Segmüller 1977, Meuli et al 1978, Heim 1982, Jupiter et al 1985).

Aims. The aims of stable internal fixation may be summarized as follows: restoration of the exact anatomical configuration of bone by precise alignment of the fragments; creation of biomechanical conditions for immediate resumption of function, since the injured bone is given back its load-carrying capacity without delay; and predictability of bony union on the basis of lasting stability.

Technique. Stable internal fixation is based on adequate metal implants of a modular system, i.e. of different sizes but applied in the same manner and with the same type of instruments (Pannike 1972, Segmüller 1976, Müller et al 1979, Pohler 1980) and on mechanical techniques generating stability by compression. These techniques must eliminate alternating or cyclic bending stresses on the metal implant or it will fatigue and then break (Pohler 1980). However, no implant will be fully effective unless used according to correct biomechanical principles. These are discussed below.

Interfragmentary compression

Interfragmentary compression, generating enough friction between the two bony fragments to withstand the local forces caused by the musculotendinous system (Segmüller 1977, Müller et al 1979, Mason 1979, Segmüller et al 1980, Jupiter 1984, Jabaley 1985), can be achieved by the following:

1. Lag screw (Fig. 14.2)
2. Lag screw plus plate (neutralization)
3. Dynamic compression plates (Heim & Pfeiffer 1982)
4. Tension-band techniques.

Tension-band techniques

Stability is supplied by an eccentric force, equal or greater than the bending forces, applied on the dorsum of the bone to neutralize the bending forces of the flexor tendons (Segmüller 1977, Massengill et al 1979, Ansorge 1980, Massengill et al 1982, Sennwald 1983, Vanik et al 1984, Black et al 1985)

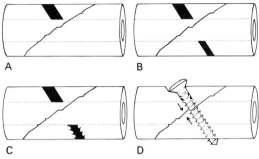

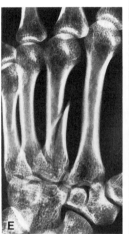

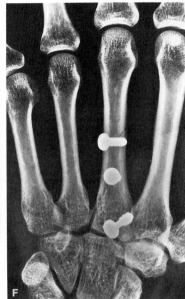

Fig. 14.2   Technique of lag-screw stabilization. (A) The gliding hole (wide calibre) is drilled in the near cortex. (B) The far cortex must be drilled to the same size as the inner diameter of the screw. (C) The far drill-hole is threaded to the same diameter as the threads of the screw. (D) The screw glides through the wide gliding-hole and is threaded into the far cortex; when it is tightened, the fragments are compressed together. (E & F) Spiral fracture of third metacarpal; cortical screw in the diaphysis and cancellous screw in the metaphysis providing permanent stability and allowing bone healing despite resumption of early activity of the hand

as shown in Figure 14.3. In a transverse fracture, some compression at the fracture site may be generated when the bending load surpasses the tensile strength of the implant and when cortical bone on the flexor side is intact and ready to serve as a fulcrum or a bony buttress. A zone of comminution, unstable single fragments or a defect on the palmar aspect would prevent an efficient

stabilizing tension-band effect. This technique does not produce permanent or invariable compression at the fracture site, but rather an intermittent pressure within those narrow limits which do not disturb primary bone healing.

This biomechanical principle is realized by: a tension-band wire alone (figure of eight-wire) on the tension side; a tension-band wire combined

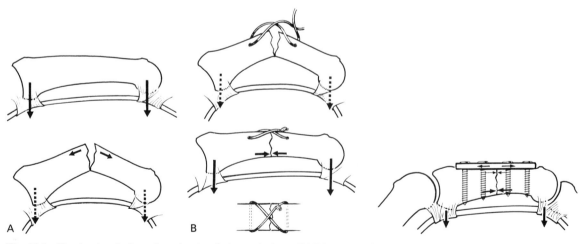

Fig. 14.3   Tension-band wire and tension-band plate technique. (A) Diagrammatic representation of the bending stress acting on the diaphysis of a phalanx. (B) A superficially placed figure-of-eight wire loop restores tensile strength on the dorsal cortex, while interfragmentary compression is provided on the flexor side by the functional load resumed after operation. (C) Tension-band plate technique. The plate is placed on the side of tension, restoring tensile strength and neutralizing rotational forces. Precondition for this technique: an anatomically obvious bending load must accompany everyday function

two parallel oblique K-wires which neutralize forces; or a tension-band plate which at one and the same time restores the tensile strength of the fractured bone and neutralizes torsional as well as shearing forces.

Adaptation and bridge techniques using plates

Neither compression nor a tension band effect can be achieved in the presence of severe comminution or bone loss unless a compression-resistant bone graft (Fig. 14.4) is used (Segmüller 1976, Segmüller 1977, Segmüller 1981). In these circumstances the internal fixation must be strictly distinguished from compression osteosynthesis. The difference lies in the fact that there is no real partnership between the bone fragments and the metal implant has to withstand, largely by itself, all muscle forces and is therefore subject to alternating bending forces. No implant in the long run can tolerate this. Internal fixation, however, may still be successful when the incipient and gradually progressing bone union diminishes the cyclic bending stresses on the implant before fatigue fracture of the implant occurs, when the implant is larger or when the postoperative functional load is substantially reduced. If this biomechanical constellation is misjudged, failure and fatigue fracture of any metal implant will occur in time.

RATIONALE OF 'RIGID' INTERNAL FIXATION IN SEVERE FRACTURE WITH OR WITHOUT BONE LOSS

Restoring endangered or lost function in the severely injured hand implies a comprehensive knowledge of the refined techniques of tendon surgery, nerve repair and skin-coverage, including free flaps. All these techniques have ceased to be performed on a macroscopic level of surgery, but rather have become routine microscopic procedures. Comprehensive treatment includes, without doubt, skeletal reconstruction in the most severe multiple-tissue injuries. Advances in the refined operative techniques of internal fixation based on sound principles, as outlined above, are now available.

Bone graft and internal fixation

Research

Earlier in this century (Bunnell 1948) solid cortical bone grafts were tailored in carpenter's fashion and used in case of non-union and malunion. A solid graft could be fitted into a compact, exactly cut-out bed in order to achieve a certain degree of stability. The only tool for fixation was the K-wire. However, revascularization and remodelling of this type of graft took years and a rather long

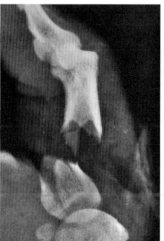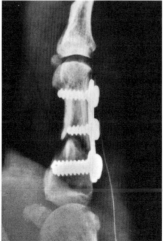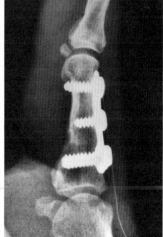

Fig. 14.4 Bridge plate: stability in the absence of compression by bridging a fracture site or a cancellous bone graft is minimal. The metal implant must withstand on its own all muscle forces and is therefore subject to alternating bending forces. During the phase of bone consolidation, the plate can withstand these stresses only if a plate of adequate mechanical properties is used and functional after-treatment is adapted

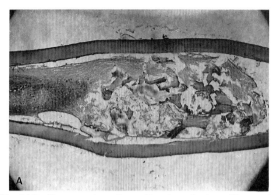

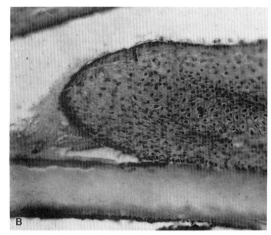

Fig. 14.5 Regeneration of cancellous bone in the millipore chamber. (A) Longitudinal section through millipore chamber: small cancellous chips in the centre, young tissue growing out towards left, millipore membrane above and below. (B) The front of proliferating connective tissue which, starting from the autogenous cancellous bone, grows out towards the periphery of the millipore chamber

period of immobilization by plaster cast was inevitable.

Significantly quicker revascularization and osteogenesis may be expected from cancellous or corticocancellous grafts. It has been shown often that cellular elements from the intertrabecular spaces of transplanted autogenous cancellous bone may survive and proliferate, laying down new bone on the surfaces of the transplanted, and therefore avascular, trabecular structures.

In our studies (Segmüller 1967, Segmüller 1977) we have observed the survival and further development of cancellous bone enclosed in a Millipore diffusion chamber which was incubated and perfused in the peritoneal cavity of the rabbit without any vascular contact between the graft and the host tissue (Fig. 14.5). Under these rather unfavourable survival conditions (comparable to the environment of a bone graft without microvascular hookup), we found that within 15 days a thick layer of cell-rich connective tissue, derived from the autogenous cancellous bone, migrated inside the diffusion chamber centrifugally towards the periphery of the chamber. After 4 weeks ample chondroid tissue in varying stages of maturity was demonstrated.

Heterotopic transplantation of cancellous bone from the iliac crest to the interosseous space of the hind-leg in a rabbit (Fig. 14.6) shows new bone formation within 20 days (Segmüller 1977), and

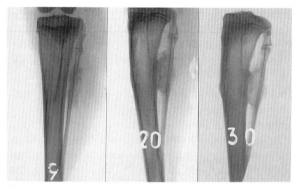

Fig. 14.6 Heterotopic transplantation of cancellous bone in the rabbit. Radiographs of tibia of the rabbit, 9, 20 and 30 days after transplantation of autogenous cancellous bone from the iliac crest onto the interosseous membrane. The structure of the graft changes, new bone formation has already started before the 20th day, and integration of the transplanted cancellous bone into the neighbouring bone structure of tibia and fibula is obvious at 30 days following transplantation

full integration and remodelling of the graft by one month. The necrotic trabeculae serve as a scaffolding ready to support the deposition of osteoid by numerous osteoblasts (Fig. 14.7).

Clinical application

Even though the time factor in the human differs to some extent, survival of the endothelial cells and the manner of proliferation and formation of new bone seems to be identical, since there is no

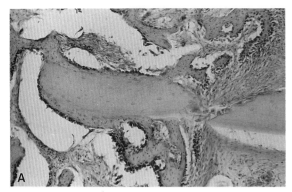 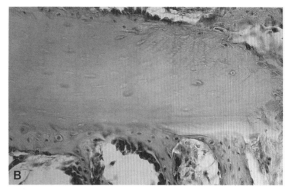

Fig. 14.7 (A) Histology of transplanted cancellous bone after 30 days. Cancellous bone trabeculae are themselves necrotic but they are covered by a cellular layer of numerous osteoblasts. (B) Higher magnification showing the 'halos' in a necrotic trabeculum: these are the empty lacunae from which osteocytes have disappeared. New trabeculae graft themselves in different directions onto the surfaces of the necrotic trabeculum

difference between the X-ray studies of cancellous bone grafts in the rabbit as compared with the human. Therefore, bone grafts are used liberally in late reconstructive procedure as well as in fresh fractures.

A prerequisite for success is perfect immobilization of the graft to abolish any movement between graft and graft bed. Even 'micro-movements' disturb vascular ingrowth and non-union of the graft may result.

Bone grafting in the hand is based on two factors, namely:

1. Neutralization of all forces acting upon the site of the graft by stable internal fixation.
2. Autogenous cortico-cancellous grafts which serve two purposes. Mechanically, a compression resistant graft permits the application of the principle of compression for stabilization. The autogenous cancellous graft also represents a biological tool, which promotes osteogenesis and remodelling remarkably and predictably.

Fractures with bone shattering or bone defects are as a rule associated with severe soft tissue injuries. Local vascularization may be poor, and a number of procedures are to be performed in the same operative session (Foucher et al 1977, Meuli et al 1978, Segmüller 1981, Meyer et al 1981), so cancellous bone grafts are preferred as the biologically most suitable transplant. Stability is maintained through the entire period of incorporation and remodelling by modern techniques of internal fixation, i.e. dynamic compression plate in the

presence of a corticocancellous compression resistant bone graft or else a bridging plate, when a purely cancellous graft was deemed to be preferable.

FRACTURES AT DIFFERENT LEVELS AND IN DIFFERENT RAYS

The surgeon must be aware of some anatomical characteristics of the hand at various levels. Unlike other areas of the body, the digits lack any muscle-endowments to surround the bones: in addition there is only a thin layer of subcutaneous tissue, closely surrounding the gliding structures of the tendons which cling to the skeleton like a glove. The skin accordingly is limited in its capacity to expand and there is little room to accommodate any oedematous swelling in the epifascial and subfascial space.

Many authors (Flatt 1966, Strickland et al 1982) have stated that substantial damage to soft tissues is almost inevitable in any fracture of the hand and that associated soft-tissue lesions may influence the final digital performance far more than the fracture itself. This is especially true with crushing injuries in which these soft-tissue structures, essential for normal function, are damaged first before the bone is shattered. Concomitant involvement of digital nerves and vessels may occur and vary from mild neurapraxia to complete disruption. Crushing injuries frequently produce multi-level fractures of the hand and according to Strickland more than

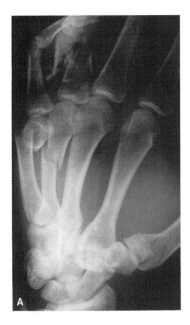
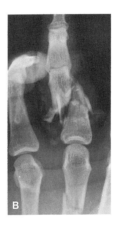
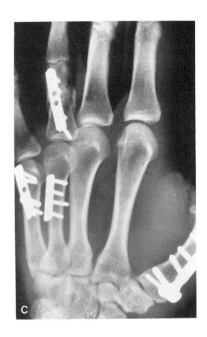
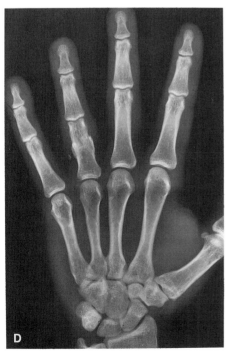
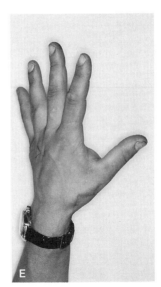
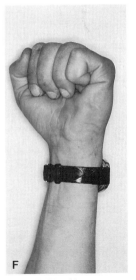

Fig. 14.8 Fractures at various levels and rays. (A & B) Fractures, stable and unstable, which were accompanied by skin contusions, skin defects and extensor tendon damage. (C & D) Radiograph after plating of all four fractures as described in the text. Final radiograph after healing of fractures and removal of plates. (E & F) Functional result. In multi-level fractures where compound fractures need internal fixation, we advocate also internal fixation of any other fractures to allow an unhindered early rehabilitation programme

50% of phalangeal fractures resulted from crushing injuries.

Operative management

Soft tissue

Soft tissue recovery must always be given priority under any circumstance. If, for any reason, a partial objective of fracture treatment has to be deferred temporarily, it is the osseous union in perfect alignment of the fragments which has to take second place. Never should the primary restoration of skin coverage take second place. This must be achieved as soon as possible, by well established techniques such as split-thickness skin-grafts, full-thickness skin-grafts and local and distant flaps; split-skin grafts will survive on any open wound that is not obviously infected. Nevertheless, soft tissue recovery is greatly enhanced by firm stabilization of the bone.

Bone fixation

Multiple unstable fractures are hardly controlled by external splints and plaster casts nor by Kirschner wire fixation, and therefore rigid internal fixation is recommended. This effectively controls all muscle forces acting upon the skeleton of the hand immediately following surgery when rehabilitation is started. Another advantage is the elimination of external immobilization to offer optimal conditions for wound healing and wound care.

The techniques to be applied in the presence of multiple fractures are: lag screw fixation; tension band plate fixation; bridging plate (strut plate); and bone grafting combined with stable internal fixation.

The use of metal implants in open wounds is not contraindicated as long as stability is maintained. However loose metal implants of any type and size do have a detrimental effect on soft tissue recovery and will, as a rule, lead to non-union, malunion or septic non-union.

This management has been used in our Hand Service for many years. An example (Fig. 14.8) may illustrate the early management and final result.

Example. A 23-year-old patient was struck by a car, incurring short oblique unstable fractures of the fourth and fifth metacarpals and an almost undisplaced fracture at the base of the first metacarpal, all with skin contusions with questionable viability and large haematoma. A comminuted, compound diaphysial fracture of the proximal phalanx of the ring finger was associated with severance of the extensor mechanism and some smaller skin defects.

The goal of the treatment was elimination of pain and early resumption of protected motion, despite a variety of stable and unstable, closed and open fractures and injuries to the soft tissue in the same hand.

Open reduction with direct visualization of all the fracture sites was done immediately. The comminuted fracture of the proximal phalanx was stabilized by a 2 mm strut plate, bridging the zone of comminution. No cancellous bone graft was necessary. Skin closure was supplemented by the use of split-skin grafts. A tension band plate protected the fracture of the base of the first metacarpal from further displacement under the pull of the abductor pollicis longus. A neutralization plate was used on the fourth metacarpal, with two screws in the centre of the plate applied as lag screws, and finally a plate was added to a separate lag screw to immobilize a short oblique subcapital fracture of the fifth.

Postoperatively the hand was immobilized for four days on a simple palmar plaster splint; then the dressing was changed and the small drainage tubing from all fracture sites are removed. A removable splint was applied on the fifth day and progressive loading of all the fracture sites encouraged by an active rehabilitation programme which was completed 5 weeks after the primary reconstruction.

In the presence of serial fractures in the transverse and/or in the longitudinal direction of the hand, all fractures, especially compound fractures, should be equally well taken care of by internal fixation in order to minimize pain when rehabilitation is started. Such an operative approach carries very little morbidity and the aftercare is fairly simple, since a complex situation is transformed into a simple closed wound situation.

FRACTURES ACCOMPANIED BY MULTIPLE SOFT-TISSUE INJURIES

In multi-structural fracture lesions functional recovery depends on more than bone stabilization. Scar formation of all tissues involved, especially of the gliding structures of tendons and joints, must be kept at a level compatible with function. A

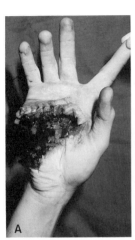

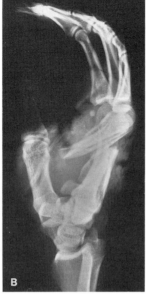

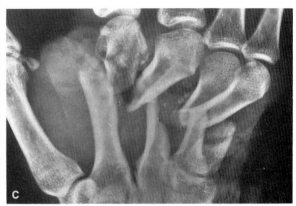

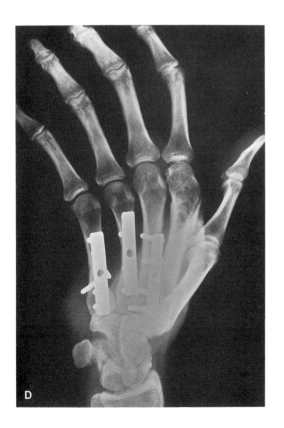

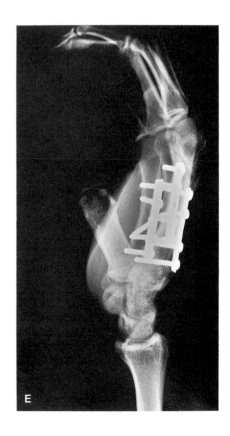

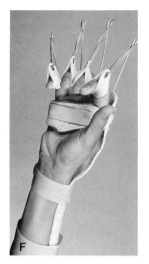
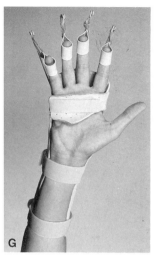
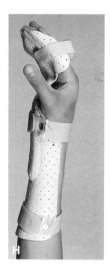
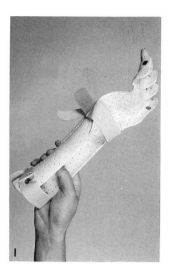

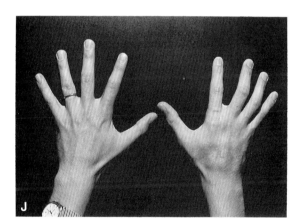
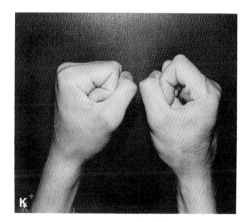

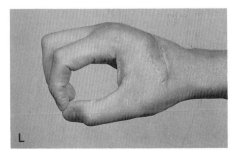

Fig. 14.9 Fractures with multiple soft-tissue damage. (A, B & C) Chain-saw injury with severance of all structures of the metacarpal level of the hand excluding the thumb. (D & E) Primary and definitive reconstruction of the skeleton by stable internal fixation. (F & G) Rehabilitation centred on re-education of extensor and flexor tendons by dynamic splints. (H & I) Passive positioning of hand and fingers on a resting splint is mandatory for more than 4 months. (J, K & L) Functional result 18 months later: full recovery of function except for precise coordination by intrinsic muscles

realistic approach in dealing with these injuries includes a number of considerations.

Aetiology

Compound, comminuted fractures of this extent are often the result of a chain-saw injury, gun-shot wound or high-velocity injuries, though many other mechanisms of injury are known.

Nature of wound

A sharp cut may be less harmful since all structures are still identifiable and viable. Following chain-saw and high-velocity injuries there is additional loss of tissue by the mechanical impact, lack of viability and avulsion.

Contamination

The danger of contamination of these wounds must be evaluated, since such injuries, by definition, extend into subcutaneous tissue and also deeper structures with questionable viability. Necrotic tissue is probably the most important single factor in generating deep infection. Under ideal conditions primary repair of all structures is still recommended as long as vascular flow is restored and maintained. With modern techniques of surgical repair it may be questioned whether tendon and nerve-repair should be deferred and await sound healing and integrity of skin and soft tissue (Bennett 1982). Not only are the techniques of restoration of arterial and venous flow well established, but also fixation of the skeleton of the hand utilizes a variety of internal and external stable fixation techniques. In selected cases of additional abrasion and avulsion injuries micro-surgical tissue transfer techniques must be considered in combination with internal fixation, repair and/or graft of tendons and nerves. Such primary integrated reconstructive surgery should be offered to the patient for minimal scar formation is still the main prerequisite for the best recovery of the human hand following trauma. Thus, stable internal fixation has become another turning point in the management of severe multi-structural trauma.

Example. A 19-year-old man (Fig. 14.9) was caught by a chain-saw on the ulnar border on his right hand at the level of the metacarpals. Soft tissue loss of between 5 and 7 mm was present in the extrinsic and intrinsic tendons, as well as in all digital nerves with the exception of the thumb. The arteries and veins were severed on the palmar and dorsal aspects of the hand. The second to fifth metacarpal bones were fractured in transverse or short oblique fashion. A small zone of comminution was present but bone loss was minimal.

The plan was to carry out definitive repair of all structures in one session, if possible, starting with internal fixation of the metacarpals. This was done with tension-band plates, neutralization plates and Kirschner wires alone in the second digit. Following this precise restoration of the skeleton, all other structures were repaired; revascularization was done and grafts were necessary for the digital nerves. Sensation, excellent tendon excursion, grip and pinch function were restored and also the appearance of the hand was acceptable to the patient and to the surgeon. The only functional impairment was the lack of fine coordination of digital performance since intrinsic muscle recovery was inadequate.

The final objective of reconstructive hand surgery is the integral reconstruction of all specialized structures of the hand in one operative session, minimizing scar formation during the postoperative course of rehabilitation.

MULTI-FRAGMENT FRACTURES WITH OR WITHOUT BONE LOSS

Among the most important indications for a rather aggressive surgical approach and stable internal fixation are multi-fragmentary fractures, closed or compound. Without operative stabilization they can hardly be controlled. The first goals in the management of this unstable type of fracture are to preserve length in conjunction with internal fixation, to create optimal conditions for bone healing and for soft tissue management, converting a complex clinical problem to a problem of soft tissue management alone (Jabaley 1985). Any method involving prolonged immobilization of the limb will further contribute to the ever-present danger of chronic swelling, a painful hand, joint stiffness and tendon adhesions.

Operative stabilization of a large fracture site, if early loading of the bone and motion of the joint is desired, implies a meticulous reduction and close contact of the fragments. We seek to compress the bone fragments for stability and assign a major

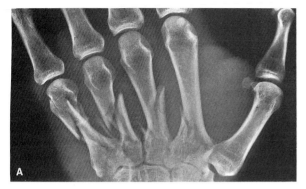

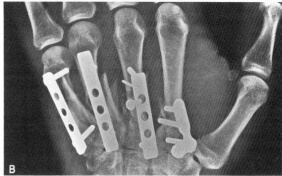

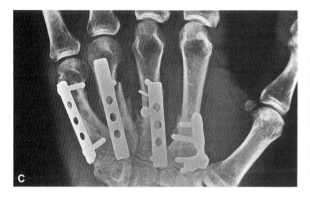

Fig. 14.10 Bridging large fracture sites without attempt of achieving compression-stability. (A) Comminuted metacarpal fractures with extensive skin contusion and devitalized fragments or fragment ends. (B) Strut plates, rather large, 2,7 mm, are used. The fragments are not further devitalized by any operative manipulation. (C) Within 16 weeks stability is established by fast bone healing. Some rotational deformity of the rays is, in these circumstances, acceptable in favour of undisturbed bone healing and healing of skin. Corrective osteotomy for rotational deformity may be considered, if necessary, one year later

portion of the load to be carried by the bridging implant. Limited external splint-immobilization optimizes primary wound healing; then external dynamic and static splints govern early protected motion, initiating the rehabilitation programme.

Primary internal fixation of a multiple-fragment fracture may be carried out in three ways.

Bridging plate

Bridging a large fracture site without any attempt to re-establish bony continuity or to apply compression is illustrated in Figure 14.10. The advantage of such a bridging or strut plate lies in the control of length and rotation of a metacarpal or phalanx, preservation of some blood supply to loose single fragments, and facilitation of wound healing under stable conditions. The fracture site must be opened but the fragments are stripped and exposed as little as possible, avoiding manipulation by instruments. Haematoma is evacuated and adequate drainage is installed. Since there is no compression, the metal implant must be big enough

to take up the mechanical load of motion without the assistance of bone beneath it. The aftercare is modified: a full functional load is not permitted for a period of three weeks, nor is mobilization against resistance. However, guided protected motion is instituted as soon as the soft tissues have healed, within the first two weeks. Fracture healing is fast and resembles fracture healing in non-operative management, as the fragments are not manipulated unduly.

Cancellous bone grafting and bridge plate

Internal fixation, in conjunction with cancellous bone chips to fill in defects left by loose fragments (Fig. 14.11), is used to replace devitalized cortical fragments of phalanges and metacarpals. Cancellous bone chips are taken from the distal end of the radius. The healing and remodelling of cancellous bone under stable conditions is a matter of less than five weeks and the mechanical properties of such bone grafts add quickly to the mechanical stability of a simple bridging plate. In this bio-

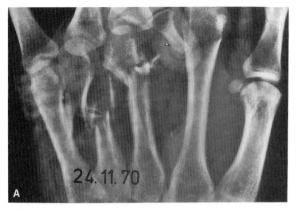

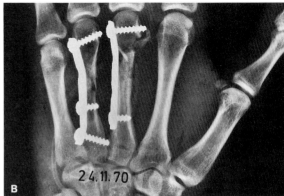

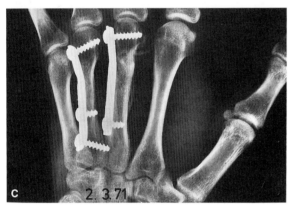

Fig. 14.11 Open multi-fragment fracture. (A) Compound subcapital metacarpal fractures with devitalized fragments. (B) Fragments removed and replaced by cancellous bone grafts; restoration of length and rotation, supported by lateral buttress plates. (C) Bone remodelling within 1 year

mechanical situation, a plate may also be applied as a buttress plate. The goals of protected wound healing and early motion are realized, but early load-bearing and mobilization against resistance are again avoided. Reconstruction as well as qualified aftercare of all additionally injured structures is encouraged simultaneously. Sequential interventions can be avoided.

Use of compression-resistant bone grafts

In this technique, stability is based on compression. Autogenous corticocancellous grafts have more osteogenic activity than cortical grafts or homogenous bank bone. Stable fixation of grafts requires, however, compression-resistant grafting material which is corticocancellous bone. For fractures with loss of bone and for large comminuted compound fractures, corticocancellous grafts of every shape

and size, taken from the iliac crest, may be used. These can be fashioned to fill in a defect or to replace a number of individual loose fragments which are removed from the fracture site. This compression-resistant graft may be stabilized by any fixation technique which produces compression, exactly as large fragments are immobilized solidly and permanently (Figs 14.12 and 14.13). The postoperative management is identical with that following open reduction and stabilization by compression.

Exercises must be started as soon as the wound has healed and everyday functional loading of the hand is encouraged. Revascularization of the grafted bone proceeds rapidly and osseous healing and remodelling is demonstrable by radiograph within 3 months. However it takes over a year to regain the full mechanical strength of the bone, so it is advisable not to remove the metal implant early.

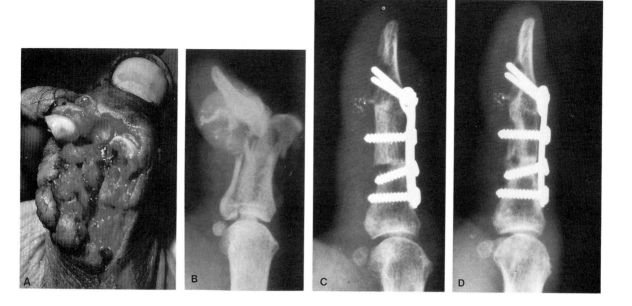

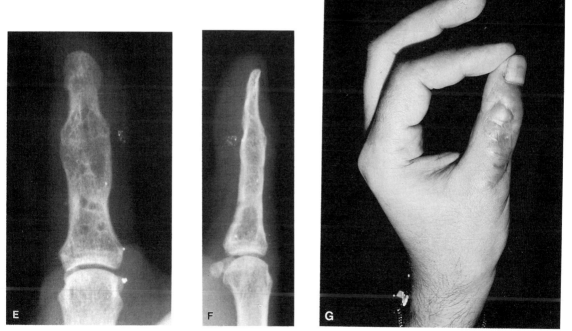

Fig. 14.12 Primary reconstruction by cortico-cancellous iliac bone graft. (A & B) Destruction of skin, extensor tendon, IP joint and proximal phalanx of the thumb. (C & D) All fragments, mostly devitalized, are replaced primarily by a pressure-resistant cortico-cancellous bone graft. The tension-band plate, in the presence of an active flexor tendon, provides perfect stability. Resurfacing of skin defects is performed by thin split-thickness grafts. The cortical component of the graft lies on the palmar aspect, providing buttressing (fulcrum). (E, F & G) Osseous union and functional results one year later

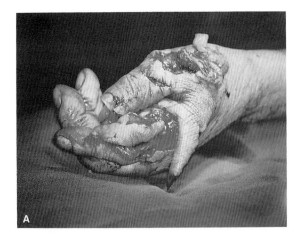

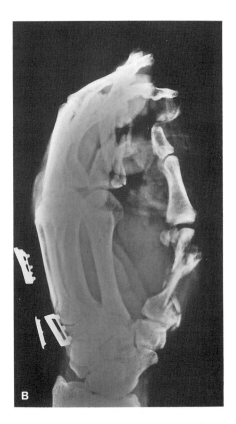

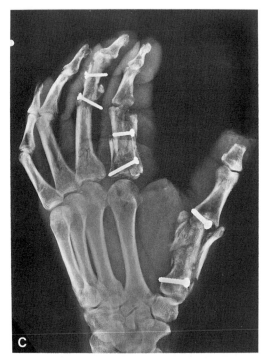

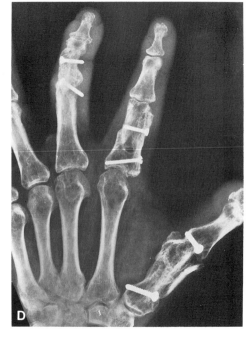

Fig. 14.13   The use of cortico-cancellous bone without metal plates. A cortico-cancellous bone graft is pressure-resistant and can therefore be used like a metal plate stabilized by lag screws, a method used when viability of skin is questionable. (A & B) Severe bone and soft tissue damage in thumb, index and middle finger. (C) Cortico-cancellous graft to bridge metacarpal and first MCP joint and also the fracture zone of the proximal phalanx of the index finger, held by screws. (D) Cortico-cancellous bone grafts healed solidly ; screw still in situ

CONCLUSION

The concepts of internal fixation and stability have been well established (Perren et al 1969a, Perren et al 1969b) and their clinical applications have become numerous. However, only a full understanding of principles, techniques and biomechanics may lead to further developments in its clinical application as applied in the hazardous subspeciality of hand surgery.

Today and in the future there will be ample scope for closed treatment of fractures in the hand, as well as for Kirschner-wire pinning, which Chase (1968), Tubiana (1971) and others considered to be the internal fixation of choice in the hand.

In mutilating injuries of the hand, skeletal reconstruction with full and primary restoration of its load-carrying function must be given the same attention as soft tissue replacement and tendon and nerve reconstruction. The postoperative rehabilitation programme need no longer be delayed or hampered by bony injuries. A biomechanically oriented osteosynthesis does not aim at taking load off the skeleton but rather offers it in a physiological way right through the phase of the rather long period of bone healing.

REFERENCES

Ansorge D 1980 Die Leistungsfähigkeit der Zuggurtungs-Osteosynthese am Handskelett. Zentralblatt für Chirurgie 105:468–474

Barton N J 1979 Fractures of the shafts of the phalanges of the hand. The Hand 11:119–133

Belsole R 1980 Physiological fixation of displaced and unstable fractures of the hand. Orthopedic Clinics of North America 11:393–404

Bennett J E 1982 Abrasion injuries of the hand. In: Strickland J W, Steichen J B (eds) Difficult problems in Hand Surgery, C. V. Mosby, Saint Louis, ch 1, p 3

Black D, Mann R J, Constine R, Daniels A U 1985 Comparison of internal fixation techniques in metacarpal fractures. Journal of Hand Surgery 10A:466–472

Brown P W 1973 The management of phalangeal and metacarpal fractures. Surgical Clinics of North America 53:1393–1437

Bunnell S 1948 Surgery of the Hand. J. B. Lippincott, Philadelphia, ch 6, p 248

Bunnell S 1953 The injured hand: principles of treatment. Industrial Medical Journal 22:251–254

Charnley J 1967 The closed treatment of common fractures (3rd edn) Churchill-Livingstone, Edinburgh

Chase R A, Laub D R 1968 Die Hand. Verlag Hans Huber, Bern

Crawford G P 1976 Screw fixation for certain fractures of the phalanges and metacarpals. Journal of Bone and Joint Surgery 58A:487–492

Flatt A E 1966 Closed and open fractures of the hand; fundamentals of management. Postgraduate Medicine 39:17

Foucher G, Merle M, Michon J 1977 Traitement 'tout en temps' des traumatismes complexes de la main avec mobilisation précoce. Annales de Chirurgie de la Main 31:1059–1063

Fyfe I S, Mason S 1979 The mechanical stability of internal fixation of fractured phalanges. The Hand 11:50–54

Heim U 1973 Indications et techniques de l'ostéosynthèse AO dans le traitement des fractures de la main. Acta Orthopaedica Belgica 39:957–972

Heim U, Pfeiffer K M 1982 Small fragment set manual: technique recommended by the ASIF group (2nd edn). Springer-Verlag, Berlin

Jabaley M E, Freeland A E 1985 Rigid internal fixation in the hand: 104 cases (In press)

Joshi B B 1976 Percutaneous internal fixation of fractures of the proximal phalanges. The Hand 8:86–92

Jupiter J B, Koniuch M P, Smith R J 1985 The management of delayed union and nonunion of the metacarpals and phalanges. Journal of Hand Surgery 10A:457–466

Kilbourne B C, Paul E G 1958 The use of small bone screws in the treatment of metacarpal, metatarsal, and phalangeal fractures. Journal of Bone and Joint Surgery 40A:375–383

Mason S M, Fyfe I S 1979 Comparison of rigidity of whole tubular bones. Journal of Biomechanics 12:367–372

Massengill J B, Alexander H, Parson J P, Schecter M J 1979 Mechanical analysis of Kirschner wire fixation in a phalangeal model. Journal of Hand Surgery 4:351–356

Massengill J B, Alexander H, Langrana N, Mylod A 1982 A phalangeal fracture model—quantitative analysis of rigidity and failure. Journal of Hand Surgery 7:264–270

Meuli Ch, Meyer V, Segmüller G 1978 Stabilization of bone in replantation surgery of the upper limb. Clinical Orthopaedics and Related Research 133:179–183

Meyer V E, Chiv D T, Beasley R W 1981 The place of internal skeletal fixation in surgery of the hand. Clinics in Plastic Surgery 8:51–64

Müller M E, Allgöwer M, Schneider R, Willenegger H 1979 Manual of Internal Fixation (2nd edn). Springer-Verlag, Berlin

Pannike A 1972 Osteosynthese in der Handchirurgie. Springer-Verlag, Berlin

Perren S M, Huggler A, Russenberger M, Straumann F, Müller M E, Allgöwer M 1969a A method of measuring the change in compression applied to living cortical bone. In: Cortical bone healing. Acta Orthopaedica Scandinavica, Suppl. No. 125 (Mungsgaard, Copenhagen)

Perren S M, Huggler A, Russenberger M et al 1969b The reaction of cortical bone to compression. In: Cortical bone healing. Acta Orthopaedica Scandinavica, Suppl. No. 125 (Mungsgaard, Copenhagen)

Pohler O E M, Straumann F 1980 Fatigue and corrosion fatigue studies on stainless-steel implant material. In: Evaluation of Biomaterials, Winter G D, Leray J L, de Groot K (eds) John Wiley & Sons, Chichester

Segmüller G 1967 Spongiosaregeneration in der Milliporekammer. Helvetica Chirurgica Acta 34:5

Segmüller G 1976 Stabile Osteosynthese in der rekonstruktiven Chirurgie der Hand. Handchirurgie 8:23–27

Segmüller G 1977 Surgical stabilization of the skeleton of the hand. Hans Huber, Bern (Distributed in the USA by Williams & Wilkins)

Segmüller G, Rimoldi M, Wiedmer U 1980 Zur Daumengrundgelenksarthrodese: Zuggurtungstechnik. Orthopädische Praxis 5:409–411

Segmüller G 1981 Stabile Osteosynthese und autologer Knochenspan bei Defekt- und Trümmerfrakturen am Handskelett. Handchirurgie 13:209–211

Sennwald G, Segmüller G 1983 L'arthrodèse métacarpo-phalangienne du pouce selon le principe du hauban: indications et technique. Annales de Chirurgie de la Main 2:38–45

Strickland J W, et al 1979 Phalangeal fractures in a hand surgery practice: a statistical review and in-depth study of the management of proximal phalangeal shaft fractures. Journal of Hand Surgery 4:285

Strickland J W, Steichen J B, Kleinman W B, Flynn N 1982 Factors influencing digital performance after phalangeal fracture. In: Strickland J W, Steichen J B (eds) Difficult problems in Hand Surgery, C. V. Mosby, Saint Louis, ch 15, p 126

Taylor I, Daniel R K 1973 The free flap: composite tissue transfer by vascular anastomosis. Australian and New Zealand Journal of Surgery 43:1–3

Taylor I 1977 Microvascular free bone transfer, a clinical technique. Orthopedic Clinics of North America 8:425–447

Tubiana R 1971 Le traitement chirurgical des fractures récentes des métacarpiens et des phalanges. In: Vilain R (ed) Les traumatismes ostéo-articulaires de la main. Expansion Scientifique Française, p 33

Vanik R K, Weber R C, Matloub H S, Sander J R, Gingrass R P 1984 The comparative strengths of internal fixation techniques. Journal of Hand Surgery 9A:216–221

Vilain R 1971 Traitement des fractures ouvertes et des pertes de substance osseuse associées à des pertes de substance cutanée. In: Les traumatismes ostéo-articulaires de la main. Expansion Scientifique Française, p 53

15 Fixation of fractures in reattachment of amputated parts

PRINCIPLES OF OSTEOSYNTHESIS

Requirements for osteosynthesis in replantation

Speed

As stabilization of the bone in replantation surgery is performed before circulation has been re-established, it is imperative that the fixation technique selected should not add significantly to the ischaemic time of the amputated digit. In addition, several digits are often involved; therefore it is vital that the surgeon choose a method of bony stabilization that does not unduly prolong an already lengthy operation.

Stability

Stabilization of the fracture as the first step in the operation means that the replant surgeon can then manipulate the digit with relative impunity to facilitate repair of the tendons, nerves, and vessels. Postoperatively, the stability protects the repaired vital structures during early mobilization of the digit. Secure fracture fixation is also more likely to enhance union and prevent malunion, thus eliminating the need for additional later procedures, such as bone grafting or osteotomy.

Early motion

As viability rates have exceeded 90% in many replantation centres, attention should now be focused on increasing the ultimate level of function (Ikuta 1978, Weiland et al 1977). One of the best methods to achieve this goal is to implement a regimen of early motion. Therefore the surgeon should select a method of fracture fixation that will enable him to feel confident enough to mobilize the replanted digit during the immediate post-operative period. Although capable of providing secure fracture fixation, some varieties of internal and external fixation hardware are excessively bulky or impinge on soft tissue structures, restricting range of motion of the affected digit.

Low morbidity

Replanted digits have experienced the ultimate vascular insult and do not readily withstand additional surgical procedures. Therefore, a technique of bony stabilization that has a low degree of associated morbidity should be chosen (Vlastov & Earle 1984). Some of the complications that commonly occur and should be avoided with fracture fixation in the hand are pain, stiffness, instability, infection, excessive dissection, extension of the fracture line, damage to the neurovascular bundle and impingement on tendon, ligament and skin.

Best chance of union

Methods of fracture stabilization that are associated with a high degree of bony union typically have maximum bony contact and stability, the latter being enhanced by compression. Dissection is kept to a minimum to avoid damaging the periosteal blood supply and care is taken to avoid sacrificing both the endosteal and periosteal vascular networks, which would leave the fracture site with minimal ability to repair itself.

Simplicity

The technique selected should ideally have a short learning curve with a relatively low degree of skill required to achieve the desired result consistently. The technical complexity of the instrumentation and the procedure itself should not be so overwhelming that it cannot be readily assimilated by an inexperienced assistant.

Adaptability

The ideal method of fixing fractures should have a wide range of clinical application, adapting easily to varying fracture patterns and locations in all age-groups (Pritsch et al 1981). This flexibility enables the surgeon to become proficient with a minimum of surgical techniques and allows the operating room to lower costs by not having to stock several different sets of instrumentation.

Durability

There is a race between fracture healing and implant failure and therefore ideal componentry will withstand the rigours of early motion before fatiguing. There should be few parts to loosen and become displaced or lost which would necessitate restabilization.

Retrievability

If the fixation fails or becomes symptomatic, the hardware should be easily removed in the clinic or in the operating room with minimal dissection.

Availability

The fixation components need to be readily available in most hospitals and should not be so esoteric as to make the acquisition of replacement parts an unnecessarily time-consuming ordeal.

Cost

In this age of escalating medical costs, it is up to the surgeon to assume a reasonable degree of fiscal responsibility and select a method of fracture fixation that not only fulfils most of the requirements outlined above but is also cost-effective.

Basic principles of bony management in replantation surgery

As outlined in the previous section on general requirements, there are many qualities that the replant surgeon must consider when selecting a particular osteosynthesis technique. Of all of these considerations, speed, stability and early range of motion are probably the most important (Lister & Kleinert 1979, Hoffmann & Buck-Gramcko 1982, Yamano et al 1982). It is imperative that thorough preoperative planning is undertaken to ensure a high rate of viability and ultimate function. Our replant sequence consists first of evaluating the digit, outside the formal operating room but underneath a microscope and observing sterile technique. If the amputated digit is suitable for replantation, the tendons and neurovascular structures are identified and tagged. Then the amputated part is subjected to thorough irrigation and debridement. The bone ends are cleansed and shortened for several reasons. There is often significant comminution and/or contamination of the fracture fragments, necessitating shortening to obtain adequate cortical apposition and to reduce the likelihood of infection. It is also advisable to shorten the bone to permit end-to-end vessels anastomoses (Urbaniak et al 1978). However, the dynamic balance of the hand must be kept in mind: it is preferable not to shorten the phalanges more than 0.5 cm and the metacarpals by 1 or 2 cm in order to preserve as much of their mechanical advantage as possible. The forearm bones and humerus can be shortened by much more without severe functional deficit.

The paramount consideration in bone shortening is that it should ensure that skin closure can be achieved and that deeper closure can be of fully-vascularised soft tissues (Tupper 1978). This is a particular problem in 'macroreplantation'; that is, where the amputated part has a significant amount of muscle. In such cases the part should be perfused before reattachment and all muscle which does not 'weep' perfusate should be ruthlessly excised (Fig. 15.1). Only then can primary healing be assured. Only then can appropriate bone resection be performed, such as to bring muscle to muscle without tension. Such shortening has the merit of allowing tension-free suture of good quality nerves

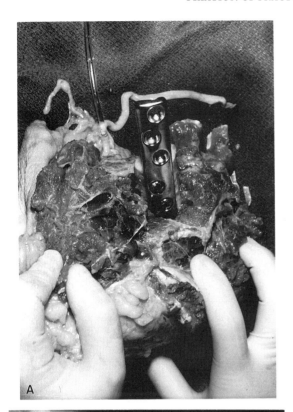

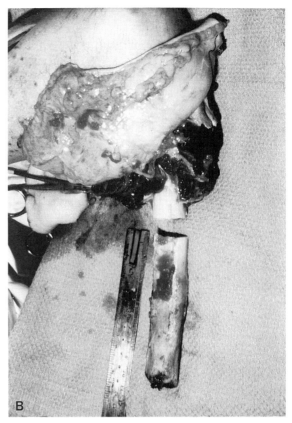

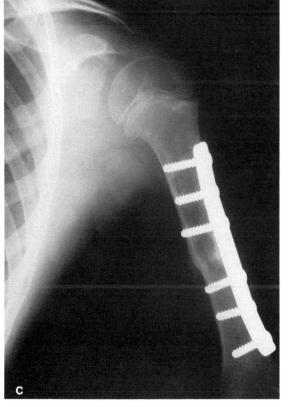

Fig. 15.1 (A) Following amputation through the mid-shaft of the humerus, the amputated part is being prepared. The catheter seen in the upper left of the photograph is in the brachial artery. The limb has been perfused with Ringer's lactate and all muscle which did not weep lactate has been excised. After bone shortening, a six-hole plate has been applied to the humerus. (B) Here, in another case, is shown the extensive bone resection deemed necessary after thorough debridement of potentially viable muscle. (C) The fracture fixation employed in (A) is seen 6 months after replantation, with satisfactory union of the humerus

and vessels. However, where it has been done in the metacarpus or phalanges, the flexor and extensor tendons should be shortened also. One may measure to do this, or better, observe the posture of the finger in flexion and extension of the wrist after placement of trial sutures.

As stated above, shortening is usually started on the amputated part. This should be done while consulting radiographs of both the hand and the part. Comminution of the bone is often an indication of the extent of severe soft-tissue damage and elimination of the comminuted segment will permit adequate debridement of that damaged tissue. Further, shortening may be undertaken simply to facilitate soft-tissue repair and therefore can be done on the hand or the part or both. Study of the radiograph will determine from where the bone is to be removed, considering joint function, tendon insertions and the placement of the selected method of osteosynthesis. For example, where an amputation is through the junction of the proximal and middle thirds of the middle phalanx, shortening the proximal segment would eliminate part of the superficialis insertion, make osteosynthesis

difficult and probably impede motion of the proximal inter-phalangeal joint. In this situation the bone should be taken from the distal segment. Shortening of phalanges can be best achieved with a fine, power-driven saw-blade. In order to avoid damage to vital structures, the periosteum should be carefully stripped back to a point 5 mm beyond the intended saw-cut, to be repaired later. Take a piece of rubber and cut a 5 mm hole in it. The rubber can then be passed over the bone (Fig. 15.2), to protect the soft tissues during the saw cut. The rubber dam can with benefit be retained while intraosseous wires are inserted and fixation completed, and removed only to repair periosteum and tendons.

After shortening, the bone is stabilized. In order to save time, some fracture fixation techniques, for example intraosseous wiring of phalanges or plating of a humerus, can be started on the amputated part before the patient is ready in the operating room (Fig. 15.3; see also Fig. 15.1A). Whenever possible,

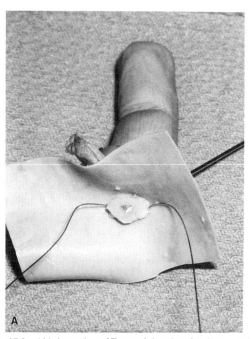

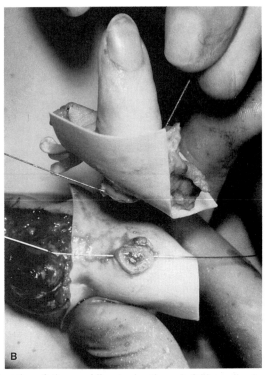

Fig. 15.2 (A) A portion of Esmarch bandage has been used to protect the soft tissues while squaring the end of this proximal phalanx and inserting the necessary monofilament wire and Kirschner pin preparatory to Type A intraosseous wiring. (B) Here, in another case (that shown in Fig. 15.3), the preparation of both ends with a rubber dam is shown. The rubber is removed by incision after bone fixation is complete

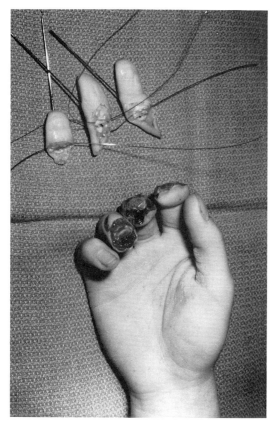

Fig. 15.3   Here the prior preparation of all three digits before replantation is shown. Type A intraosseous wiring is intended for all three

the periosteum is then repaired, both to reduce adhesions and improve osteogenesis.

Although speed is important, the surgeon must guard against any tendency to accept imperfect fixation of the bone. Angular and rotational malalignment will be a source of considerable functional disability to the patient long after the wounds have healed. Anything other than rigid fixation will prevent the institution of early motion, as will transfixation of a joint or, less widely appreciated, the presence of a Kirschner wire through the skin over a joint.

TECHNIQUES OF OSTEOSYNTHESIS

Splints, cast and traction

These forms of fracture management do not fulfil the basic criterion of stability capable of withstand-

ing early motion of the injured part. Furthermore, they achieve stability by constriction or longitudinal pull, both of which are contraindicated in microvascular procedures. Because of these and other shortcomings, splints, casts and the various form of traction are not employed as the primary means of bony stabilization in replant surgery and will not be discussed further.

Kirschner pin fixation

Indications

Kirschner pin fixation is best suited for transverse diaphyseal fractures through the shaft of the phalanges and metacarpals, the latter especially in children (Fig. 15.4). The technique is also well suited to bony stabilization of amputations through the carpus. The method is quick, corrects the deformity, is easy to learn, adaptable, easily retrieved, readily available and cheap. The three basic variations of this technique are the longitudinal (Schlenker 1979), single oblique and crossed

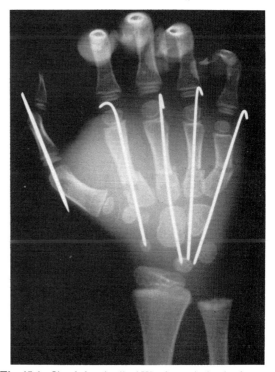

Fig. 15.4   Simple longitudinal Kirschner pin fixation has been employed in this transmetacarpal amputation in an 8-year-old child

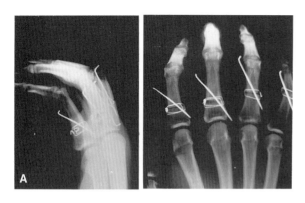

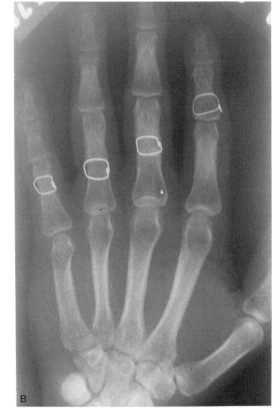

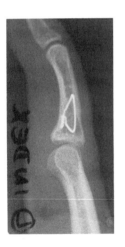
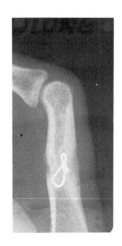

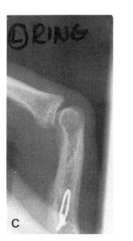
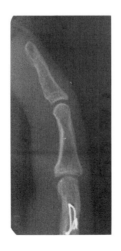

Fig. 15.5 (A) Type A intraosseous wiring has been used in all four fingers in this four-finger replantation: for osteosynthesis in the index, middle and ring and for arthrodesis in the little finger. (B & C) The results of Type A intraosseous wiring in another four-finger replantation are seen here in the antero-posterior view and lateral views. Firm union has been achieved with good alignment. The Kirschner pins have been long since removed

configurations. The latter has been shown to be the most stable pattern of the three, rivalling that of intraosseous wires and plates with screws (Fyfe & Mason 1979). Although the crossed configuration is stable, it has been stated that it holds the fracture fragments in distraction and not in compression. Although the Kirschner pin is generally associated with low morbidity, the surgeon must take care to decrease the incidence of pin-tract infection by avoiding undue traction on the skin, and to avoid the loss of motion caused by impaling the joint or tendon. Kirschner pins which emerge through the skin over a joint limit motion both mechanically and because they are painful—if the part is sensate. Where motion is achieved nonetheless, the incidence of pin-tract infection is very high. Not only does this predispose to osteitis (Green & Ripley 1984), but the necessary premature removal of the pin may lead to non-union or loss of motion, or both. To avoid these problems, pins should only be left sticking out through the skin where the skin will certainly remain immobile. In all other circumstances, the pin should be cut flush with the bone.

Technique

For replantation of amputated digits, the open retrograde technique of K-pin fixation is the most feasible (Edwards et al 1982). It is helpful to place a preview pin over the dorsal cortex of the reduced fracture to assure accurate pin placement in both the near and far cortices. Smooth, trocar-tipped K-pins ranging in size from 0.028 to 0.065 inch (0.7 to 1.6 mm) are used, depending on the size of the bone to be stabilized. (The 0.028–0.065 inch (0.7–1.6 mm) sizes are seldom employed.) It is helpful to place a hypodermic needle (14–18 gauge) over the pin to serve as a guide, to protect the soft tissues, and to enhance the purchase of the pin on the inner surface of the cortex. It is recommended that the distal fragment be pinned first, as the adjacent fingers can be flexed out of the way of the distally protruding pins. Especially with proximal phalangeal fractures, the neighbouring rays tend to block the path of the proximally protruding pins and it is often impossible to reattach the drill in this area.

Using a power-driven drill, the K-pin is inserted into the medullary canal of the distal fragment and directed obliquely across the cortex in the coronal plane at the angle determined by the preview pin. The pin is advanced distally through the skin until enough length is exposed to permit reattachment to the drill. The pin is then backed out distally until the proximal tip is flush with the fracture. A second pin is then drilled obliquely in a similar fashion through the opposite side of the distal fragment in the coronal plane, slightly anterior or posterior to the first pin. Final reduction is performed and the fragments are compressed by hand while both pins are drilled proximally across the fracture and barely through opposite cortices in the proximal fragment. Stability of the fracture fixation is tested in all planes, correct alignment is confirmed and the digit is put through a full passive range of motion to rule out intra-articular penetration or tethering of the extensor mechanism.

The pins can be cut off flush with the cortex or left exposed to facilitate removal, according to the tenets outlined above. If the latter course is chosen, it is imperative that the protruding pins do not interfere with motion of the digit. As much as possible, the periosteum is closed over the fracture site to decrease the incidence of tendon adhesions.

Intraosseous wiring

Indications

Intraosseous wiring (Lister 1978) has become our method of choice for transverse phalangeal fractures and intra-articular fractures at the metacarpal and phalangeal levels. Intraosseous wiring is not recommended for metacarpal shaft fractures where mini-compression plates are more effective.

This technique is quick, offers good stability, allowing early motion, and has low morbidity. It readily corrects the deformity and maintains the correction. High rates of union are achieved with this method (Fig. 15.5), it is relatively simple, is reasonably durable and cheap and the components are readily available. It is not quite as adaptable as K-pin fixation to various fracture patterns. It cannot be used when there is comminution or missing fragments, except in conjunction with an intramedullary pin (*see below*). The wire can be difficult to retrieve at times. The technique we

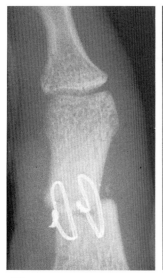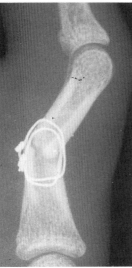

Fig. 15.6   Here a double loop antero-posterior (sagittal) wiring has been employed in replantation. Non-union with deformity has resulted

employ is the Type A wiring which combines the monofilament wire with a Kirschner pin. The double-loop sagittal wiring without Kirschner pin has proved less stable and has led to some non- and malunion (Fig. 15.6).

Technique

Whereas Type B wiring is for intra-articular fractures, Type A wiring is for arthrodesis and transverse fractures and will be discussed first.

The bone ends are prepared in standard fashion. Transverse drill-holes are made in the coronal plane on both sides of the fracture line, using a 0.035 inch K-pin (0.9 mm). These holes are parallel to the bone ends, approximately 5 mm from them, and somewhat dorsal to the axis. 20-gauge needles are passed through the holes. An 0 monofilament wire is passed through the needles to form a box-like configuration, in such a way that the twist of the wire will be on the non-contact side of the digit. More specifically, avoid placing the bulk of the wire on the radial side of the index, middle or ring fingers and the ulnar side of the thumb or little finger. The 0.035 inch (0.9 mm) K-pin is then driven obliquely across the intramedullary

canal of the amputated digit, emerging through the skin in a retrograde fashion. Once again it is helpful to utilize the 'preview' pin technique in order to determine the correct angle for the oblique K-pin. A 16-gauge hypodermic needle can be employed as a guide and to provide purchase on the endosteal surface of the bone. The surgeon then reduces the two bone ends under direct vision and holds them firmly together while his assistant drives the K-pin into the proximal fragment until it is embedded in cortical bone. Only then are the ends of the intraosseous wire twisted around one another (by convention in a clockwise direction), cut to about 1 cm in length, grasped with a heavy needle-holder and tightened down.

Tightening down the wire involves two distinct manoeuvres. The wire is first pulled to snug it on to the bone on the opposite cortex and then it is twisted to tighten it. The K-pin is usually left protruding from the skin over the distal fragment and bent over on itself to form a small loop to make it easier to remove. An 0.045 inch (1.1 mm) K-pin is used to drill a small hole through one cortex close to the twisted end of the monofilament wire, which is then turned down into the hole to avoid a potentially painful prominence.

Although rarely applicable in replantation surgery, there are occasional instances where the amputation passes through a joint, removing a small fragment of articular surface that is amenable to Type B intraosseous wiring. The fracture is exposed, reduced and held in place with forceps to check the congruity of the articular surfaces. Two parallel holes are then drilled with a 0.035 inch (0.9 mm) K-pin at right angles to the fracture and across it. This task is facilitated by leaving the first K-pin in place as a pilot for the second. A 20-gauge hypodermic needle is inserted along both tracts to facilitate passage of the 0 monofilament wire. The wire is tightened and embedded in the same way as the Type A.

Intramedullary rod

Indications

The main indications for the intramedullary Steinmann rod described below are significant comminution and or bone loss where it is desirable to maintain overall alignment and some semblance of the original length (Grundberg 1981). Other techniques in this general category have been described, such as intramedullary screws and the intramedullary bone dowel (Leung & Kok 1981) and porcelain peg. However, we feel that there are faster and equally secure techniques for stabilizing the relatively transverse fractures for which these methods have been recommended.

The Steinmann rod method is swift and, when used in conjunction with an intraosseous or tension band wire as it commonly is, can provide enough stability to implement early range-of-motion exercises. The best results are obtained when there is enough diaphyseal bone stock remaining to grasp the rod securely. This technique can also be employed when only a small metaphyseal cap remains, but it is imperative that there is no intra-articular component to the fracture which might allow violation of the joint space by the implant. The procedure has low morbidity and it avoids deformity. The device is simple, durable, readily available and cost-effective. On the other hand, because of the commonly associated comminution, union can be a problem and it is recommended that primary bone grafting be undertaken if the wound is reasonably clean. In fractures not associated with amputation, the rod is not very suitable unless there is significant bone loss or comminution, because it is very difficult to insert the rod into the intramedullary canal. In replantation, this difficulty does not arise and the rod can be inserted easily. The most significant drawback is the inability to retrieve the implant once healing has taken place.

Technique

During the initial operative exposure it is important to preserve the soft-tissue structures, particularly the periosteum and extensor mechanism, as much as possible. One should also take considerable care to keep the soft-tissue attachments on small, comminuted fragments as they will be pulled into reasonable alignment through a ligamentotaxis effect during the soft tissue closure. If there is significant bone loss, the ends can be shortened to permit adequate cortical apposition.

The medullary canal is reamed with drills or graduated Steinmann rods until a snug fit is achieved. The length of the rod is then determined by measuring and adding together the amount that fits into the proximal and distal fragments. The largest diameter rod in the length previously determined is selected or, in the case of an intramedullary canal that is relatively flat, two thinner rods are employed for increased stability. The rod is cut to length, eliminating the sharpened point. Two transverse holes parallel to the fracture-line are then drilled in the frontal plane, with a 0.035 inch (0.889 mm) K-pin of approximately 5–10 mm from the fracture surface. An 0 monofilament stainless steel wire is then passed through the drill-holes, in either a box or figure-of-eight configuration, but not tightened. The Steinmann rod is inserted into the intramedullary canal of both the proximal and distal fragment and manually impacted. If there is good cortical apposition, and thus no reason to expect further collapse, the spurs on the ends of the cut-off Steinmann rods can be left intact in anticipation that they might provide increased rotational stability in the cancellous bone. If there is significant comminution and further collapse is to be expected, it is advisable to file the sharp ends smooth to diminish the likelihood of intra-articular penetration. The wires are tightened and cut to leave a 1 cm tail which is bent over and embedded into a hole drilled with an 0.045 inch (1.1 mm) K-pin into the non-contact surface of the bone. Finally, the periosteum and extensor mechanism are repaired, which helps to reduce the fragments if there is severe comminution.

Plate and screws

Indications

The principal indication for the use of plates and screws in replantation surgery of the hand is for transverse fractures of the metacarpal shafts and for the forearm bones and humerus (Ikuta & Tsuge 1974, Irigaray 1980, Meuli et al 1978, Riggs & Cooney 1983) (*see Fig. 15.1c*). Only oblique and spiral fractures have enough overlap to allow interfragmentary compression with screws alone and plates in the phalanges are generally too bulky to be of any practical use. An axial interfragmentary compression plate provides rigid fixation and thus the freedom to institute early motion. The implants correct the deformity, promote union and are very durable. On the negative side, they are more time-consuming to implant than other methods and require more extensive soft-tissue dissection to apply them and consequently a more involved operation to remove them. The technique is not simple, not readily adaptable to many clinical replant situations, not always available and very expensive.

Technique

The technique described will be that recommended by the Swiss Association for the Study of Internal Fixation, abbreviated to ASIF (Segmüller 1977: see also Chapter 14 of this book, by the same author). Once again, basic principles of fracture preparation should be observed; specifically as little soft-tissue dissection as possible because this would further compromise the blood-supply.

The most common plates utilized on the metacarpal will be the 2.7 mm dynamic compression plate and the quarter-tubular plate, both of which can be employed in such a way as to produce axial interfragmentary compression. As provisional fixation with reduction forceps or K-pins is difficult, the reduction may be held in place by the assistant with his fingers. A plate is selected which is long enough to have at least two holes on either side of the fracture and bent to fit the dorsal surface of the metacarpal. The first hole is drilled with a 2.0 mm drill in the smaller fragment, usually the amputated part, and the plate is fixed to this bone with the first 2.7 mm screw, after tapping the drill-hole. After this initial critical screw has been inserted, the plate can be used to aid in the reduction while the axial alignment is checked. The second screw is then inserted in the amputated metacarpal shaft.

Now attention is turned to the other side of the fracture; the larger, usually proximal, fragment. An eccentric hole is made and the screw inserted in such a way that compression is applied. The remaining screw or screws are introduced and the periosteum closed as much as possible.

External fixation

Indications

The technique of percutaneous pin fixation secured with an external frame has found widespread use in the management of many fracture patterns and locations in the upper extremity (Pritsch et al 1981, Riggs & Cooney 1983). Most common are comminuted fractures in the distal forearm, carpus, metacarpus and phalanges which are not amenable to open reduction and internal fixation because of the multiplicity of fragments. However, in the replant situation, many of these fractures are best managed by shortening for the reasons outlined previously and thus are stabilized by internal means. External fixators are bulky and often adversely affect positioning of the amputated extremity when performing delicate microvascular procedures. The percutaneous fixation pins may skewer vital structures such as nerves, veins or arteries and may impinge on the skin or tether the extensor mechanism and thus restrict motion. For these and other reasons, external fixators are rarely employed in the management of the bone in replant surgery.

Comparison and selection of techniques

Each of the above techniques has its merits and drawbacks when viewed in the light of the requirements set out initially. These are summarized in Table 15.1. The preferred method differs according to the level of injury (Table 15.2). In general, we favour the Kirschner pin alone in the distal phalanx, Type A intraosseous wiring in the proximal and middle phalanges, and plates and screws for metacarpals and the more proximal long bones. In the distal phalanx of the thumb especially, the Kirschner pin may be inserted retrograde through the tip and only advanced into the proximal fragment after the vessel repairs are complete (Fig. 15.7).

Interfragmentary screw fixation alone is rarely used in replantation because bone shortening usually squares the ends. Where, however, length must be maintained for complex architectural reasons (Fig. 15.8) screws may find a place.

Table 15.1 Qualities of different types of fixation

	Cast, splint, traction	Kirschner pin	Intraosseous wiring	Intramedullary rod	Plate and screws	External fixation
Speed	+	+	+	+	−	±
Stability	−	±	+	±	+	+
Early movement	−	±	+	±	+	+
Low morbidity	−	+	+	+	±	+
Avoids deformity	±	±	+	±	+	±
Promotes union	±	±	+	±	+	±
Simplicity	+	+	+	+	−	±
Adaptability	−	+	−	−	−	+
Durability	−	−	±	±	+	+
Retrievability	+	+	±	−	−	+
Availability	+	+	+	+	−	−
Cost	+	+	+	+	−	−

Table 15.2 Techniques of fracture fixation: preferred methods of fixation by fracture level

Fracture site	Method of fixation			
	Kirschner pin	Intraosseous wiring	Intramedullary rod	Plate and screws
Distal phalanx	+	±	−	−
Middle phalanx	+	+	±	−
Proximal phalanx	+	+	±	−
Metacarpal	±	±	+	+
Carpal	+	−	−	−
Forearm	−	−	±	+
Humerus	−	−	±	+

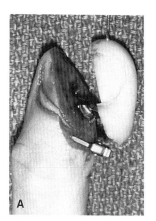
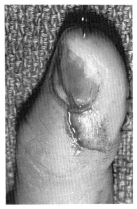
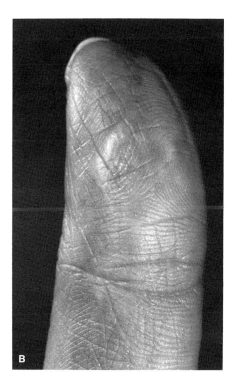

Fig. 15.7 Replantation at the level of the distal phalanx is commonly fixed by a Kirschner pin, but applied in an unusual manner. Here in (A) the Kirschner pin has been passed into the distal phalanx. The skin was then sutured, vessel repair undertaken, and only then was the fracture reduced and the Kirschner pin advanced. In this way the vessels on the palmar aspect of the distal phalanx could be repaired in a comfortable position. The eventual result is full survival (B) (surgery largely by Dr Luis Scheker)

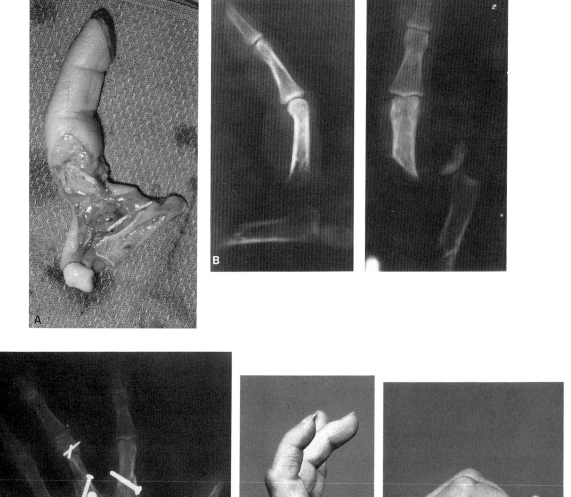

Fig. 15.8 (A, B & C) This amputation of an index finger was sustained in a frame cutter. It can be seen that a significant segment of the proximal phalanx of the adjacent middle finger and part of the metacarpophalangeal joint were removed plus the entire index finger. For this reason, single digit replantation at the proximal phalanx was undertaken. Internal fixation with interfragmentary screws was employed and relatively good function was achieved (D & E)

Silicone block spacer

Indications

Although not a method of fracture fixation, we have had experience with a unique method of managing the patient with severe bone loss in the hand. On occasions, one will encounter a replant situation, such as transmetacarpal amputation, wherein, for example, there may coexist adequate bone stock in the first and second metacarpals with severe loss of bone stock in the fourth and fifth metacarpals. In this situation, it may be advantageous to preserve length on the ulnar side of the hand by filling the gap with a biologically compatible spacer until the wounds have declared themselves and the defect can be filled with autogenous bone graft.

Technique

After the defect has been defined, a template is fashioned from a piece of Esmarch bandage or sterile foam, and a 0.5 inch piece of silicone is carved to fit the gap. The silicone spacer is secured with multiple K-pins which are passed easily through bone into the rubber block. After the wounds have healed without evidence of infection, the spacer can be removed surgically and the defect grafted with a corticocancellous strut. It is interesting to note that an apparent inflammatory response around the silicone creates a smooth tube of fibrous tissue, not unlike periosteum, which is an ideal bed for the autogenous bone graft.

MANAGEMENT OF THE DESTROYED JOINT

Primary arthroplasty

Indications

The indication for primary silicone interpositional arthroplasty in replantation surgery (Wray et al 1984) is a destroyed joint with sufficient bone stock to support the prosthesis and a functional need to maintain length or motion (Fig. 15.9). Where a choice between arthrodesis and arthroplasty exists, joint implants are used in joints which are usually supported laterally during function: all the meta-carpophalangeal joints of the fingers, the proximal interphalangeal joints of the middle and ring fingers and the basal joint of the thumb.

Technique

By virtue of the amputation, the approach has already been made for the surgeon. As much of the ligamentous anatomy as possible is preserved during preparation of the bone ends. Reaming of the medullary cavity on both sides of the joint is undertaken and the appropriate size of prosthesis selected.

Primary arthrodesis

Indications

Fusion is preferable, where sufficient bone length is available, in those joints which commonly function without lateral support: the distal interphalangeal joints, the proximal interphalangeal joints of the index and little fingers and the joints of the thumb other than the basal. Unlike the non-replant situation, the shortening which typically accompanies joint fusion is a benefit.

Technique

Our preferred technique is that of intraosseous wiring, as previously described. For arthrodesis, the bony surfaces are prepared by osteotomizing the contiguous surfaces of the joint into flat surfaces or, shaping them, into a 'spike and cone' as recommended by Carroll and Hill (1969).

The correct position is determined by observing the normal 'cascade' of the uninjured hand. A slight variation of the boxed intraosseous wire technique is to utilize a tension-band wire that passes through the bone in the distal fragment but is looped around the proximal end of the two parallel intramedullary K-pins in a figure-of-eight fashion. Another variation of traditional arthrodesis techniques is to employ the Harrison peg (Harrison & Watson 1980). The intramedullary Harrison polypropylene peg comes in three sizes with angles varying from 20 to 50°. The medullary canals are 'reamed' with a small osteotome or similar rectangular object and then the bone ends

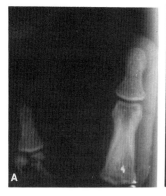
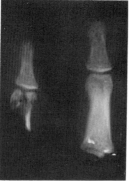
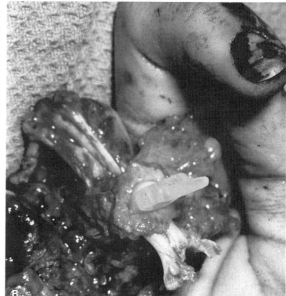
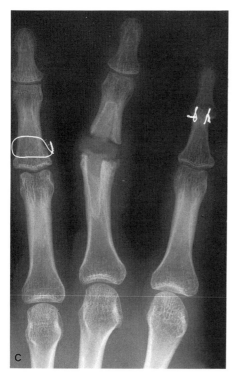

Fig. 15.9 (A) Radiograph of the amputated parts show that the middle finger has been amputated through the proximal interphalangeal joint. (B) Immediate silicone arthroplasty can maintain length and give some promise of motion. The implant is inserted in the usual manner, taking care to preserve as much periosteum and palmar plate as possible to ensure stability. The flexor tendons were subsequently debrided and shortened in order to maximize function. (C) In another case, three types of fixation have been employed: type A intraosseous wiring, immediate silicone arthroplasty, and double sagittal wiring

are impacted over the ends of the peg. No additional fixation is required. Like the intramedullary nail, it is much easier to put in when dealing with an amputation or near-amputation than is an ordinary arthrodesis. Although a pseudarthrosis does occur in a significant percentage of cases, it is not significant. The method is quick and effective.

REHABILITATION

The postoperative period can be divided into three phases: immediate, intermediate, and late. *Imme-*

diately after the operation the replanted extremity is immobilized in a bulky dressing which helps to diminish swelling and pain and provides protection from the routine trauma of daily ward activities. The goal of replantation is not survival alone, but restoration of function; therefore, from the beginning in uncomplicated replantation, the patient is started on gentle active range-of-motion exercises. After the dressing is first changed on the fifth day, the patient is encouraged to remove his protective splint three times a day for 15 minutes of active therapy. When not actively exercising, the injured extremity is immobilized in the 'safe' position—45° of wrist extension, 70° of metacarpophalangeal joint flexion and no greater than 5° of interphalangeal flexion (*see Chapter 3*). As both flexor and extensor mechanisms are involved, early therapy is gradual and never includes passive stretching.

The *intermediate* period commences after six weeks with implementation of dynamic splinting during the day. The dynamic splinting is alternated between the flexion and extension modes and the replanted extremity is placed in a static splint during the night.

The *later* period is the time for assessing the functional outcome of the replantation to date and the potential need for secondary procedures. Although rising technical expertise has provided high viability rates, there has not been the same dramatic rise in ultimate function. This has caused us to become more aggressive with respect to early therapy.

COMPLICATIONS

Complications have been reviewed by Leung (1980).

Infection

By definition, all amputation fractures are Grade 3 open wounds which might have a poor prognosis. However, in spite of the severe nature of these wounds, the incidence of acute and chronic osteomyelitis is relatively low. Our management consists of premedication cultures followed by a preoperative bolus of cephalosporins which are then continued for 3–5 days. If the wounds are severely contaminated (especially farm injuries) the patient is given triple antibiotic therapy, consisting of a penicillin and an aminoglycoside in addition to the cephalosporin. Obviously, basic principles governing management of osteomyelitis in the long bones also apply to the management of a similar disease process in the small bones of the hand. These are immediate incision and drainage, intravenous antibiotics and sequestrectomy or reamputation if indicated.

Non-union

In spite of the compromised vascular status of the amputation, non-union is reported to be less than

10% in most series (Kuwata et al 1984, Snelling & Hendel 1979). The principles of ideal fixation should be observed at all times to ensure a rate of high union (Fig. 15.10). A technique of fracture fixation that is rigid and provides compression will give the most consistent results. Primary bone-grafting is rarely indicated except in the cleanest of wounds. The surgeon should be aggressive with secondary bone-grafting as an impending non-union could severely retard the patient's rehabilitative efforts.

Malunion

The temptation is to be rather cavalier about the seemingly low priority that bony stabilization has in the sequence of replantation surgery. However, little time is lost by ensuring that angulatory and rotatory alignment is correct. If malunion occurs, it will in most instances impair function and will require correction.

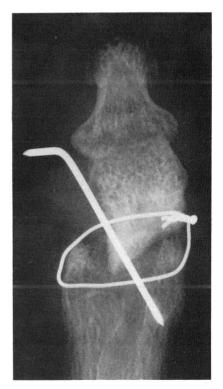

Fig. 15.10 Haste in replantation can lead to improper bony fixation and resultant malaligned non-union. From this radiograph it is evident that the bone ends were improperly prepared in this radically shortened replantation performed in 1975. Non-union resulted

REFERENCES

Carroll R E, Hill N A 1969 Small joint arthrodesis in hand reconstruction. Journal of Bone and Joint Surgery 51A:1219–1221

Edwards G S, O'Brien E T, Heckman M M 1982 Retrograde cross-pinning of transverse metacarpal and phalangeal fractures. The Hand 14:141–148

Fyfe I S, Mason S 1979 The mechanical stability of internal fixation of fractured phalanges. The Hand 11:50–54

Green S A, Ripley M J 1984 Chronic osteomyelitis in pin tracks. Journal of Bone and Joint Surgery 66A:1092–1098

Grundberg A B 1981 Intramedullary fixation for fractures of the hand. Journal of Hand Surgery 6:568–573

Harrison D H, Watson J S 1980 Use of the polypropylene peg for immediate stabilization in digital replantation. Journal of Hand Surgery 5:253–259

Hoffmann R, Buck-Gramcko D 1982 Osteosynthesis in digital replantation surgery. Annales Chirurgiae et Gynaecologiae 71:14–18

Ikuta Y 1978 Method of bone fixation in reattachment of amputations in the upper extremities. Clinical Orthopaedics and Related Research 133:169–178

Ikuta Y, Tsuge K 1974 Micro-bolts and micro-screws for fixation of small bones in the hand. The Hand 6:261–265

Irigaray A 1980 New fixing screw for completely amputated fingers. Journal of Hand Surgery 5:381

Kuwata N, Kawai S, Doi K 1984 Clinical and experimental studies of bone union in reimplantation of digits: a preliminary report on ischemic interval. Microsurgery 5:30–35

Leung P C 1980 An analysis of complications in digital replantations. The Hand 12:25–32

Leung P C, Kok L C 1981 Use of an intramedullary bone peg in digital replantations, revascularization, and toe-transfers. Journal of Hand Surgery 6:281–284

Lister G D 1978 Intraosseous wiring of digital skeleton. Journal of Hand Surgery 3:427–435

Lister G D, Kleinert H E 1979 Replantation. In: Grabb W C, Smith J W (eds). Plastic surgery (3rd edn), Little Brown, Boston

Meuli H, Meyer V, Segmüller G 1978 Stabilization of bone in replantation surgery of the upper limb. Clinical Orthopaedics and Related Research 133:179–183

Pritsch M, Engel J, Farin I 1981 Manipulation and external fixation of metacarpal fractures. Journal of Bone and Joint Surgery 63A:1289–1291

Riggs S A, Cooney W P 1983 External fixation of complex hand and wrist fractures. Journal of Trauma 23:332–336

Schlenker J D 1979 Single K-wire in thumb replantation. (Letter to the Editor.) Annals of Plastic Surgery 3:387

Segmüller G 1977 Surgical stabilization of the skeleton of the hand. Williams and Wilkins, Baltimore

Snelling C F T, Hendel P M 1979 Avascular necrosis of bone following revascularization of the thumb. Annals of Plastic Surgery 3:77–87

Tupper J 1978 Techniques of bone fixation and clinical experience in replanted extremities. Clinical Orthopaedics and Related Research 133:165–168

Urbaniak J, Hayes M, Bright D 1978 Management of bone in digital replantation: free vascularized and composite bone grafts. Clinical Orthopaedics and Related Research 133:184–194

Vlastou C, Earle A S 1984 A simple method of controlling rotation in replanted digits. Journal of Reconstructive Microsurgery 1:147–148

Weiland A J, Villarreal-Rios A, Kleinert H E, Kutz J E, Atasoy E, Lister G D 1977 Replantation of digits and hands: analysis of surgical techniques and functional results in 71 patients with 86 replantations. Journal of Hand Surgery 2:1–12

Wray R C, Young V L, Weeks P M 1984 Flexible-implant arthroplasty and finger replantation. Plastic and Reconstructive Surgery 74:97–99

Yamano Y, Matsuda H, Nakashima K, Shimazu A 1982 Some methods for bone fixation for digital replantation. The Hand 14:135–140

SECTION

Wrist fractures

2

PART

A

Fractures of the carpus

Robert A. Dickson

16 Scaphoid fractures: conservative management

The carpal scaphoid is the commonest of the carpal bones to be fractured (Dunn 1972, Leslie & Dickson 1981) and accounts for between 1% and 2% of all fractures presenting to accident departments (Scott 1956). It is the commonest injury to befall the wrist of a working man and in military service it is more frequent than Colles's fracture (Perkins 1950). One-sixth of all scaphoid fractures present as established non-unions (Scott 1956). Recommended methods of treatment vary enormously and opinions concerning diagnosis, treatment, prognosis and disability are conflicting. Moreover, most of the controversial statements about failure to diagnose or failure to treat immediately have not been substantiated by careful analyses of large numbers of patients (Russe 1960, London 1961, McLaughlin & Parkes 1969, Dunn 1972, Leslie & Dickson 1981). Despite the overwhelming evidence, traditional attitudes prevail. A recent editorial (British Medical Journal 1981) stated that teaching dogma about immobilization of injured wrists need not, however, be revised. The annual report of the Medical Defence Union (1983) went even further backwards when making the following statement: 'Failure to diagnose a fracture of the scaphoid continues to result in claims which are almost always indefensible; even if the clinical diagnosis is not confirmed by X-ray examination the wrist should be treated in plaster of Paris; failure to diagnose and therefore treat adequately may result in permanent weakness and osteoarthritis.' Such views cannot now remain unchallenged.

In order to understand the rationale behind the management of scaphoid fractures and resolve some of the controversies, the following points

need to be addressed—mechanism of injury, radiographic features, site and direction of fractures, the presence of associated injuries, the time to union, the outcome in relationship to the injury and factors concerning non-union.

MECHANISM OF INJURY

Three-quarters of patients sustain their injuries as a result of a fall on the outstretched hand while a further 15% sustain their injury as a result of a longitudinal force in the first web (crank-handle kick-back, motorcycle handlebar or steering wheel) (Leslie & Dickson 1981). These two chief injury mechanisms produce different fracture patterns and prognoses very much according to the local anatomy. The radial and proximal surfaces of the scaphoid form a convexity which articulates with a reciprocal concavity on the distal end of the radius. The proximal three-fifths of the scaphoid are covered with articular cartilage but the distal two-fifths, including the base of the tubercle, are extra-articular and provide attachment for strong ligaments (Dickison & Shannon 1944). The distal half of the scaphoid is secured to the trapezium and the trapezoid bones by strong and dense ligaments while the proximal half has a very strong ligamentous attachment to the lunate. Any force on the midcarpal joint area will also occur in the region of the waist of the scaphoid and indeed waist fractures have been called a continuation of the intercarpal joint line (Dickison & Shannon 1944). Moreover, the internal structure of the scaphoid is cancellous and the waist region is markedly constricted. All these factors contribute to the high prevalence rate of waist fractures. In a fall on the outstretched hand, the wrist is both hyperextended and radially deviated and in this position the scaphoid is fixed in the concavity of the articular surface of the radius. Any further movement of the intercarpal joint will tend to fracture the scaphoid waist, referred to as 'snapped waist' (Todd 1921, Grace 1929). Precisely where the fracture occurs in the scaphoid depends on the amount of radial deviation of the wrist: the less the radial deviation, the more proximal the fracture. Falls on the outstretched hand in ulnar deviation produce avulsion fractures of the tubercle.

Obletz and Halbstein (1938) demonstrated that the scaphoid receives its blood supply from two sources: (1) ligaments about the tubercle; and (2) ligaments attached to the dorsal surface. In 13% of the 297 cadavers that they dissected there was no arterial foramen proximal to the mid-waist of the scaphoid and in 20% only one. Two-thirds of patients therefore had two or more arterial foramina in the proximal half of the scaphoid. In one-third of waist fractures there will therefore be some avascular change (Fig. 16.1).

A more significant force applied to the first web in a longitudinal fashion by crank-handle, motorcycle handlebar or steering wheel produces fracturing through the proximal part of the scaphoid, often in a vertical oblique direction with considerable instability and local disruption of soft tissues, accounting for their more serious prognosis.

SITE AND DIRECTION OF FRACTURES

An analysis of 1105 fresh fractures of the scaphoid derived from six large studies (Stewart 1954, Russe 1960, London 1961, Margo & Seely 1963, Leslie & Dickson 1981) revealed the following site of fracture–tuberosity 10%; distal third 11%; waist 72%; proximal pole 6% (Fig. 16.2). Russe (1960) further divided his waist fractures into three directions—horizontal oblique (35%), transverse (60%) and vertical oblique (5%). Horizontal oblique and transverse fractures were caused either by a fall on the outstretched hand or a blow to the extended wrist, while the less common but more serious vertical oblique fracture was caused by a shearing force directed longitudinally up the first cleft. The importance of dividing waist fractures by direction has since been confirmed (Leslie & Dickson 1981). Thus, when the mechanism of injury is considered in relation to the anatomy of the scaphoid and the site and direction of the fracture, a clear pattern of prognosis emerges. As the fracture line moves in distal to proximal direction, both time to union and rate of non-union increase.

RADIOGRAPHIC FEATURES

Recent statements concerning the adverse effects of failure to diagnose a scaphoid fracture (editorial, British Medical Journal 1981; Medical Defence Union 1983) grossly exaggerate the situation. Moreover, reports of large series of scaphoid fractures produce quite the opposite opinion and there are several important reports (Russe 1960, London 1961, McLaughlin & Parkes 1969, Dunn 1972, Leslie & Dickson 1981), in particular the study by Leslie and Dickson (1981), which address this problem. Four views, and often more, are

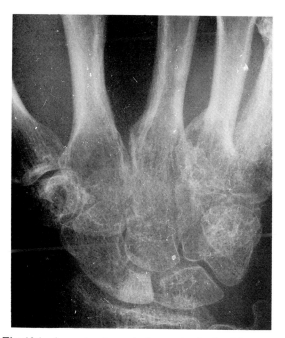

Fig. 16.1 Avascular change in the proximal pole of the scaphoid three months after a horizontal oblique fracture of the waist. The fracture has united perfectly and increased radiodensity can be expected in at least one-third of cases

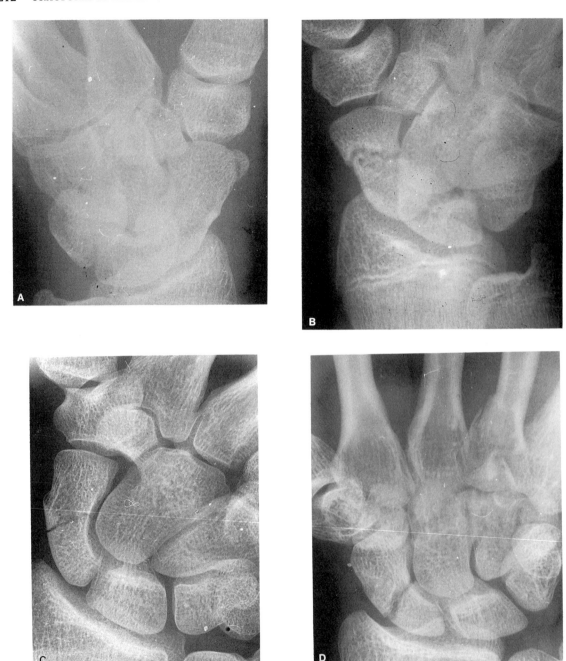

Fig. 16.2 (A) Avulsion fracture of the tuberosity of the scaphoid. (B) Horizontal oblique fracture of the scaphoid waist. (C) Transverse fracture of the scaphoid waist. (D) Vertical oblique fracture of the scaphoid waist

necessary to diagnose a fractured scaphoid (Russe 1960). In addition to a postero-anterior view and a lateral view, there should also be semi-pronated and semi-supinated views. Russe (1960) recommended that the oblique views should be in 25° of pronation and of supination but the views taken now in X-ray departments are $45°$ of pronation and $45°$ of supination (Leslie & Dickson 1981). These four views, then, constitute the 'standard views' and are the minimum requirement when a patient presents with pain located to the radial side of the wrist and tenderness in the anatomical snuffbox as a result of injury.

If only these four views are taken, the following statistics apply. 95% of scaphoid fractures are recognized as such by the casualty officer (Leslie & Dickson 1981). The casualty officer in the UK, and in many other parts of the world, is a senior house officer or at best a junior registrar with little experience of musculo-skeletal injuries. Indeed it is precisely to acquire some of this experience that these individuals are appointed and only rarely do they stay in post for more than six months (that being the time required to satisfy Royal Colleges of Surgeons). Against that background, 95% is a remarkably high figure and in many accident departments (probably the majority) the inexperienced casualty officer receives the medico-legal back-up of a radiologist scrutinizing the films of all patients seen in the accident department who have not been admitted to the hospital within 48 hours of injury. When experienced radiologists or orthopaedic surgeons scrutinize the same films, 98% of scaphoid fractures are clearly visible on these four standard views (Leslie & Dickson 1981). This gives a figure of 2% of scaphoid fractures not being visible on presentation and Russe (1960) pointed out that this slight figure can be reduced somewhat by the taking of oblique projections at different angles of rotation and the use of a magnifying glass when there is strong clinical suspicion of a fracture. The views which should be particularly scrutinized are the postero-anterior and semi-pronated views, as in only six cases out of 222 was the fracture not seen on either of these views (Leslie & Dickson 1981). Further views in differing degrees of pronation can help to reduce this figure (Russe 1960). The lateral view is merely of value in excluding a concomitant carpal dislocation (Fig. 16.3). Moreover, as two-thirds of fractures occur in the waist of the scaphoid, this area of the bone should be carefully scrutinized.

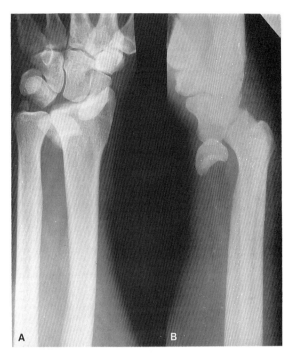

Fig. 16.3 (A) The PA radiograph shows the lunate and most of the scaphoid overlapping the lower radius. This striking appearance is not usually so clear on the PA view. Note also the fractured ulnar styloid strongly suggesting wrist instability. The casualty officer was quite understandably confused. (B) The lateral radiograph reveals all. The lunate has turned through 180 degrees and lies in front of the lower radius. The scaphoid and rest of the carpus has subluxed forwards and proximally

The crucial question is 'What are the characteristics of the fractures in those 2% or less which are not visible at presentation?' Two investigations have studied this aspect (McLaughlin & Parkes 1969, Leslie & Dickson 1981). Fractures that are not visible at presentation but become so during

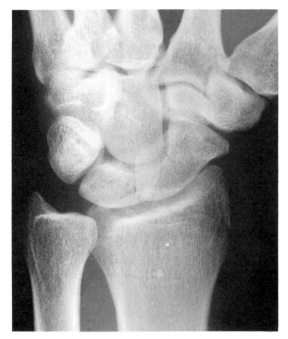

Fig. 16.4 A scaphoid infraction—an incomplete fracture on the compression side of the scaphoid—which is the only fracture of the scaphoid which is sometimes not visible on the initial radiographs and which will heal under any circumstances, whether immobilized or not

the first 2–3 weeks following injury are scaphoid 'infractions': incomplete fractures on the compression side of the waist of the scaphoid (Fig. 16.4). McLaughlin and Parkes (1969) performed a fascinating study in which they aspirated the local articulations at presentation and explored some. The scaphoid infractions were not only incomplete fractures but were surrounded by an intact, or substantially so, shell of articular cartilage and subchondral bone as well as ligament and it was quite clear to them at the time, and confirmed at follow-up, that these fractures would heal under any circumstances, whether immobilized or not. These important findings have been confirmed (Leslie & Dickson 1981). The old-fashioned dogma of a fracture not being visible on the first radiograph becoming visible by bone absorption around the fracture site and then going on to non-union because it has been neglected has no substance whatsoever. Indisputably, however, there is an onus on casualty officers and those in charge of accident departments to ensure that someone with

experience does look at the films of all outpatient musculo-skeletal injuries so that fractures visible at presentation are actually seen. There is a trend, in one-third of cases, for the fracture to become more obvious radiographically during the first few weeks following injury. Those in whom the fracture continues to be more obvious, and those which develop cystic change (Fig. 16.5), have a statistically higher probability of proceeding to non-union (Leslie & Dickson 1981).

ASSOCIATED INJURIES

This is an important matter as one-eighth of all patients with a scaphoid fracture have another significant injury. One-third of these associated injuries are in the nature of a multiple injury pattern, whereas two-thirds are fractures in the same upper extremity, of which fractures of the radial styloid, distal radius and ulnar styloid are

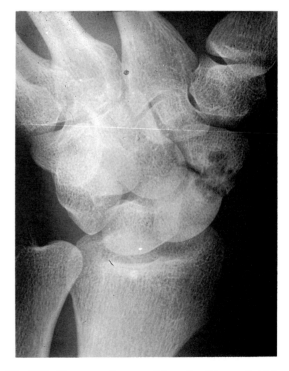

Fig. 16.5 Transverse fracture of the waist of the scaphoid 6 weeks after injury showing a more obvious fracture line with cystic change—not a good prognostic sign

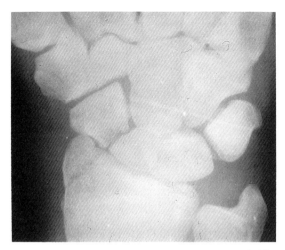

Fig. 16.6 Transverse fracture of the waist of the scaphoid with a fracture of the radial styloid—not an uncommon injury pattern

the commonest (Fig. 16.6). In a patient with multiple injuries, unless all sites of discomfort are carefully examined and radiographed where necessary, a scaphoid fracture can be overlooked, only to become the problem in the medium to long term when the other injuries have healed. Concomitant fractures of the same upper extremity indicate violence of a more severe or multifocal nature and the presence of a fractured ulnar styloid should always raise the suspicion of another fracture close by, which is sometimes overlooked (Medical Defence Union 1983).

TIME TO UNION

Union should always be considered radiologically and occurs when bony trabeculae are seen to cross the fracture line or a sclerotic band is present at the site of the fracture (Fig. 16.7) (Russe 1960). When all fractures are considered, the average time to bony union is nine to ten weeks (Dunn 1972, Leslie & Dickson 1981). However, there is considerable variation around this mean and the two most important factors are the site of the fracture and the age of the patient. We have already seen that union takes longer the more proximal the fracture, ranging from a mean of 39 days for tuberosity fractures to 93 days for proximal pole fractures. In patients between the ages of 10 and 14 years, fractures of the waist of the scaphoid unite in six weeks, whereas it takes twice as long in those aged 20–24 years. The mechanism of injury also has

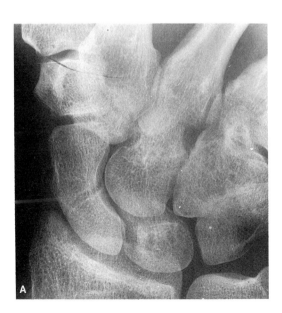

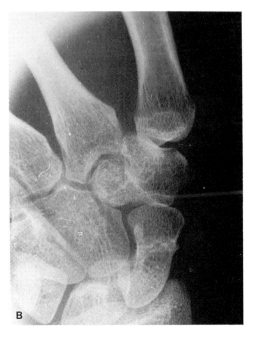

Fig. 16.7 Radiological union. (A) Trabeculae cross the fracture line. (B) There is a sclerotic band at the site of the fracture

Table 16.1 Type of fracture and time to union

Type of fracture	Radiological union (days)	Clinical union (days)	Duration of plaster (days)	Time as outpatient (days)
Tuberosity	39	33	30	42
Distal pole	44	50	47	64
Waist				
horizontal oblique	57	55	49	76
vertical oblique	72	75	65	90
transverse	67	84	64	109
Proximal pole	93	79	64	142

some effect here: while transverse fractures of the waist caused by falls take between eight and nine weeks to unite, the same fracture caused by a longitudinal force up the first web takes almost 12 weeks. Therefore by paying attention to variables which affect the time to bony union, the duration of plaster immobilization can be more accurately determined (Table 16.1). There can be little to recommend suggestions that if scaphoid fractures are not united by two months they should be screwed (Fisk 1982, Leyshon et al 1984) when a significant number will not have united by then, as would be entirely expected, the great majority of which would do so in a further month whether plastered or not.

FACTORS RELATED TO NON-UNION

This is another crucial matter. Most large series, of several hundred cases, report a consistent non-union rate of 5% (Stewart 1954, Russe 1960, London 1961, Leslie & Dickson 1981) though in one study of more than 100 cases the non-union rate was as low as 2% (Kessler et al 1963). Smaller series tend to provide a non-union rate of about 10% (Cobey & White 1963, Margo & Seely 1963, Dunn 1972) but these smaller numbers are less reliable statistically. Some series report a surprisingly high rate of non-union, in excess of 20% (Codman & Chase 1905, Barr et al 1953), but in these studies immobilization was often for less than 8 weeks and was frequently prescribed for only one week; clearly therefore too short a period of immobilization for those that really need it. Waist fractures in the young adult increase the non-union rate and those surgeons who routinely prescribe a period of 3 months in plaster followed by mobilization, whether the fracture has healed

or not, report the acceptable 5% non-union rate (London 1961, Dawkins 1967).

The most frequently reported feature of scaphoid fractures which is associated with an increased non-union rate is displacement of the fragments (Soto-Hall & Haldeman 1934, Dickison & Shannon 1944, Murray 1946, Sashin 1946, Luck et al 1948, Barr et al 1953, McLaughlin 1954). Some go as far as to say that reduction is a prerequisite for union (Murray 1946) or that displacement requires immediate bone grafting (Sashin 1946). This, however, is incorrect. The important distinction is between those that are initially mildly displaced but do not displace further during treatment, and those that displace during the period of immobilization (Leslie & Dickson 1981). Those which *do* displace during the period of immobilization, and those with gross displacement at presentation, are part of a more serious carpal instability pattern for which immediate operative treatment is necessary (*see Fig. 16.3*). Approximately 5% of scaphoid fractures are mildly displaced on the initial films (Fig. 16.8) but do not displace further and, although a further month of immobilization is required to secure union, there is no increased tendency for non-union (Mazet & Hohl 1963, Leslie & Dickson 1981). However, less than one-fifth of those fractures that do displace during immobilization go on to non-union and therefore, while prompt operative treatment has its proponents, increasing displacement *per se* cannot be recommended as the criterion. If the fracture becomes more obvious during the second month of immobilization with continued displacement, then the likelihood of securing sound union diminishes considerably (Leslie & Dickson 1981). Therefore a number of variables have to be taken into consideration before operative treatment should be prescribed.

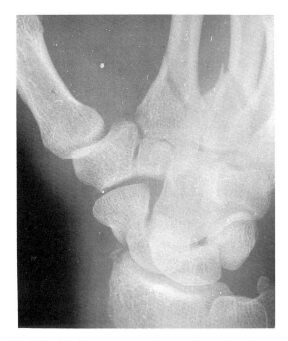

Fig. 16.8 Displaced transverse fracture of the waist of the scaphoid with fractures of both radial and ulnar styloids and separation of the scaphocapitate joint. There are also fractures of the second and the third metacarpal bases. All fractures united uneventfully with 3 months in plaster

The important age group to watch for in the development of non-union is the young man between the ages of 16 and 30 with a fracture of the proximal pole or a transverse or vertical oblique fracture of the waist (Table 16.2). For reasons that are not clear, significantly more right-sided scaphoid fractures go on to non-union (Leslie & Dickson 1981).

CONSERVATIVE TREATMENT

Acute injury

It is a sensible policy to prescribe a period of plaster immobilization of the wrist until the time when a fracture in that site, in that age group, with that mechanism of injury would be expected to unite. Most authors recommend a below-elbow cast, but the variation of opinion about the precise position of the wrist is extraordinary. Extension in radial deviation is favoured by most (Berlin 1929, Hosford 1931, Friedenberg 1949, Fisk 1982). However, London (1961) has found eight different recommended positions of the wrist, each at considerable variance with the next, so that it was clear to him that the precise position of the wrist did not matter. Although an above-elbow cast is recommended by some (Verdan 1960), there is no difference in the time to healing or non-union rate whether an above or below-elbow cast is prescribed (Dunn 1972). Interestingly, while most accident departments prescribe a below-elbow cast incorporating the proximal phalanx of the thumb, this appears to be unnecessary. Bohler's experience of more than 700 scaphoid fractures immobilized with the thumb left entirely free indicates that thumb immobilization is not necessary (Jahna 1954). On balance, the best cast is probably a below-elbow one with the wrist slightly extended and radially deviated. Whether the thumb is immobilized depends upon the courage of the plasterer. The cast should be left on until that fracture is expected to unite and then removed to permit an accurate radiological appraisal of the fracture. If trabeculae have crossed the fracture site, then the fracture has united. If

Table 16.2 The prognosis of scaphoid fractures in relation to age

	5–9	10–14	15–19	20–24	25–29	30–39	40–49	50–59	60+
				Age group (years)					
Number (%) of patients	1(0.4)	20(9)	53(24)	56(25)	30(14)	26(12)	18(8)	10(4.3)	8(3.3)
Duration of plaster (days)	29	35	51	55	64	60	70	45	52
Time to clinical union (days)	29	38	58	80	73	76	76	59	56
Time to radiological union (days):									
all fractures	29	42	56	78	67	79	73	53	52
waist fractures only	0	42	60	79	69	70	67	56	66
Duration as an outpatient (days)	49	51	76	111	94	95	93	70	61
Time off work (weeks)	0	0	5	6	3	5	5	2	0.4
Incidence of non-union (%)	0	0	7.5	9	6.6	0	0	0	0
Number (%) with symptoms still present	0	4(21)	7(15)	6(24)	2(20)	2(20)	3(21)	1(12)	0

after three months radiological union has not been achieved, there is no advantage in continued immobilization. Although there is probably no need to immobilize a scaphoid infraction to achieve union, it is important to treat the patient and not the radiographs (London 1961). Even scaphoid infractions are painful and the patient expects to be, and should be, treated symptomatically.

Scaphoid non-union

Again it is important to treat the wrist and not the radiographs (London 1961). The number of individuals with scaphoid non-unions who are asymptomatic or minimally symptomatic is probably considerable and it is not known what proportion are sufficiently disabled to present for treatment (Scott 1956). Although it is customary for surgical treatment to be recommended for the symptomatic non-union, there is a conservative alternative. 'The ununited neglected fracture can be coaxed back to health by plaster of Paris' (Speed 1935). In a series of 436 scaphoid fractures, 99 were

old and 73% of these united with plaster immobilization (Stewart 1954). Similarly, in another series, seven out of nine old fractures (including five with avascular necrosis) also united with plaster immobilization (Dehne et al 1964). Prolonged immobilization of the wrist, however, particularly the dominant one, is disabling in itself and long-term immobilization, for three months or more, clearly has its drawbacks. Nonetheless, there would appear to be nothing wrong with the strategy of prescribing, say, six weeks of plaster immobilization followed by repeat radiographs in order to determine if union looks likely. Thus, the fracture line becoming less visible, cystic change filling in, avascular increased density becoming more normal would all be considered favourable radiological features and a policy of six weeks' immobilization would certainly spare some patients the need and uncertainties of surgical intervention. Furthermore, in some, although the radiographic features of non-union might not change, the patient may become asymptomatic and that, after all, is one aim of treatment.

REFERENCES

Barr J S, Elliston W A, Musnick H, Delorme T L, Hanelin J, Thibodeau A A 1953 Fracture of the carpal navicular (scaphoid) bone. Journal of Bone and Joint Surgery 35A:609–625

Berlin D 1929 Position in the treatment of fracture of the carpal scaphoid. New England Journal of Medicine 201:574–579

British Medical Journal 1981 Editorial: Fractures of the carpal scaphoid. 283:571–572

Cobey M C, White R K 1963 An operation for non-union of fractures of the carpal navicular. Journal of Bone and Joint Surgery 45A:1321–1322

Codman E A, Chase H M 1905 The diagnosis and treatment of fracture of the carpal scaphoid and dislocation of the semilunar bone. Annals of Surgery 41:321

Dawkins A L 1967 The fractured scaphoid: a modern view. Medical Journal of Australia 1:332–333

Dehne E, Deffer P A, Feighney R E 1964 Pathomechanics of the fracture of the carpal navicular. Journal of Trauma 4:96–114

Dickison J C, Shannon J G 1944 Fractures of the carpal scaphoid in the Canadian army. Surgery, Gynaecology and Obstetrics 79:225–239

Dunn A W 1972 Fractures and dislocations of the carpus. Surgical Clinics of North America 52:1513–1538

Fisk G R 1982 Injuries of the wrist. In: Wilson J N (ed) Watson-Jones Fractures and Joint Injuries (6th edn). Churchill Livingstone, Edinburgh, p 721

Friedenberg Z B 1949 Anatomic considerations in the treatment of carpal navicular fractures. American Journal of Surgery 78:379–381

Grace R V 1929 Fracture of the carpal scaphoid. Annals of Surgery 89:752–761

Hosford J P 1931 Prognosis in fractures of the carpal scaphoid. Proceedings of the Royal Society of Medicine 24:92–94

Jahna H 1954 Behandlung und Behandlungsergebnisse von 734 frischen einfachen Brüchen des Kahnbeinkörpers der Hand. Wiener medizinische Wochenschrift 104; 1023–1024

Kessler I, Heller J, Silberman Z, Pupko L 1963 Some aspects in nonunion of fractures of the carpal scaphoid. Journal of Trauma 3:442–452

Leslie I J, Dickson R A 1981 The fractured carpal scaphoid. Journal of Bone and Joint Surgery 63B:225–230

Leyshon A, Ireland J, Trickey E L 1984 The treatment of delayed union and non-union of the carpal scaphoid by screw fixation. Journal of Bone and Joint Surgery 66B:124–127

London P S 1961 The broken scaphoid bone. Journal of Bone and Joint Surgery 43B:237–244

Luck J V, Smith H M A, Lacey H B, Shands A R 1948 Orthopaedic surgery in the Army Air Forces during World War II. Recurrent dislocation of the shoulder and un-united fractures of the carpal scaphoid. Archives of Surgery 57:801–817

McLaughlin H L 1954 Fracture of the carpal navicular (scaphoid) bone. Journal of Bone and Joint Surgery 36A:765–774

McLaughlin H L, Parkes J C 1969 Fracture of the carpal

navicular (scaphoid) bone : gradations in therapy based upon pathology. Journal of Trauma 9 : 311–319

Margo M K, Seely J A 1963 A statistical review of 100 cases of fracture of the carpal navicular bone. Clinical Orthopaedics 31 : 102–104

Mazet R, Hohl M 1963 Fractures of the carpal navicular. Journal of Bone and Joint Surgery 45A : 82–112

Medical Defence Union 1983 Annual report. p 30–31

Murray G 1946 End results of bone grafting for non-union of the carpal navicular. Journal of Bone and Joint Surgery 28 : 749–756

Obletz B E, Halbstein B M 1938 Non-union of fractures of the carpal navicular. Journal of Bone and Joint Surgery 20 : 424–428

Perkins G 1950 Fracture of the carpal scaphoid. British Medical Journal 1 : 536–537

Russe O 1960 Fracture of the carpal navicular. Journal of Bone and Joint Surgery 42A : 759–768

Sashin D 1946 Treatment of fractures of the carpal scaphoid. Archives of Surgery 52 : 445–465

Scott J H S 1956 Assessment of ununited fractures of the carpal scaphoid. Proceedings of the Royal Society of Medicine 49 : 961–962

Soto-Hall R, Haldeman K O 1934 Treatment of fractures of the carpal scaphoid. Journal of Bone and Joint Surgery 16 : 822–828

Speed K 1935 Fractures of the carpus. Journal of Bone and Joint Surgery 17 : 965–968

Stewart M H 1954 Fractures of the carpal navicular (scaphoid). Journal of Bone and Joint Surgery 36A : 998–1006

Todd A H 1921 Fractures of the carpal scaphoid. British Journal of Surgery 9 : 7–26

Verdan C 1960 Fractures of the scaphoid. Surgical Clinics of North America 40 : 461–464

T. J. Herbert

17 Scaphoid fractures: operative treatment

Traditionally, operative treatment of scaphoid fractures has been limited to the management of non-union and its complications such as avascular necrosis and degenerative arthritis. More recently the value of surgery in the management of acute fractures of the scaphoid has been given more thought.

Cooney et al (1980) and others (Taleisnik 1982, O'Brien 1984) have drawn attention to the problems associated with *unstable* acute fractures of the scaphoid and the need to consider internal fixation in the management of these cases. McLaughlin (1954) advocated this approach over 30 years ago, but pointed out the technical problems involved in achieving satisfactory fixation. Maudsley and Chen (1972) and Huene (1979) have reported excellent results in limited series of acute fractures, using more refined techniques of internal fixation. O'Brien and Herbert (1985) emphasized the rapid restoration of wrist function associated with primary internal fixation of acute fractures. In spite of these reports, the vast majority of acute scaphoid fractures are still treated by the time-honoured method of immobilization in plaster, with little or no attempt being made to assess the severity of the injury or the degree of instability present. A fracture of the scaphoid signifies major trauma to the wrist, and it is unfortunate that radiographs do not indicate the amount of damage to the articular cartilage and carpal ligaments associated with this injury. Indeed, the initial films may even fail to show a fracture, although there has, in fact, been sufficient trauma to produce carpal instability and subsequent displacement of the bone fragments (Fig. 17.1).

The scaphoid bone, acting as it does as a stabilizing link between the two rows of the carpus, fractures in response to a disruptive force across the midcarpal joint. Whilst this becomes obvious in the case of a trans-scaphoid perilunate fracture dislocation (see Fig. 17.6), it may be that most scaphoid fractures occur as a result of transient subluxation of the midcarpal joint. An understanding of this mechanism of injury must increase one's awareness of the likelihood of instability and other complications. As pointed out by Weber (1980), scaphoid fractures are analogous to fractures of the femoral neck. As with other intra-articular fractures, one would expect that open reduction, to restore joint congruity, and internal fixation, to allow early motion, would produce better results than treatment in plaster. Why then has surgery never been accepted as the treatment of choice for scaphoid fractures? There appear to be three reasons for this.

1. The traditional teaching that 95% of acute scaphoid fractures will unite with adequate conservative treatment. However this does not apply to all types of scaphoid fracture. Cooney et al (1980) reported a union rate of 54% for displaced scaphoid fractures, and my own experiences have been similar. Malunion (Fig. 17.2), though seldom recognized, is also common. These problems will only be recognized by long-term and critical follow-up, which should include radiographs of both wrists at least a year after injury. It is not good enough to claim that union has occurred by, say, six weeks simply because the radiograph appears to show union of the fracture. This brings us to the second point.

2. There are problems associated with radiographic examination of the wrist. It is well known

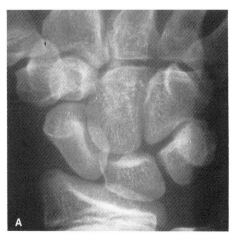 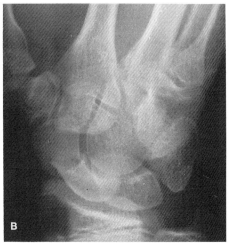

Fig. 17.1   (A) Initial radiograph following hyperextension injury to wrist in a 15-year-old boy. There does not appear to be any fracture of the scaphoid. (B) Radiographs of the same wrist, taken six weeks later, show a displaced fracture of the scaphoid with carpal instability

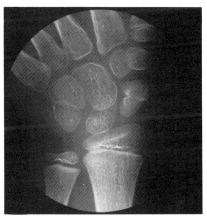 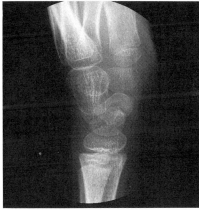

Fig. 17.2   Scaphoid fracture in an 8-year-old boy: radiographs following immobilization in plaster for three months show fibrous union with marked anterior angulatory deformity at the fracture site. The lateral view shows the scaphoid deformity and the associated carpal subluxation with dorsiflexion of the lunate

that radiographs may fail to show an acute scaphoid fracture. However, it is less well known that a fracture which appears radiologically united may, in fact, be un-united (Fig. 17.3). Similarly, standard views commonly fail to demonstrate instability of the acute fracture. In all cases, it is necessary to have high quality films and views should include PA (postero-anterior) in full ulnar and full radial deviation, 45° PA obliques and true laterals with the wrist in neutral position. Identical films of the opposite wrist should be taken for

comparison, since it is only in this way that minor differences in carpal alignment may be detected. There may well be a place for cineradiography or even arthrography in the management of acute scaphoid fractures.

3. The third reason relates to the problems of surgery and the difficulty in achieving satisfactory internal fixation. With the advent of the Herbert Scaphoid Bone Screw System (Fig. 17.4), it appears that some of these problems have been overcome (Herbert 1982, Herbert & Fisher 1984).

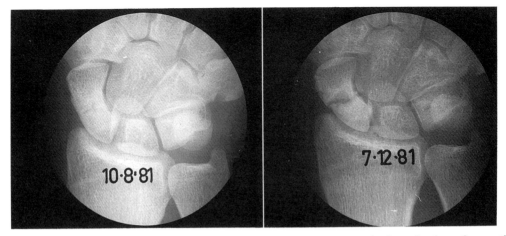

Fig. 17.3 This patient sustained a fractured scaphoid in March 1981. Following treatment in plaster for almost five months, radiographs (10.8.81) were reported as showing union. Four months later (7.12.81) there are clear signs of established non-union

Thus, an awareness of the high complication rate of conservative treatment, aided by precise diagnostic and operative methods, should lead to a new approach to the management of these troublesome fractures, with surgery becoming the treatment of choice in many instances.

ACUTE FRACTURES

Before embarking on surgery for acute scaphoid fractures it is essential that the surgeon is completely familiar with the instrumentation and operative techniques, as well as the anatomy of the wrist joint; familiarization through the use of cadavers is strongly recommended. Lack of experience is no reason to condemn the patient to non-operative treatment. If one is not proficient at this sort of surgery, the patient should be referred to someone who is.

Indications for surgery (in acute fractures)

The classification used is shown in Figure 17.5.

Unstable fractures (Type B).
1. Distal oblique (B1);
2. Mobile waist fractures (B2);
3. Proximal pole fractures (B3);
4. Fracture–dislocations (B4);
5. Comminuted and multiple fractures (B5).

Fractures showing signs of delayed union or displacement during treatment in plaster (Type C). Displacement of the fracture during treatment in plaster indicates unrecognized instability with a high likelihood of malunion or non-union. Similarly, the persistence of clinical and radiological signs of fracture following six weeks treatment in plaster is an indication to abandon conservative treatment. In these circumstances plaster should be removed and active mobilizing exercises of the wrist and hand commenced. Surgery should be delayed until joint stiffness and osteoporosis have

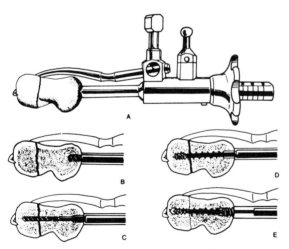

Fig. 17.4 Herbert scaphoid fixation system. (A) guiding jig clamps over scaphoid, holding fragments reduced and guiding instruments; (B) short drill for trailing screw thread; (C) long drill for leading screw thread; (D) tap for leading thread; (E) double threaded screw, inserted through jig on hexagonal driver. Compression produced by differing pitches on screw threads, the trailing thread being self-tapping

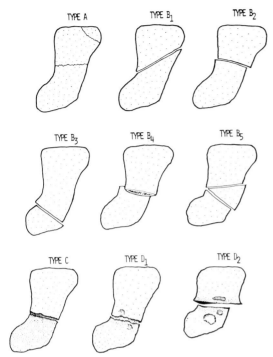

Fig. 17.5 Classification of scaphoid fractures according to their radiographical appearance. Type A: acute stable. Type B: acute unstable. Type C: delayed union. Type D: established non-union. (From Herbert & Fisher 1984)

been reversed; this normally takes at least two to three weeks.

Economic and social reasons. Given the choice, many patients would prefer to have their fracture treated by primary internal fixation, to avoid the limitations imposed on them by the use of plaster.

Surgical principles

1. Adequate exposure of fracture(s)
2. Atraumatic surgical technique
3. Anatomical reduction and restoration of articular surfaces
4. Rigid internal fixation
5. Careful repair of soft tissues, allowing
6. Early mobilization of the joint

Operative technique

Incision. The incision should be planned to allow adequate access to the fracture. The standard anterior approach, incising the capsule immediately beneath the flexor carpi radialis tendon, is normally the best approach to the scaphoid.

However, for small proximal pole fractures (i.e. less than 25% of the bone) a direct, dorsal approach is preferable. A transverse or curved longitudinal skin incision is used for this approach: the extensor pollicis longus tendon is mobilized and retracted, and the capsule is incised directly over the proximal pole of the scaphoid, which is easily palpable when the wrist is palmar-flexed.

For a simple trans-scaphoid perilunate fracture–dislocation, a long 'S' shaped anterior incision is employed, which will provide adequate access both to the scaphoid and to the carpal tunnel. For complex fracture–dislocations, two or more incisions may be required (Green 1982); the lower end of the radius may be exposed through an extended anterior incision or a lateral incision, whilst the rest of the carpus is best exposed from the dorsum.

Reduction of fracture. In most acute fractures, a haemarthrosis is present, so that a fine sucker must be used before one can visualize the fracture and adjacent bones. Reduction of the fracture can be difficult. Oblique fractures of the scaphoid are extremely unstable and reduction can only be achieved and held by the use of a Kirschner wire. If the fracture is comminuted, and the loose fragments cannot be reduced, it may be necessary to remove them and insert a bone graft in order to achieve a stable reduction.

If the midcarpal joint is dislocated, this can normally be reduced by gentle manipulation and traction prior to surgery. If this is not possible, the use of force should be avoided and open reduction is indicated. In all fracture–dislocations the carpal tunnel should be opened and the median nerve decompressed. There is frequently a large haematoma present, and this should be removed. The transverse tear in the anterior capsule is clearly seen in the floor of the carpal tunnel and the lunate may have dislocated through this. Following reduction, the tear should be repaired, using a fine non-absorbable suture.

Internal fixation. The use of a temporary Kirschner wire is of great benefit in achieving and holding an accurate anatomical reduction of the fracture. This should be placed as far ulnarwards as possible so that it does not interfere with insertion of the compression screw.

Occasionally, the fracture may appear unsuitable for compression fixation, in which case a second

K-wire should be used. However, postoperative plaster immobilization is always required in such cases, so that stiffness is likely. Furthermore, a second procedure to remove the wires is required.

The use of standard bone screws, whether of the cortical or cancellous type, is not normally recommended for this type of surgery. They can be very difficult to insert, fixation is usually inadequate, and the protruding screw head may cause problems.

The Herbert bone screw has proved to be satisfactory for fixation of such fractures (Herbert 1986). When the anterior approach has been used, the guiding jig should be applied to facilitate insertion of the screw. This requires mobilization of the scapho-trapezial joint, and it is important that the fracture will be stable on compression with the jig. If compression is likely to produce shearing displacement (oblique fractures) or collapse (comminuted fractures) stability can be achieved by the use of K-wires or bone graft (Fig. 17.6). Once the jig has been satisfactorily applied, drilling and tapping are carried out in the normal manner and the screw is inserted before the jig is removed. The wrist capsule should then be carefully repaired using a suitable fine suture, such as 4/0 Ethibond.

For proximal pole fractures of the scaphoid, exposed dorsally, and for most other carpal fractures, the jig cannot be used and the screw must be inserted freehand. The drill guide should be removed from the jig and held in the handle provided with the instrument set (Fig. 17.7A). The fracture should be compressed as firmly as possible by manual pressure and the drill guide aligned perpendicular to the fracture. It is important to realize that the axis of the scaphoid lies approximately 45° from the horizontal and 45° radially. Following instrumentation, a screw of appropriate length (16–18 mm) is inserted through the guide and a check radiograph is taken (Fig. 17.7B). Again, the wrist capsule is carefully repaired, using a fine non-absorbable suture.

Postoperative management

With good surgical technique, anatomical reconstruction of the carpus and satisfactory stability of both the fracture and the capsuloligamentous structures should have been achieved. A supportive dressing of wool and bandage is applied and a

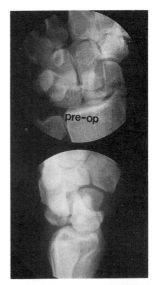
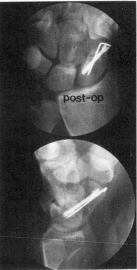

Fig. 17.6 An acute transcaphoid perilunate fracture dislocation. At operation, a K-wire was used to hold the reduction and to prevent shearing displacement of the fracture under compression from the screw

plaster front-slab is applied to hold the wrist in approximately 20° of dorsiflexion. The dressings are reduced as soon as practicable, and it is normally possible to start gentle assisted mobilizing exercises of the wrist within a few days; the more severe the injury, the sooner the mobilization should be started. Once the wound has healed, the patient is usually fitted with a light removable front-splint which is used to protect the wrist from further

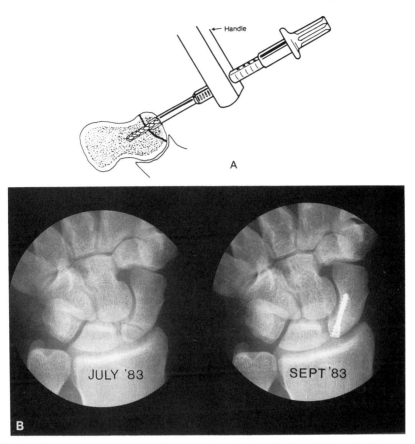

Fig. 17.7 (A) Freehand insertion of screw—when jig cannot be used, the guide is held by hand and is pushed firmly to compress the fracture. (B) Radiographs showing retrograde screw fixation of unstable proximal pole fracture (type B3)

trauma during the healing period. However, active use and exercise, including swimming, are encouraged and most patients are able to return to work within a few weeks of surgery.

Summary

Excellent results can be achieved using these techniques in the management of acute scaphoid fractures, although the risk of avascular necrosis in certain cases remains (O'Brien & Herbert 1985). However, such surgery is technically demanding and it behoves the surgeon to be familiar with the anatomy of the wrist and with the instrumentation before undertaking this form of treatment.

FIBROUS UNION

Two observations lead me to believe that fibrous union (Type D1) is a relatively common occur-

rence following conservative treatment of scaphoid fractures.

The first observation is that a very significant number of patients presenting with painful non-union, give a history of a previous acute fracture treated conservatively with an apparently successful outcome. That is to say, following treatment in plaster, the wrist became relatively (but seldom completely) symptom-free, and radiographs appeared to show reasonable bony union. Usually as a result of further injury to the wrist, the patient then develops symptoms and signs of non-union, and subsequent films show the presence of an established pseudarthrosis (*see Fig. 17.3*). The implication is that the original fracture must have healed by a fibrous union.

The second observation is that, when one operates on a scaphoid fracture which is developing radiological signs of non-union following conservative treatment, one is often surprised to find apparent union of the fracture. Quite frequently, the articular cartilage appears to have healed and it may be difficult to demonstrate any mobility at the fracture site. However, once the fracture has been identified and prised open, a fibrous union is discovered with cysts extending into both fragments. Interestingly enough, there are often synovial adhesions to the fracture site, presumably an attempt by the body to immobilize the fracture. Could it be that the synovium grows between the fracture surfaces, producing a fibrous union?

The natural history of fibrous union is not yet fully understood. It may be that prolonged immobilization will lead to bony union, albeit at the price of considerable wrist stiffness. At the other extreme, it appears that some cases of fibrous union progress quite rapidly into a mobile pseudarthrosis. What does seem certain is that fibrous union is more common than previously suspected and that it renders the wrist unduly susceptible to further injury, leading to the development of pseudarthrosis and later osteoarthritis. The best way to avoid these problems is to maintain a high index of suspicion and to improve follow-up procedures after conservative treatment. Ideally, all patients should be re-examined after a year. The persistence of swelling and tenderness around the scaphoid, together with discomfort on forced dorsiflexion of the wrist should raise the suspicion of a fibrous union. Radiographs will normally show an indistict fracture line with variable cystic changes, but no obvious deformity or carpal instability (Fig. 17.8A). In cases of doubt, one may need to consider tomography or CT scan.

Until the natural history of this condition is better understood, the best method of treatment must remain speculative. However, it is difficult to justify prolonged immobilization in plaster, in view of the incapacity that this causes the patient. It would seem more logical to immobilize the fracture by means of internal fixation. However, in the author's experience, compression screw fixation of a fibrous union does not always lead to sound bone union (Fig. 17.8B). It may be that the intact cortex has prevented sufficient compression, and I now believe that all fibrous tissue should be removed and the fracture bone-grafted, in order to encourage union.

Indications for surgery (in Type D1 fractures)

Absolute: persistent symptoms with obvious radiological changes.

Relative: continued doubt about union, particularly in younger patients.

Surgical principles

1. Free all synovial adhesions at fracture site
2. Open up fracture site and carefully remove all fibrous tissue and cysts
3. Cancellous bone grafting

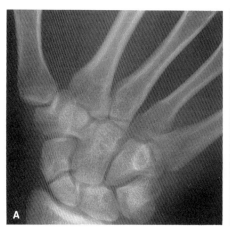
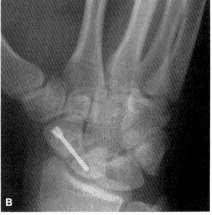

Fig. 17.8   (A) Fibrous union with no obvious instability or deformity; note presence of cysts in distal fragment. At operation the articular cartilage appeared healed and the fracture was left undisturbed. (B) Persistent non-union following compression screw fixation with loosening around the screw thread. This fracture should have been bone-grafted

4. Stabilize fracture, preferably by compression screw fixation
5. Early mobilization to prevent recurrent adhesions

Operative technique

Approach. The anterior approach should be used for all but small proximal pole fractures, which are best approached dorsally. The adherent capsule and synovium will need to be carefully freed in order to expose the fracture site.

Preparation of fracture. In the presence of a slightly mobile fibrous union without significant radiological changes, it may be justifiable to carry out compression fixation without disturbing the fracture. In all other cases the fracture line must be prised open, and fibrous tissue should be completely cleared. All cysts demonstrated on X-ray examination should be identified and carefully curetted. Small islands of sclerotic bone at the fracture line should also be removed. Fresh cancellous bone chips harvested from the iliac crest, should then be packed into all defects and into the fracture line.

Fixation. Kirschner wire fixation is contra-indicated, particularly when a bone graft has not been carried out, since it fails to produce compression. Similarly, the use of standard bone screws is unlikely to produce sufficient rigid fixation to ensure union.

These cases are an ideal indication for using the Herbert Bone Screw System. The jig is normally very simple to apply, and excellent compression and stability can be achieved, so that no postoperative immobilization is required. Care should be taken to ensure that the jig is applied in such a way that the screw will lie perpendicular to the line of the fracture. In the case of a small proximal pole fracture, where the screw is inserted freehand via a dorsal approach, it is most important to ensure that the fracture has been sufficiently well prepared to allow firm manual compression of the two fragments.

Other techniques. Most bone grafting techniques will achieve success when applied to fibrous union. The disadvantage of bone grafting without internal fixation is the need for postoperative immobilization in plaster, although this may be required only for relatively short periods if the fracture is stable.

PSEUDARTHROSIS

In the presence of established non-union or pseudarthrosis (Type D2) of the scaphoid, the fracture is usually completely mobile and unstable, although occasionally there may be a loose fibrous union present. In these circumstances the midcarpal joint is unsupported, leading to progressive carpal collapse and anterior angulatory deformity at the fracture site. The fracture surfaces become increasingly hard and sclerotic, and the proximal fragment tends to wear down and may reach a stage where there is a major discrepancy in size between the two fragments. Recent studies (Mack et al 1984, Ruby et al 1985) have shown that the natural history of scaphoid pseudarthrosis is one of progressive collapse and deformity, leading to radiocarpal osteoarthritis.

Whilst it is true that some patients may remain relatively asymptomatic for many years, wrist function is seldom normal, and there is a high susceptibility to further injury. Examination of the wrist nearly always reveals significant swelling and tenderness over the scaphoid. Wrist movements, particularly dorsiflexion, are usually restricted, except in patients with ligamentous laxity. Loss of dorsiflexion is usually associated with angulatory deformity of the scaphoid and in advanced cases, restriction of movement may be marked. Radiographs (Fig. 17.9) demonstrate instability at the fracture site with sclerosis of the bone faces and variable cystic changes. Deformity is best appreciated by comparing the length of the scaphoid in the PA view with the opposite, uninjured wrist. Carpal collapse is apparent in the lateral films and if the outline of the scaphoid can be traced, the deformity of the fragments is clear. This deformity may also be demonstrated nicely by means of lateral tomography.

There are three primary aims of treatment for scaphoid pseudarthrosis.

To relieve symptoms. This is best achieved by obtaining sound union, although stabilization of the fracture by internal fixation may produce temporary relief. When symptoms are due to

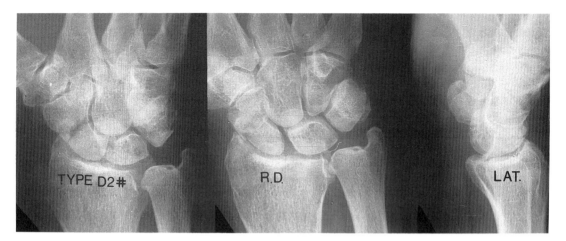

Fig. 17.9 Pseudarthrosis of scaphoid. *Note* mobility of fracture, with sclerosis of fracture faces. There is carpal instability with dorsiflexion of the lunate, anterior angulatory deformity of the scaphoid (apparent on RD view) and early degenerative osteoarthritis

degenerative arthritis, other operative techniques are required (see 'Other procedures').

To stabilize the carpus. With union of the scaphoid, progressive carpal collapse is prevented.

To correct carpal deformity. In the ideal case, it is possible to reconstruct the scaphoid and at the same time correct the carpal deformity. When this can be achieved, the range of dorsiflexion of the wrist will be considerably improved. However, full correction may not be possible, depending on the degree of soft tissue contracture.

When one considers these aims, it becomes clear that there is no place for plaster immobilization, electrical stimulation or internal fixation without bone grafting, in the management of pseudarthrosis of the scaphoid, except to produce short-term symptomatic relief. Treatment involves reconstructive surgery of the carpus.

Indications for reconstruction of the scaphoid

1. Symptomatic non-union
2. Asymptomatic non-union in younger patients at risk of developing increasing deformity

Contraindications

1. Necrosis of proximal fragment
2. Insufficient bone stock
3. Degenerative changes throughout the wrist, especially if the wrist is stiff; in these cases, an

alternative procedure is usually indicated (see 'Other procedures')

Surgical principles

1. Complete resection of pseudarthrosis, back to healthy bone
2. Reconstruction of scaphoid, using corticocancellous bone graft
3. Correction of carpal deformity
4. Stabilization of the scaphoid, to allow protected mobilization

Operative technique

Careful preoperative planning is required. The degree of deformity and shortening of the scaphoid should be determined by comparison with radiographs of the normal wrist. The opposite iliac crest should be prepared as the donor site for bone grafting.

Approach. Ideally, the scaphoid should be exposed by the standard anterior approach, since this permits complete visualization of both fragments and correction of the anterior angulatory deformity. Fisk (1978) prefers a lateral approach with excision of the radial styloid which is used as a bone graft. Others tend to prefer a dorsal approach, although the anterior approach was recommended by Russe (1960), whose technique remains the most popular one at the present time.

Fracture preparation. Whichever method of bone grafting is chosen, it is essential that the pseudarthrosis is resected sufficiently to expose healthy cancellous bone in each fragment. If, after resection, either fragment still appears sclerotic, a decision will need to be made as to whether it is reasonable to continue with bone grafting, or whether replacement arthroplasty or some other procedure is indicated. Provided there appears to be any possibility of revascularization, however, an attempt should be made to reconstruct the scaphoid.

For a volar inlay or Russe type graft, a gutter is then cut in the anterior cortex of both fragments which are hollowed out using a small curette. The cavities are packed with cancellous bone, and the fracture is stabilized by inserting two strips of corticocancellous bone, back to back and tightly impacted within the gutter to provide stability (Green 1985). Reasonable correction of the deformity may be achieved using this technique, although prolonged postoperative plaster immobilization is normally required.

The author's preferred technique (Fig. 17.10) involves excision of both fracture faces using a small osteotome. The cuts are made perpendicular to the long axis of the scaphoid so that the sandwich graft will be stable when inserted.

An attempt is made to preserve a soft tissue hinge posteriorly. Any residual pockets of sclerotic bone or fibrous tissue are carefully removed and the cavities packed with cancellous bone graft. The wrist is then forcibly dorsiflexed, a maneuvre which tends to correct the carpal deformity and open out the defect in the scaphoid to full length. A block of corticocancellous bone, of sufficient size to fill the defect, is then removed from the iliac crest. The bone graft should not be soaked in saline, but prepared and inserted as quickly as possible. The graft is carefully shaped, using small bone cutters and rongeurs, so that it fits accurately, the cortex lying flush with the anterior surface of the scaphoid (Fig. 17.10). The graft should be sufficiently wide to prevent any collapse when compression is applied. The graft is firmly impacted using a small punch and should be quite stable at this stage.

In the case of a small proximal pole fracture, it is not normally feasible to attempt elongation of the scaphoid. Cancellous bone graft is normally sufficient, and preparation of the proximal fracture face is kept to a minimum, in order to preserve sufficient bone for screw fixation.

Internal fixation. As with other types of scaphoid fracture, compression screw fixation provides maximum rigidity, so that early mobilization of the wrist may be commenced. Using the Herbert Bone Screw Instrumentation, application of the jig is usually relatively straightforward, provided the deformity has been adequately corrected and the scaphotrapezial joint sufficiently mobilized. It is important to appreciate that the scaphoid bone lies at approximately $45°$ to the horizontal plane, so that the tip of the blade should be directed as far posteriorly as possible. The jig should be applied in such a way that the screw will cross perpendicular to the line of the fracture. The jig should be compressed as firmly as possible, and at this stage the graft should be tightly locked between the two bone fragments. Drilling and tapping are then carried out by hand in the normal manner and a screw of appropriate length inserted. After removal of the jig, the screw is tightened a further one to two turns, thus providing maximum compression and ensuring that the leading thread lies entirely within the proximal fragment (see Fig. 17.11). The graft is carefully checked for stability and any prominences are trimmed with a rongeur until flush with the surface of the scaphoid. At this stage, wrist movements are checked; the range of dorsiflexion should be recorded and stability of fixation again noted. The capsule is then repaired using a fine non-absorbable suture.

Postoperative management

Provided that satisfactory fixation has been achieved, no postoperative immobilization is required and the patient is encouraged to commence early mobilizing exercises of the wrist. At the same time he is advised to avoid contact sports, or any other activity which could disrupt the repair, for a period of at least three months. With this regimen, union appears to be accelerated and function of the

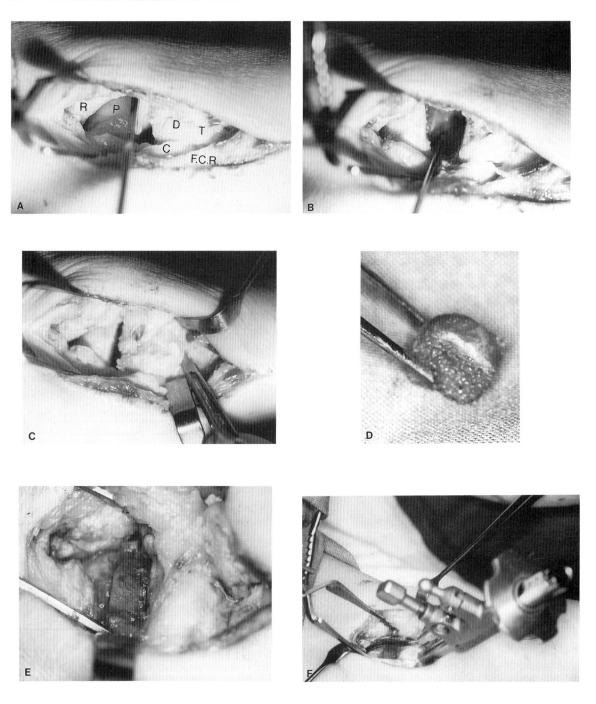

Fig. 17.10 Operative technique of scaphoid reconstruction: left wrist, anterior approach. (A) Resection of proximal fracture face with osteotome. (R = radius, P = proximal fragment, D = distal fragment, T = trapezium, C = capsule, FCR = Flexor Carpi Radialis tendon). (B) Defect left following resection of pseudarthrosis and forced dorsiflexion of wrist to correct deformity. *Note* intact soft-tissue hinge posteriorly. (C) Incision of capsule of scaphotrapezial joint. The distal end of the scaphoid should be mobilized sufficiently to allow easy application of the jig. (D) Block of corticocancellous bone graft from outer table of iliac crest. (E) Graft inserted; cortex lies flush with anterior surface of scaphoid, providing stability on compression. (F) Jig has been applied; *note* that graft has been tightly compressed and will be transfixed by screw

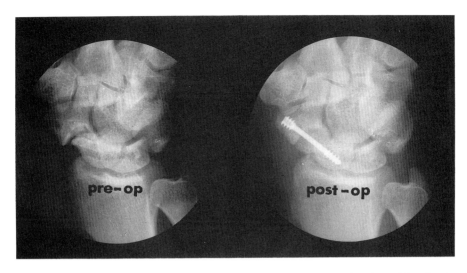

Fig. 17.11   Radiographs before and after reconstruction of scaphoid: *note* correction of deformity and firm fixation of graft by compression screw. Postoperative plaster not required

wrist, including range of movement, improves rapidly.

It is often difficult to be certain when union has occurred. With satisfactory technique, the fracture surfaces should not be visible on the initial postoperative radiograph (*see* Fig. 17.11). In successful cases, the graft remains fully incorporated; failure of union is indicated by resorption of the graft or loosening of the screw. Should this occur, and provided that the initial operation was carried out correctly, it is reasonable to assume that one or other of the scaphoid fragments is ischaemic and has lost the potential for regeneration. Under these circumstances, there is no point in carrying out further bone grafting. The patient may well remain asymptomatic for as long as the screw is stabilizing the two fragments. However, he should be warned that his wrist is unduly susceptible to further injury. If symptoms recur, then an alternative procedure will need to be considered.

OTHER PROCEDURES

Radial styloidectomy

This can be a useful procedure in the management of scaphoid non-union. Quite commonly, there may be deformity or degenerative change, localized to the articulation between the styloid process of the radius and the distal pole of the scaphoid.

Characteristically, an impingement type of pain occurs on radial deviation and palmar flexion of the wrist, and both these movements may be restricted. Under these circumstances, it is reasonable to carry out a limited radial styloidectomy, excising just enough bone to prevent impingement between the distal pole of the scaphoid and the radius (Fig. 17.12).

In the case of a scaphoid pseudarthrosis with secondary radiocarpal osteoarthritis, I prefer to carry out scaphoid reconstruction first, since elongation of the bone may relieve the radiocarpal impingement. Radial styloidectomy is usually reserved for the occasional patient in whom symptoms persist following successful reconstruction.

Operative technique

An incision 3 cm long is made directly over the radial styloid process. Care is taken to preserve the cutaneous branches of the radial nerve and the dorsal branch of the radial artery as it crosses the scaphoid distally. The wrist is held in ulnar deviation, and the periosteum over the lower end of the radius is incised between the first and second dorsal compartments. The periosteum and wrist capsule are elevated sufficiently to expose the joint between the styloid process of the radius and the scaphoid. Using a fine osteotome, directed approx-

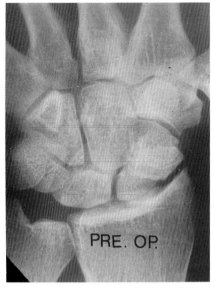
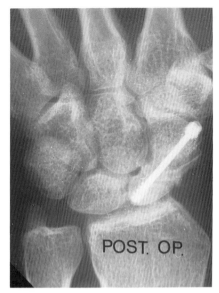

Fig. 17.12 Before and after limited radial styloidectomy following scaphoid reconstruction for longstanding non-union, with angulatory deformity and secondary radiocarpal osteoarthritis

imately 45° distally, just sufficient bone is removed to ensure that there is no impingement on full radial deviation and palmar flexion. The raw bone surface is plugged with bone wax and the soft tissues are repaired with a fine non-absorbable suture. With this technique, the radiocarpal ligaments remain intact, and there is no risk of instability. Following operation, a plaster front slab is used for 2–3 weeks, after which time it is normally safe to mobilize the wrist without further support.

Scaphoid replacement arthroplasty

Excision of part or all of the scaphoid should be avoided whenever possible in view of its strong ligamentous attachments and the role that the scaphoid plays in stabilizing the carpus. However, in the case of pan-scaphoid osteoarthritis, or when there is insufficient bone for reconstruction, symptoms may be relieved by inserting a silicone rubber scaphoid implant (Swanson 1970). In order to stabilize the carpus and to avoid overloading the prosthesis, one should consider carrying out a limited carpal fusion at the same time. If degenerative changes extend to the capitate–lunate joint, this should be fused (Watson 1980). If not, one may consider a triquetro-hamate fusion, which

preserves a greater range of wrist motion than the former.

Normally, it is only the proximal pole of the scaphoid which undergoes avascular necrosis, or which may need to be replaced following a failed bone grafting procedure. In order to preserve a smooth articulation, and prevent further collapse following excision of the proximal pole, the use of a stabilized Silastic hemi-prosthesis is recommended (Herbert 1984). A size 1 Silastic scaphoid prosthesis is cut down sufficiently to replace the excised fragment of bone only, leaving a large square peg which is locked into a suitable cavity prepared in the distal fragment (Fig. 17.13). This technique seems to impart significant stability to the implant, so that late collapse and dislocation have not been a problem. However, there is no doubt that Silastic implants do tend to wear down, particularly under loading and this may lead to the development of synovitis and cystic change in the adjacent bones. There is obviously a need for a more suitable material for arthroplasty of the scaphoid; allografts may prove to be the answer to this problem.

Partial wrist fusion

As mentioned above, there may occasionally be a place for limited fusion of the wrist in the management of un-united fractures of the scaphoid, particularly when degenerative changes involve the midcarpal joint. Scapholunate fusion has been recommended as a method of treatment for avascular necrosis of the proximal pole of the scaphoid. However, this is a very difficult procedure which is likely to result in significant loss of motion of the wrist. For this reason, I prefer to treat avascular necrosis by partial Silastic replacement, reserving scapholunate fusion for the correction of rotary dislocation of the scaphoid.

Arthrodesis of the wrist

There is no question that this is an extremely satisfactory procedure in the right circumstances. When the wrist is stiff and painful, as a result of generalized degenerative changes, or following previous unsuccessful surgery, most patients will be best served by arthrodesing the joint. In spite of the loss of movement, pain relief will result in significant improvement in hand function and grip strength. The wrist should usually be fused in 20°–30° of dorsiflexion.

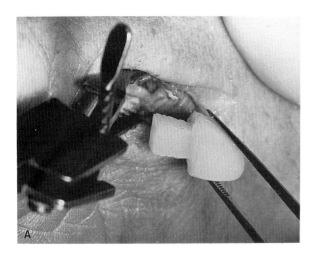
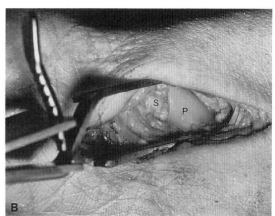
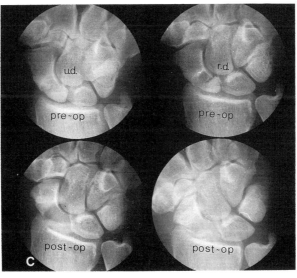

Fig. 17.13 Avascular necrosis of the scaphoid: partial Silastic replacement. The cut down Swanson implant, showing square stem which locks into suitable cavity prepared in distal fragment (A). Following insertion of prosthesis, note stable fit (B). Radiograph showing hemisilastic replacement for avascular necrosis (C). *Note* improved range of motion and stability of implant

Operative technique

A curved dorsal incision is used, extending from the midshaft of the third metacarpal distally, across the scapholunate junction, to 6 cm proximally over the shaft of the radius. The extensor retinaculum is divided and the tendons retracted. The joints between the radius, lunate, capitate, scaphoid, trapezoid and trapezium are excised and packed with cancellous bone. The ulnar carpal and carpometacarpal joints need not be disturbed unless they are involved in the degenerative process. If there has been a previous Silastic arthroplasty, the prosthesis should be removed and the space filled with a block of cancellous bone. The wrist should be placed in approximately 25° of dorsiflexion with neutral deviation, and any remaining gaps between the bones tightly packed with graft. A slab of corticocancellous bone graft, taken from the outer border of the iliac crest, is laid over the dorsum of the wrist and firmly impacted in position (Fig. 17.14).

Internal fixation is then carried out. The use of an AO condylar 'T' plate, with 3.5 mm screws, is preferred. The plate can be accurately contoured to fit the bone and hold the wrist in the correct amount of dorsiflexion. The distal end of the plate is carefully curved over the bases of the second and third metacarpals and is fixed to each of these using cortical screws of appropriate length. At least three screws should be inserted proximally into the

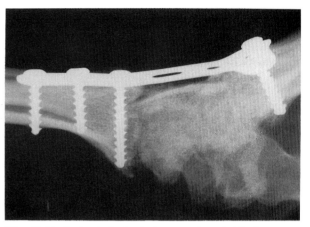

Fig. 17.14 Arthrodesis of wrist in approximately 25° of dorsiflexion, using AO 'T'-plate; the vertical limb of the plate is fixed to the radius and the cross-bar to the bases of the second and third metacarpals, using 3.5 mm cortical screws. *Note* the cortico-cancellous bone graft wedged between the radius and carpus

radius (*see* Fig. 17.14). The extensor carpi radialis longus tendon, having previously being detached from its insertion, is sutured over the plate to cover the screw heads. The extensor pollicis longus tendon is relocated in its normal position and the extensor retinaculum is repaired. The use of a small suction drain is strongly recommended, and the wrist is protected in a light, Colles-type plaster for approximately four weeks. The plate is normally removed, as soon as the fusion is sound.

REFERENCES

Cooney W P, Dobyns J H, Linscheid R L 1980 Fractures of the scaphoid: a rational approach to management, Clinical Orthopaedics and Related Research 149:90–97

Fisk G R 1979 Surgery of the Wrist. In: Rob and Smith's Operative Surgery, Orthopaedics Pt 2, Butterworth, London, p 540–543

Green D P 1982 Carpal Dislocations. In: Green D P Operative Hand Surgery Vol 1, Churchill Livingstone, Edinburgh, p 725–730

Green D P 1985 The effect of avascular necrosis on Russe bone grafting for scaphoid non-union. Journal of Hand Surgery 10A:597–605

Herbert T J 1982 The Herbert Scaphoid Bone Screw System. Technical Publication, Zimmer Inc, Warsaw, Indiana

Herbert T J 1984 Avascular necrosis of the scaphoid: partial replacement using a stabilised silicone implant. Journal of Bone and Joint Surgery 66-B:776

Herbert T J 1986 Use of the Herbert bone screw in surgery of

the wrist. Clinical Orthopaedics and Related Research 202:79–92

Herbert T J, Fisher W E 1984 Management of the fractured scaphoid using a new bone screw. Journal of Bone and Joint Surgery 66-B:114–123

Huene D R 1979 Primary internal fixation of carpal navicular fractures in the athlete. American Journal of Sports Medicine 7:174–177

Mack G R, Bosse M J, Gelberman R H, Yu E 1984 The natural history of scaphoid non-union. Journal of Bone and Joint Surgery 66-A:504–509

McLaughlin H L 1954 Fracture of the carpal navicular (scaphoid) bone. Journal of Bone and Joint Surgery 36A:765–774

Maudsley R H, Chen S C 1972 Screw fixation in the management of the fractured carpal scaphoid. Journal of Bone and Joint Surgery 54-B:432–441

O'Brien E T 1984 Acute fractures and dislocation of the

carpus. The Orthopaedic Clinics of North America 15(2):237–258

O'Brien L, Herbert T J 1985 Internal fixation of acute scaphoid fractures: a new approach to treatment. The Australian and New Zealand Journal of Surgery 55:387–389

Ruby L K, Stinson J, Belsky M R 1985 The natural history of scaphoid non-union. Journal of Bone and Joint Surgery 67-A:428–432

Russe O 1960 Fracture of the carpal navicular: diagnosis, non-operative treatment, and operative treatment. Journal of Bone and Joint Surgery 42-A:759–768

Swanson A B 1970 Silicone rubber implants for the replacement of the carpal scaphoid and lunate bones. Orthopaedic Clinics of North America 1:299–309

Taleisnik J 1982 Fractures of the carpal bones. In: Green D P Operative Hand Surgery Vol 1, Churchill Livingstone, Edinburgh, p 669–702

Watson H K 1980 Limited wrist arthrodesis. Clinical Orthopaedics and Related Research 149:126–136

Weber E R 1980 Biochemical implications of scaphoid waist fractures. Clinical Orthopaedics and Related Research 149:83–89

Glenn A. Buterbaugh and Andrew K. Palmer

18 Other carpal fractures

The scaphoid is the carpal bone that is most frequently fractured, but fractures involving the other bones of the carpus are not uncommon. The doctor assessing an injured wrist must have a thorough understanding of the anatomy of the carpus, including the geometry of each carpal bone, as well as the ligamentous supports and vascularity as they relate to the rest of the carpus. The examiner must also be aware of the different types of carpal fractures due to the subtle nature of these injuries and the difficulty in their diagnosis. A high index of suspicion, based on the knowledge of a particular fracture, is important in the initial assessment. Subsequent X-ray evaluation based on the clinical suspicion includes standard wrist views as well as special oblique and carpal tunnel views, tomography and CT (computerized tomography) scans. Once the diagnosis is established, treatment can then commence and then vary from simple immobilization for undisplaced injuries to open reduction and internal fixation for displaced fractures, particularly in the case of articular involvement.

FRACTURES OF THE LUNATE

Anatomy

The lunate, anatomically and functionally, is the intercalated segment in the wrist. Proximally it articulates with the lunate fossa and distally its semilunar shape articulates with the head of the capitate and hamate. On the radial side there is a small articulating surface with the scaphoid, as well as the attachment of the strong scapholunate interosseous ligament. On the medial side of the lunate, a small articulating surface is present for the triquetrum, as well as the attachment of the strong lunotriquetral ligament. The anterior aspect of the lunate provides the attachment for the radioscapholunate ligament, as well as vascular foramina. The dorsal surface also bears multiple vascular foramina at the attachment of a dorsal radiocarpal ligament.

The vascularity of the lunate has been well described by Gelberman et al (1980) who have shown a profuse system of dorsal and palmar vessels feeding the carpal vascular plexus. From this plexus, nutrient vessels enter the lunate from its non-articular dorsal and palmar poles. Significant interosseous anastomoses were noted in all specimens.

As an intercalated segment, the lunate reacts to the motion of the scaphoid and triquetrum. This can be well seen in examining the wrist as one progresses from radial to ulnar deviation. In radial deviation, the lunate is palmar-flexed with the scaphoid; as ulnar deviation commences, the lunate progressively dorsiflexes in response to the changing position of the triquetrum and scaphoid.

Mechanisms of injury

Fractures of the lunate can occur as an isolated event or in association with Kienböck's disease. They can result from a single injury or multiple repetitive stresses. A lunate fracture does not necessarily lead to avascular necrosis of the lunate.

Isolated lunate fractures most frequently involve the dorsal and palmar poles. *Palmar pole fractures* have been attributed to avulsion of the attachments of the radioscapholunate and radiolunotriquetral ligaments (Dobyns et al 1982). Non-union of the fracture will frequently result if the fragments are significantly displaced. *Dorsal pole fractures* (Fig. 18.1) occur as an impaction injury on the dorsal lip of the distal radius caused by severe wrist dorsiflexion or as an avulsion injury of the dorsal capsular attachment by palmar flexion. With severe injury, dorsal pole fractures can be associated with tears of the scapholunate ligament and a dorsiflexion instability pattern (DISI) as shown in Figure 18.2.

The aetiology of Kienböck's disease is unknown but generally felt to be secondary to repetitive trauma with resultant small compressive fractures and an interruption in the anastomotic blood supply of the lunate. It is associated with the ulnar minus variant in the majority of cases (Beckenbaugh et al 1980).

Clinical evaluation

Most patients describe either isolated trauma or, occasionally, repetitive trauma causing pain over the dorsal aspect of the wrist. On physical examination there is localized tenderness over the

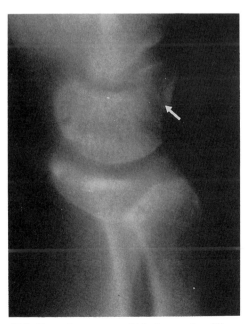

Fig. 18.1 Lateral tomogram which shows a dorsal lip fracture of the lunate not visible on the standard lateral wrist films

fracture, most notably on the dorsal aspect of the wrist, and pain on movements of the wrist.

Radiolographical evaluation

The diagnosis of lunate fractures can sometimes be made on standard wrist radiographs in the lateral or oblique views but, due to bony overlap of the scaphoid, triquetrum and distal radius, tomography may be required to make the diagnosis.

Kienböck's disease is a radiographic diagnosis of avascular necrosis of the lunate. The radiographic stages of the disease have been identified by Lichtman et al (1982). In Stage I radiographs show a lunate that is not fragmented or collapsed. Linear fractures or sclerosis may be present but the lunate itself is maintained. In Stage II there is fragmentation of the lunate but no carpal collapse (Fig. 18.3). In Stage III, there is, in addition to fragmentation of the lunate, carpal collapse with instability: in particular, on the lateral radiograph, one will note lunate dorsiflexion with scaphoid palmar-flexion and a scapholunate angle approaching 90°. In Stage IV one begins to see osteoarthritis in association with collapse of the lunate (Fig. 18.4).

Treatment

Fractures. The treatment of lunate fractures usually consists of cast immobilization for 4–6 weeks. With large dorsal pole fractures, the lunate may dorsally translate and tilt palmarward (*see Fig. 18.2*). If a large fragment exists and is displaced, open reduction and internal fixation have, according to some reports, been used with success. Occasionally non-union of the dorsal pole fracture results in persistent wrist pain: with continued symptoms, excision of the non-union will frequently result in relief of pain.

Kienböck's disease. The treatment depends on the severity of the changes. Prior to the onset of degenerative changes, many different methods have been recommended: these procedures have included radial shortening (Almquist & Burns 1982, Simmons & Dommisse 1975), ulnar lengthening (Armistead et al, 1982), scaphotrapezial-trapezoid arthrodesis (Watson et al 1985), capito-hamate arthrodesis (Chuinard 1980), lunate

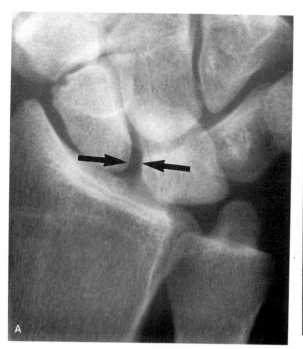

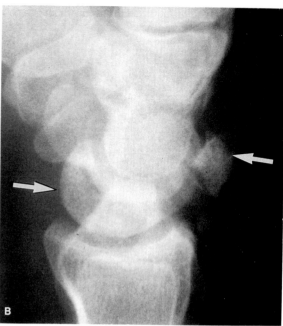

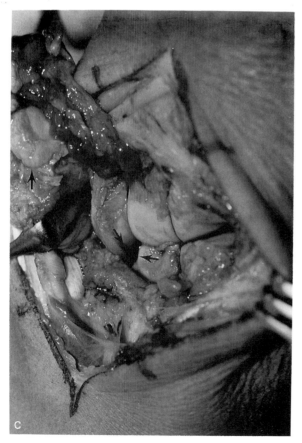

Fig. 18.2 Fracture of the dorsal pole of the lunate associated with marked dorsiflexion instability of the wrist. (A) On the PA film *note* the scapholunate diastasis whose appearance at operation reveals disruption of the scapholunate ligament (C) (arrows); there is also a fracture of the pole of the lunate attached to the dorsal capsule (arrow on left). (B) On the lateral radiograph, *note* the dorsiflexed and palmarly displaced lunate (arrow on left) with the large dorsal pole fracture (arrow on right)

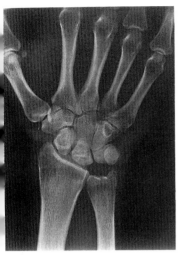
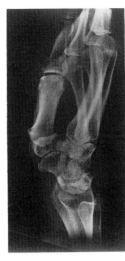

Fig. 18.3 PA and lateral radiographs show Stage II Kienböck's disease. *Note* the sclerosis, cyst formation, and fragmentation of the lunate. There is minimal collapse. Also *note* the ulnar-minus variance

excision and silicone arthroplasty (Stark et al 1981). With the onset of severe degenerative changes, proximal row carpectomy (Inglis & Jones 1977) or arthrodesis of the wrist (Graner et al 1966) are suggested.

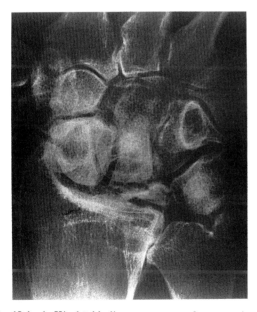

Fig. 18.4 As Kienböck's disease progresses, fragmentation and collapse of the lunate and degenerative arthritis occur. This radiograph shows severe lunate collapse with early degenerative changes consistent with Stage IV Kienböck's disease

Our preferred method of treatment for Stage I is no treatment. For Stage II or III we do a joint levelling procedure (radial shortening or ulnar lengthening) for patients with an ulnar-minus variance, and scaphotrapezial-trapezoid or scapho-capitate arthrodesis for patients with a neutral or ulnar-plus variance. In Stage IV, we recommend salvage procedures such as a limited or complete wrist fusion, depending on the amount of arthritic involvement.

FRACTURES OF THE TRIQUETRUM

Anatomy

The triquetrum is a triangular bone on the medial end of the proximal row, that articulates with the lunate and the hamate. It also articulates with the pisiform palmarly. The triquetrum has strong ligamentous supports, including a strong inter-osseous ligament between the triquetrum and lunate and the radiolunotriquetal ligament. The articulation between the triquetrum and hamate is firmly fixed by the ulnar branch of the arcuate ligament. The geometrical relationship between the triquetrum and the hamate plays an important role in the biomechanics of the wrist, most easily visualized on radial and ulnar deviation, when the inclined planes of the triquetrum and hamate are responsible for alteration in the position of the triquetrum, lunate and scaphoid.

Mechanisms of injury

Fractures of the triquetrum are the third most common carpal fractures, and can occur as flake fractures, most commonly of the dorsal and ulnar aspects. Since the triquetrum is shrouded by the strong ligamentous attachments, both palmar and dorsal chip fractures result from avulsion of ligamentous attachments (Dobyns et al 1982): for example dorsal flake fractures, caused by a fall on a palmar-flexed wrist.

Compression fractures of the triquetrum have also occurred and have been attributed to two mechanisms. In an anatomical and clinical study by Levy et al (1979), it was felt that the tip of the ulnar styloid acted as a chisel on the postero-medial aspect of the triquetrum. In dorsiflexion, the wrist is ulnarly deviated and the styloid strikes the triquetrum on its dorso-ulnar aspect, pushing it volarward, and a chip fracture results. Bryan et al (1980) stated that compression fractures of the triquetrum can occur in hyperextension and ulnar deviation of the wrist which forces the hamate against the posterior projection of the triquetrum and shears it off.

Fractures of the body may be seen with major carpal injuries such as trans-triquetral perilunate dislocations.

Clinical evaluation

Examination of the patients with triquetral chip fractures shows localized tenderness over the triquetrum dorsally, and pain on the ulnar side of the wrist with wrist motion.

Radiographical evaluation

This must include oblique radiography to bring the triquetrum clear of the lunate to identify the triquetral fracture (Fig. 18.5). A complete wrist series, including PA, lateral and oblique views, is necessary to determine if a major ligamentous injury exists (Fig. 18.6).

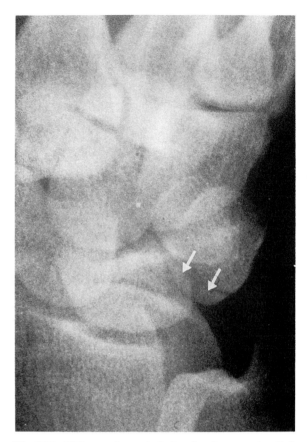

Fig. 18.5 Oblique radiograph placing the triquetrum in relief and thus showing an undisplaced fracture of the radial aspect of the triquetrum. This fracture healed clinically after cast immobilization for 4 weeks

Treatment

Bonnin and Greening (1944) reviewed 60 triquetral fractures and recommended three weeks of cast immobilization for traction injuries and a longer period of immobilization for compression injuries. They also noted clinical healing consistently preceded radiographic union. Bartone and Grieco (1956) reviewed their experience of 44 cases and stated that avulsion fractures of the triquetrum often do not unite, whereas fissure or comminuted fractures of the triquetral body almost always unite. They report no cases of avascular necrosis.

Fractures of the triquetrum associated with perilunate dislocations are major wrist injuries. Following reduction, the anatomy and displacement of the fracture are generally more apparent on the standard radiographs but evaluation must include assessment of the carpal alignment for instability patterns and further reduction with

internal fixation is required to improve fracture alignment and carpal position.

FRACTURES OF THE PISIFORM

Anatomy

The pisiform is a sesamoid bone that articulates with the triquetrum in an oval articulating surface. It is surrounded by ligamentous structures which include the palmar carpal and carpometacarpal ligaments. It provides the tendon insertion of the flexor carpi ulnaris, as well as the origin of the abductor digiti minimi. The pisiform is stabilized by the flexor carpi ulnaris, as well as the pisohamate, pisotriquetral, pisometacarpal and transverse car-

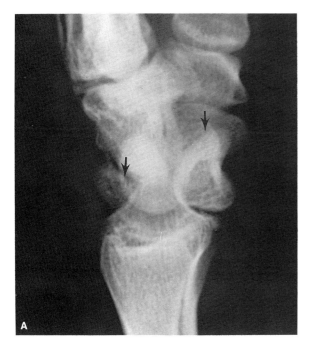
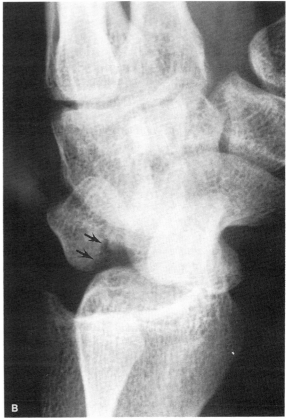

Fig. 18.6 Fractures of the triquetrum can occur in major ligamentous injuries to the wrist such as a transtriquetral perilunar dislocation. *Note* the lunate dislocation, as well as the fracture involving the triquetrum, shown on these lateral (A) and oblique (B) radiographs

pal ligaments. The ulnar nerve, as it courses across the wrist, is close to the radial side of the pisiform .

Mechanisms of injury

Fractures of the pisiform are usually due to direct trauma, as in a fall on the outstretched hand, but have also been attributed to ligamentous avulsion.

Clinical evaluation

Clinically, patients exhibit pain and tenderness over the pisiform. The evaluation must include specific testing of the ulnar nerve and its motor branch: Howard (1961) reported on six ulnar nerve palsies secondary to wrist fractures, one of which was a fractured pisiform.

Radiographical evaluation

The radiological diagnosis of pisiform fractures can be difficult and require appropriate positioning of the hand. The pisiform and pisotriquetral joint are best brought into relief by an oblique 10–30° view from the lateral with the thumb up and out and the ulnar side down. The carpal tunnel view can also show the pisiform well (Fig. 18.7). The radiographical aspects of the pisiform are well described by Vasilas et al (1960). The fracture pattern of the pisiform may be linear or show evidence of comminution.

Treatment

The treatment of pisiform fractures consists of splinting for 3–4 weeks. If persistent pain or non-union results, excision of the pisiform is indicated.

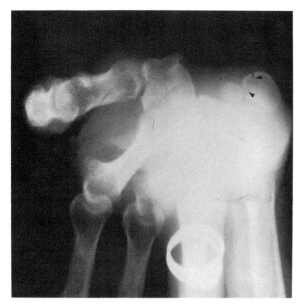

Fig. 18.7 A pisiform fracture is displayed on this carpal tunnel view

FRACTURES OF THE TRAPEZIUM

Anatomy

The trapezium is a pentagonal bone with articular surfaces on five sides. The trapezium articulates with the scaphoid proximally and the trapezoid medially. Distally, it articulates with the base of the second metacarpal and with the thumb metacarpal. Radially the trapezium is non-articular. On the palmar surface of the trapezium is the trapezial ridge, which provides attachment for the transverse carpal ligament, as well as providing a tunnel for the passage of the flexor carpi radialis.

Trapezial body fractures

Mechanisms of injury

Fractures of the body have been frequently reported in the literature (Dobyns et al 1982, Bryan & Dobyns 1980). They occur with a direct blow on the adducted thumb and a fall with the wrist dorsiflexed and in radial deviation, pressing the trapezium between the thumb metacarpal and the radial styloid.

Radiographical evaluation

Fractures of the body are best seen radiographically by an oblique lateral wrist radiograph with the ulnar aspect of the hand down and the forearm in $20°$ of pronation.

Treatment

Displaced fractures have been treated by open reduction and internal fixation with Kirschner wires (Cordrey & Ferrer-Torells 1960) or a small cancellous lag screw through a dorsal radial approach (Freeland & Finley 1984). Each report recommended accurate articular reduction and stabilization of the first carpometacarpal joint, and claims good results following accurate anatomical reduction.

Trapezial ridge fractures

Mechanisms of injury

A fall on a dorsiflexed wrist may cause direct trauma to the palmar ridge of the trapezium (Fig. 18.8). This also causes flattening of the palm as the

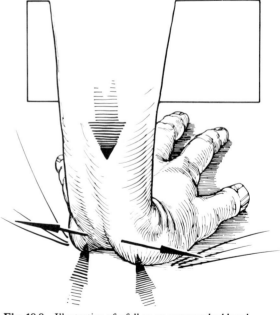

Fig. 18.8 Illustration of a fall on an outstretched hand, whereby the load is applied to the trapezial ridge either through direct impact or through tension applied by the transverse carpal ligament as the thenar and hypothenar eminences diverge

thenar and hypothenar eminences are displaced laterally, which tenses the transverse carpal ligament (flexor retinaculum) and may lead to its avulsion with its point of insertion on the ridge of the trapezium.

Clinical evaluation

Clinically there is marked tenderness over the palmar ridge of the trapezium, accentuated by active wrist flexion.

Radiographical evaluation and treatment

The fracture is best seen radiographically on the carpal tunnel view (Fig. 18.9). Palmer (1981) reviewed three cases of trapezial ridge fractures and described two types (Fig. 18.10). Type 1 is at the base of the trapezial ridge and Type 2 near its

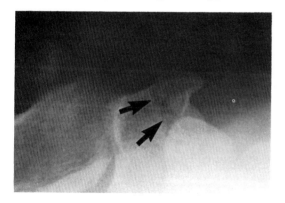

Fig. 18.9 Carpal tunnel view showing a fracture of the base of the trapezial palmar ridge

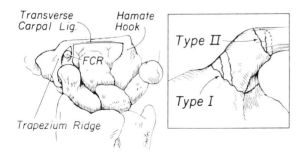

Fig. 18.10 View through a carpal tunnel, with the tendon of the flexor carpi radialis cradled by the palmar ridge of the trapezium. The insert illustrates the two types of fracture: type one at the base of the palmar ridge of trapezium (direct loading) and type two fracture at the tip (avulsion)

tip. The patient with the Type 1 fracture went on to union with cast immobilization, whereas both Type 2 patients developed non-union despite adequate immobilization. McClain and Boyes (1966) reported four cases requiring excision of the trapezial ridge fragment and a carpal tunnel release, with improvement and return to work.

FRACTURES OF THE TRAPEZOID

Anatomy

The trapezoid articulates with the scaphoid, capitate, trapezium, and second metacarpal. It is firmly fixed to the neighbouring carpus by strong ligamentous supports. There is minimal motion occurring at this second metacarpal joint and fractures of the trapezoid are rare due to strong ligamentous attachments.

Mechanisms of injury

Occasionally trapezoid fractures can occur and are associated with fracture-dislocations of the carpometacarpal joints of the index and middle fingers. These injuries generally occur with violent trauma to the hand and wrist.

Clinical evaluation

There is marked tenderness over the trapezoid, with significant hand swelling. Occasionally numbness in the thumb, index, middle and ring fingers can occur secondary to median nerve compression as it courses through the carpal canal.

Radiographical evaluation

Fractures of the trapezoid can frequently be seen on standard AP, lateral and oblique views of the hand and wrist (Fig. 18.11), but occasionally tomograms are required.

Treatment

Fractures of the trapezoid associated with fracture-dislocations of the index metacarpal require reduction and internal fixation (Fig. 18.12). If a

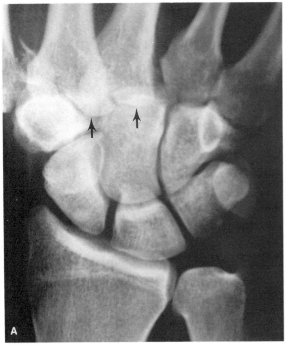

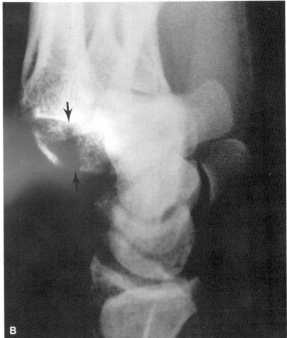

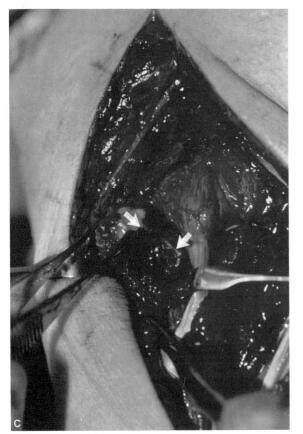

Fig. 18.11 Dislocations of the carpometacarpal joints of the index and middle fingers can be seen on the PA film (A) and the lateral shows these are associated with an intra-articular fracture of the trapezoid (B). This can be seen on the photograph taken at operation through a dorsal approach : *note* the dorsal trapezoid fragment in the forceps (C) and the arrows identifying the intra-articular line of fracture

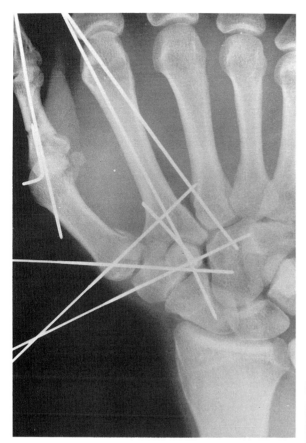

Fig. 18.12 Trapezoid intra-articular fracture and its associated metacarpal dislocations which were reduced and internally fixed with Kirschner wires

significant intra-articular component is present, open reduction is required with internal fixation to restore articular congruity and provide a stable carpometacarpal joint. This is most frequently done through a dorsal approach. Occasionally late arthritis of the trapezoid/second metacarpal joint occurs and fusion of this joint is the treatment of choice.

FRACTURES OF THE CAPITATE

Anatomy

The capitate is the largest of the carpal bones and has strong dorsal and palmar ligamentous attachments. It articulates with the hamate, lunate, trapezoid, scaphoid and base of the second, third and fourth metacarpals. The capitate is constricted into a waist just distal to the proximal articular surface and distally the bone expands. There are multiple strong ligamentous attachments to the palmar surface of the capitate, most notably the radioscaphocapitate ligament which runs from the radius across the waist of the scaphoid to the capitate. The arcuate ligament also attaches to the capitate and provides stability between the triquetrum, hamate and capitate.

Mechanisms of injury

Fractures of the capitate either involve the body of the capitate alone (Fig. 18.13) or are associated with a scaphoid fracture (scaphocapitate syndrome or trans-scaphoid trans-capitate perilunate dislocation). A displaced fracture of the capitate can only occur if there is also significant ligamentous

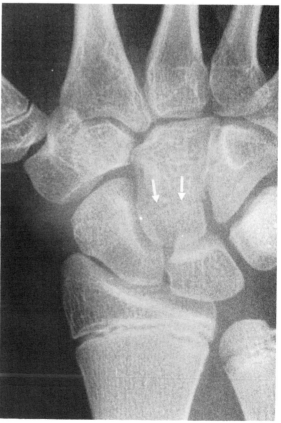

Fig. 18.13 Fractures of the body of the capitate can occur from dorsiflexion injuries. This PA radiograph of a child shows an undisplaced fracture which healed uneventfully after four weeks

injury. The scaphocapitate syndrome is a severe injury to the carpus consisting of displaced fractures of the scaphoid and capitate, as well as a ligamentous injury.

Various mechanisms of injury have been reported. Fenton (1956) described a mechanism where the radial styloid acts as a chisel impinging on the scaphoid; the scaphoid then fractures and with progression of the severe force, the capitate fractures too. Subsequently the proximal pole of the capitate rotates through 180°. Stein and Siegel (1969) reviewed this mechanism of injury and observed that in radial deviation the radial styloid comes up to the trapezium and not the scaphoid. They felt that with severe dorsiflexion, there is a tension force on the scaphoid and the dorsal lip of the radius forcibly strikes the head of the capitate causing it to fracture. The wrist then continues into an extremely dorsiflexed position and the proximal pole of the capitate rotates 90°. When the wrist returns to a neutral position, the proximal fragment rotates another 90° further to its final position. Vance et al (1980) reviewed seven cases of combined scaphoid and capitate fractures, in addition to the previous literature. They defined six patterns of fracture-dislocation and found that although some patients had sustained severe dorsiflexion injuries, others had suffered a blow on the back of the palmar-flexed wrist.

Clinical evaluation

Patients with fractures of the capitate have localized tenderness over that bone as well as pain on motion of the wrist.

Radiographical evaluation

Capitate fractures can be seen on standard radiograph views of the wrist, especially the lateral. In the scaphocapitate syndrome, the proximal pole of the capitate is rotated 180°. The lateral film identifies this injury, although the findings are subtle and easily missed (Fig. 18.14).

Treatment

Isolated undisplaced capitate fractures are best treated with cast immobilization for about six

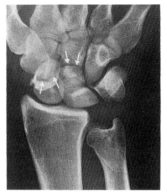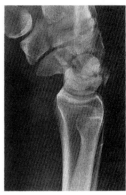

Fig. 18.14 Fractures of the scaphoid and capitate indicate a severe ligamentous injury to the carpus. These PA and lateral radiographs show the grossly malpositioned scaphoid fracture with the proximal capitate fragment rotated through 180°

weeks (Adler & Shaftan 1962). Once the local tenderness resoves, motion of the wrist can begin. The treatment of displaced capitate fractures consists of accurate reduction and coaptation of the fracture fragments. For the scaphocapitate syndrome and proximal fragment rotation, many methods of reduction have been advocated. Alternatively, some favour observation of the fragment and excision of the proximal fragment if pain exists.

Long-term follow-up of capitate fractures has been reported by Rand et al (1982). They reviewed 13 patients with capitate fractures or non-union. After a mean follow-up of five years, they found four cases of avascular necrosis of the proximal fragment and a high incidence of post-traumatic arthritis in patients with longer follow-up. Non-union of the capitate has also been reported by Freeman and Hay (1985) and can occur with isolated capitate fractures or in the scaphocapitate syndrome. Non-union can present with pain or occasionally with symptomatic wrist instability due to snapping at the non-union site.

We recommend cast immobilization for six weeks for isolated undisplaced capitate fractures. For displaced capitate fractures, we advise accurate reduction with reduction of the fracture fragments. In the scaphocapitate syndrome with rotation of the proximal capitate fragment, open reduction and internal fixation are needed to re-establish the bony anatomy.

FRACTURES OF THE HAMATE

Anatomy

The hamate is triangular, with an apex proximally widening to a large distal base. At the distal end of the palmar surface, the hook of the hamate protrudes forwards for 8 mm. Proximally, the apex of the hamate is completely concealed by the triquetrum. The hamate articulates with the triquetrum proximally and ulnarly, with the capitate radially and with the fourth and fifth metacarpals distally.

The hamate is stabilized in the carpus by the ulnar branch of the palmar arcuate ligament and three dorsal ligaments. Distally, there are strong ligamentous attachments to the ring and little finger metacarpal bases. The transverse carpal ligament, the pisohamate ligament and the origin of the short flexors and opponens to the little finger have their origin from the hook of the hamate. The ulnar nerve is in close proximity to the hook of the hamate as it courses through Guyon's canal giving off its motor branch.

Mechanisms of injury

Fractures of the hamate hook have been well described in the literature and over 50 cases have been reported. The typical mechanism is the swing of a golf club interrupted by hitting the ground (Torisu 1972) or the similar swing of a tennis racket, baseball bat, cricket bat or similar other implement which is halted by a sudden impact. When both hands are used to grip the handle, the fracture is commonly observed to occur in the wrist nearer the end of the handle, e.g. the left wrist in right-handed batters or golfers (Stark et al 1977).

Fractures of the body of the hamate frequently involve the distal articular surface and are associated with carpometacarpal dislocation of the ring and little fingers. The fracture involves the dorsal lip of the hamate which is attached to the dislocated bases of the fourth and fifth metacarpals.

Clinical evaluation

Patients with hook fractures present with diffuse pain on the ulnar side of the hand, often not well localized over the hook due to the significant hypothenar fat pad. Since the ulnar nerve and the little finger flexor tendons are anatomically close to the hamate hook, nerve and tendon function must be specifically tested. Reports of flexor tendon rupture, ulnar nerve neuropathy, ulnar artery, and carpal tunnel syndrome have been noted following hamate hook fractures (Howard 1961, Carter et al 1977, Ogunro 1983, Cameron et al 1975). Patients with carpometacarpal dislocations associated with distal dorsal hamate lip fractures present with a dorsal ulnar prominence over the hamate with this fracture dislocation. They have marked tenderness and weakness with firm grasp.

Radiographical evaluation

Occasionally the fracture can be seen on PA views (Fig. 18.15) but frequently, carpal tunnel views

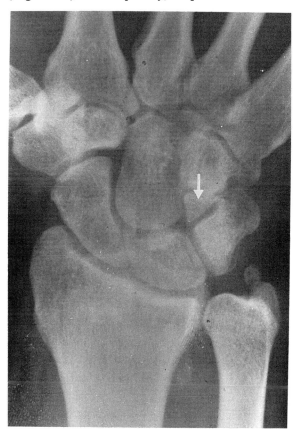

Fig. 18.15 When fractures of the hamate hook involve a large portion of the hamate, the fracture line can appear on the PA radiographs. This patient's fracture was of the proximal triangle of the hamate

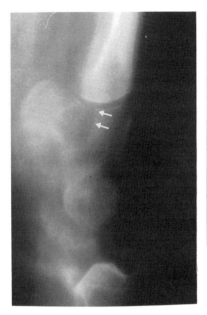

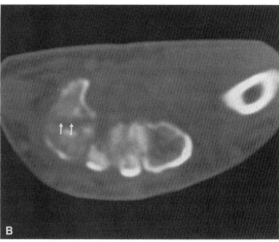

Fig. 18.16   (A) Lateral tomogram shows the extent of the fracture. (B) Excellent visualization of the hamate hook fracture on the CT scan

are needed. Further work-up should include tomograms (Fig. 18.16) and computerized tomography (Fig. 18.16b) to help visualize the fractures (Egawa & Asai 1983). Fractures of the dorsal lip of the distal end of the hamate, which are usually associated with carpometacarpal dislocations, can be visualized radiographically. They may not be evident on the lateral view (Fig. 18.17), but can be revealed on the oblique view (Fig. 18.18). Here again, lateral tomography is occasionally required to define the fracture and the joint incongruity (Fig. 18.19).

Treatment

Fresh fractures of the hook of the hamate should be immobilized in cast for 4–6 weeks. In cases where a hamate hook fracture was overlooked and the patient seen later with symptomatic non-union, the treatment is excision of the hook; even in patients without symptoms. Excision has been recommended due to the possibility of late flexor tendon rupture (Stark et al 1977). We prefer that

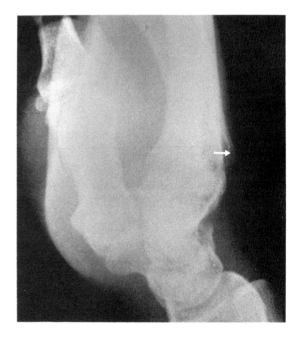

Fig. 18.17   Radiograph showing evidence of a dislocated little finger metacarpal, with the metacarpal base prominent on the lateral film

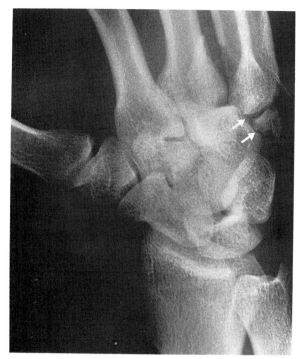

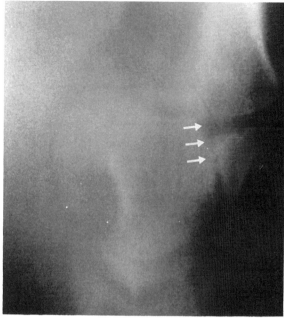

Fig. 18.19 Lateral tomogram providing the only clear evidence of dislocation of the bases of the fourth and fifth metacarpals with an intra-articular fracture of the hamate (arrow)

Fig. 18.18 On oblique radiographs the hamate and little finger metacarpal are put in relief and the fracture which accompanies the dislocation can be seen, as in this example

patients without symptoms should be advised that there is a possibility of late flexor tendon rupture, but our recommendation is to follow these patients until symptoms occur. In these cases, although there is a risk of delayed flexor tendon rupture, there is also a risk of ulnar nerve palsy from the surgical exposure, as well as associated risks with surgical intervention.

Recent fractures associated with carpometacarpal dislocation require either closed or occasionally open reduction and internal fixation to maintain reduction of the carpometacarpal joint.

In cases where the patient is seen late, carpometacarpal fusion is recommended (Clendenin & Smith 1984) and results in minimal functional problems due to the intrinsic mobility of the triquetral hamate joint.

CONCLUSION

In the evaluation of patients with wrist pain, a high index of suspicion must be maintained to be successful in the diagnosis of carpal bone fractures. The clinical examination is very important because frequently the diagnosis is not apparent on plain or routine X-ray studies and special views, tomograms or CT scans are required: it is the clinical findings which enable one to order the appropriate views. Attention must also be given to carpal bone position and possible wrist instability patterns.

Once the diagnosis is made, appropriate treatment can begin. In many instances, cast immobilization is curative although open treatment may be required in cases of articular involvement, wrist instability or non-union.

REFERENCES

Adler J, Shaftan G 1962 Fractures of the capitate. Journal of Bone and Joint Surgery 44A: 1537–1547

Almquist E, Burns J 1982 Radial shortening for the treatment of Kienböck's disease. A 5- to 10-year follow up. Journal of Hand Surgery 7: 348–352

Armistead R, Linscheid R, Dobyns J, Beckenbaugh R 1982 Ulnar lengthening in the treatment of Kienböck's disease. Journal of Bone and Joint Surgery 64A: 170–178

Bartone N F, Grieco R V 1956 Fractures of the triquetrum. Journal of Bone and Joint Surgery 38A: 353–356.

Beckenbaugh R, Shives T, Dobyns J, Linscheid R 1980 Kienböck's disease: the natural history of Kienböck's disease and consideration of lunate fractures. Clinical Orthopaedics 149: 98–106.

Bonnin J, Greening W 1944 Fractures of the triquetrum. British Journal of Surgery 31: 278–283

Bryan R, Dobyns J 1980 Fractures of the carpal bones other than lunate and navicular. Clinical Orthopaedics 149: 107–111

Cameron H, Hastings D, Fournasier V 1975 Fracture of the hook of the hamate. Journal of Bone and Joint Surgery 57A: 276–277

Carter P, Eaton R, Littler J 1977 Ununited fracture of the hook of the hamate. Journal of Bone and Joint Surgery 59A: 583–588

Chuinard R 1980 Kienböck's disease: an analysis and rationale for treatment by capitate-hamate fusion. Orthopaedic Transactions 4: 18

Clendenin M, Smith R 1984 Fifth metacarpal/hamate arthrodesis for post-traumatic osteoarthritis. Journal of Hand Surgery 9A: 374–378

Cordrey L J, Ferrer-Torells M 1980 Management of fractures of the greater multangular. Journal of Bone and Joint Surgery 42A: 1111–1118

Dobyns J, Beckenbaugh R, et al 1982 Fractures of the hand and wrist. In Flynn J E, Hand Surgery, Williams and Wilkins, Baltimore, Maryland, USA

Egawa M, Asai R 1983 Fracture of the hook of the hamate: Report of six cases and the suitability of computerized tomography. Journal of Hand Surgery 8: 393–398

Fenton R 1956 The naviculo-capitate fracture syndrome. Journal of Bone and Joint Surgery 38A: 681–684

Freeland A, Finley J 1984 Displaced vertical fracture of the trapezium treated with a small cancellous lag screw. Journal of Hand Surgery 9A: 843–845

Freeman B, Hay E 1985 Nonunion of the capitate. A case report. Journal of Hand Surgery 10A: 187–190

Gelberman R, Bauman T, Menon J, et al 1980 The vascularity of the lunate bone and Kienböck's disease. Journal of Hand Surgery 5: 272–278

Graner O, Lopes E, Carvalho B, Atlas S 1966 Arthrodesis of the carpal bones in the treatment of Kienböck's disease, painful ununited fractures of the navicular and lunate bones with avascular necrosis, and old fracture-dislocations of carpal bones. Journal of Bone and Joint Surgery 48A: 767–774

Howard F 1961 Ulnar-nerve palsy in wrist fractures. Journal of Bone and Joint Surgery 43A: 1197–1201

Inglis A, Jones E 1977 Proximal-row carpectomy for diseases of the proximal row. Journal of Bone and Joint Surgery 59A: 460–463

Levy M, Fischel R, Stern G, Goldberg I 1979 Chip fractures of the os triquetrum. The mechanism of injury. Journal of Bone and Joint Surgery 61B: 355–357

Lichtman D, Alexander A, Mack G, Gunther S 1982 Kienböck's disease—update on silicone replacement arthroplasty. Journal of Hand Surgery 7: 343–347

McClain E T, Boyes J H 1966 Missed fractures of the greater multangular. Journal of Bone and Joint Surgery 48A: 1525–1528

Ogunro O 1983 Fracture of the body of the hamate bone. Journal of Hand Surgery 8: 353–355

Palmer A 1980 Trapezial ridge fractures. Journal of Hand Surgery 6: 561–564

Rand J, Lischeid R, Dobyns J 1982 Capitate fractures. A long-term follow-up. Clinical Orthopaedics 165: 209–216

Simmons E, Dommisse I 1975 The pathogenesis and treatment of Kienböck's disease (abstract). Clinical Orthopaedics 105: 300

Stark H, Jobe F, Boyes J, Ashworth C 1977 Fracture of the hook of the hamate in athletes. Journal of Bone and Joint Surgery 59A: 575–582

Stark H, Zemel N, Ashworth C 1981 Use of a hand-carved silicone-rubber spacer for advanced Kienböck's disease. Journal of Bone and Joint Surgery 63A: 1359–1370

Stein F, Siegel M W 1969 Naviculocapitate fracture syndrome. A case report: new thoughts on the mechanism of injury. Journal of Bone and Joint Surgery 51A: 391–395

Torisu T 1972 Fracture of the hook of the hamate by a golfswing. Clinical Orthopaedics 83: 91–94

Vance R M, Gelberman R H, Evans E 1980 Scaphocapitate fractures. Patterns of dislocation. Mechanisms of injury and preliminary results of treatment. Journal of Bone and Joint Surgery 62A: 271–276

Vasilas A, Grieco R, Bartone N 1960 Roentgen aspects of injuries to the pisiform bone and pisotriquetral joint. Journal of Bone and Joint Surgery 42A: 1317–1328

Watson H, Rju J, DiBella A 1985 An approach to Kienböck's disease: triscaphe arthrodesis. Journal of Hand Surgery 10A: 179–187

Fractures of the distal radius

B

19

Smith's and Barton's fractures

The anatomical nature of many of the more troublesome fractures and dislocations about the wrist was clearly identified prior to discovery of the X-ray. Yet, up to the early 19th century, most surgeons diagnosed post-traumatic wrist deformity as dislocation unless they could elicit false motion or crepitation.

Among the first to distinguish the impacted distal radius fracture from wrist dislocation was Pouteau of Lyon. In a book published posthumously in 1783, Pouteau described several wrist fractures that did not elicit crepitus with manipulation.

In 1814, Abraham Colles, Professor of Surgery at Trinity College in Dublin, clearly identified dorsally displaced fractures that lay 'about an inch-and-a-half above the carpal extremity of the radius.' He noted that these fractures often had been misdiagnosed as anterior dislocation of the distal ulna. At about the same time, Dupuytren also described common fractures of the distal radius and differentiated them from dislocations; this was included in a book of his lectures published in 1832.

Goyrand (1832, 1836) of Aix substantiated his clinical observations of distal radial fractures with post-mortem examinations of 47 patients (Fig. 19.1). Of these, 45 were displaced dorsally and two in a volar (anterior) direction. Goyrand noted that an intact fibrocartilage between the radius and ulna limited the displacement of the distal fragment of a fractured radius. After severe trauma, if the fibrocartilage were ruptured, displacement of the fracture fragment would be more severe. Goyrand described an intra-articular fracture of the volar lip of the distal radius and noted that the carpus

dislocated volarly with the fracture fragment. Often this displacement was severe.

In the USA, John Rhea Barton of Philadelphia also described intra-articular fractures of the distal radius. In 1838 he reported dorsal lip fractures of the distal radius with 'a subluxation of the wrist consequent to fracture through the articular surface of the carpal extremity of the radius.' He also noted that some patients sustained volar lip fractures with volar displacement of the carpus. Barton cautioned against confusing the intra-articular fractures of the distal radius with the more proximal extra-articular fractures of the radius and ulna.

Robert W. Smith was a junior colleague of Abraham Colles and assumed his chair as Professor of Surgery after Colles's death.* In his treatise on 'Fractures and Dislocations' (1847) Smith described an injury of 'exceedingly rare occurrence' that 'causes displacement of the lower fragment [of the radius] along with the carpus forward, and the head of the ulna backward' (Fig. 19.2). He believed the fracture to be caused by a fall upon the back of the hand. He dissected no specimens, but identified the fracture 'from half an inch to an inch above the articulation.' Smith carefully differentiated these injuries from volar dislocation of the carpus and from dorsal displacement of the distal end of the radius but he offered no advice as to its treatment.

Thus, in the 65 years from Pouteau's posthumous report of fractures of the distal radius, the dorsal and volar displaced extra-articular and intra-articular fractures of the distal radius were described on both sides of the Atlantic and on both

* Smith actually carried out the post-mortem on Colles.

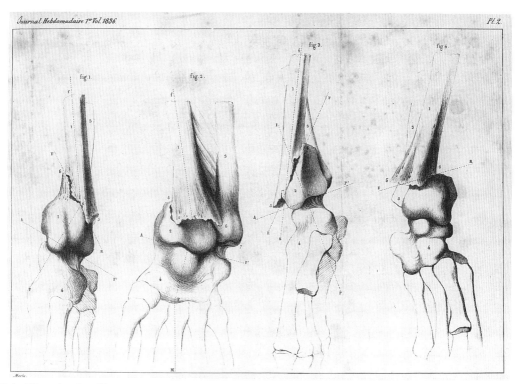

Fig. 19.1 These drawings illustrate the relationship of the fracture fragments in injuries of the distal radius with volar and dorsal displacement of the distal fragment as reported from post-mortem examination (Goyrand 1836)

sides of the English Channel. That several authors independently described the same injuries was due, no doubt, to the limited circulation of some of the published works. It remained for investigators late in the 19th century to verify the earlier clinical descriptions by post-mortem examinations of injured hands, and then by radiological examination of acute fractures (Roberts 1897). More recently, fractures of the distal radius have been further studied in order that we might better understand the pathomechanics of the forces producing these injuries (Frykman 1967). Each of the fractures has

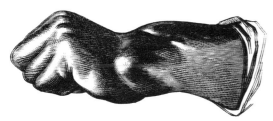

Fig. 19.2 This drawing illustrates the characteristic deformity of injuries associated with fractures of the distal radius with volar displacement of the lower fragment (Robert W. Smith 1847)

been given one or more eponyms and each has been classified. Unfortunately, some of the eponyms are inaccurate and some of the classifications confusing, yet our understanding of these difficult fractures has improved.

SMITH'S FRACTURES

Classification

Although Robert Smith's original description of the distal radius fracture 'with displacement of the lower fragment forward' clearly localized the site of injury at 0.5–1 inch (12–25 mm) from the distal end of the radius, F B Thomas (1957) broadened the eponym 'Smith's fractures' to include also the volarly displaced intra-articular fracture of the volar lip of the distal radius and fractures of the cortex of the distal radial metaphysis. He described four different types of Smith's fracture and his classification will be used in this chapter. Paterson (1966) extended this classification still further to include volarly-displaced greenstick and epiphyseal fractures of the distal radius of adolescents.

Smith's type I fracture

This fracture corresponds to the original description published by William Smith in the 19th century. It is also known as a 'reversed Colles's fracture.' The fracture is located at the lower cancellous end of the radius and is displaced volarly. The volar cortex is frequently comminuted. There may also be a fracture of the ulnar styloid. The Smith's I fracture is more frequent in older patients, particularly women.

Mechanisms of injury

The Colles's fracture, with dorsal displacement of the distal radial fragment, is caused by a fall on the palm of the outstretched hand. It therefore might appear reasonable to suppose that the 'reversed Colles's' or 'Smith's I' fracture, which is characterized by a volar displacement of the distal radial fragment, would be due to a fall on the back of the hand. But such is *not* the case. People rarely fall on the dorsum of the hand. Our natural tendency, whether falling forward or backward, is to protect the body by throwing out the dorsiflexed hand so that the palm and fingers strike the ground first. Few patients with Smith's I fracture recall falling

on the back of the hand. Rarely does one see bruises, lacerations or abrasions to suggest such an injury. Most patients with Smith's I fracture have fallen onto the palm of the hand. Why, then, do some patients who have fallen on the palm of the hand sustain a volarly displaced Smith's fracture while others sustain a dorsally displaced Colles's fracture? How do similar injuries cause opposite deformities?

In order to understand the mechanism of injury causing these fractures, we must carefully examine the motion that occurs at the distal radioulnar joint. This joint permits motion only in one plane: rotation. The sigmoid notch of the radius rotates about the ulnar head through an arc of almost $180°$. The axis of rotation is at the centre of the ulnar head at the distal end of the forearm and *not* at the midline of the radius. At the elbow, by contrast, the axis of rotation is within the radial head. At the wrist, almost all forearm pronation and supination involves rotation of the radius about the ulna.

Now consider the distal 1 inch (25 mm) of the radius as though it were detached from its shaft after a fracture (Fig. 19.3). If the hand is held firmly to the table with the palm down, as the forearm supinates the proximal radius will rotate

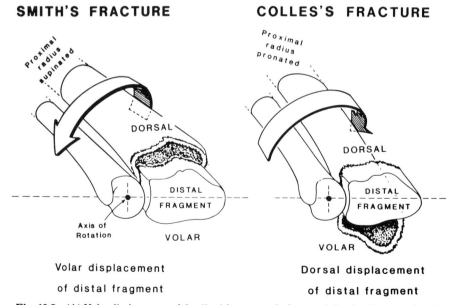

Fig. 19.3 (A) Volar displacement of the distal fragment of a fractured distal radius is produced by supination of the proximal radius about the ulna (Smith's fracture). (B) Dorsal displacement of the distal fragment is produced by pronation of the proximal radius (Colles's fracture)

dorsally about an axis of rotation within the ulnar shaft. As the proximal radius rotates dorsally, the position of the distal fragment remains fixed so that it comes to lie volar to the shaft. By contrast, if the forearm pronates, the proximal portion of the radius rotates volarly about an axis within the ulnar shaft. The distal fragment will lie dorsal to it when rotation is completed. In both cases, the hand has been dorsiflexed. In the first case, however, the distal fragment is displaced volar to the radial shaft because the forearm has supinated. This is the Smith's I fracture. In the second case, the distal fragment is supinated relative to the proximal forearm and lies dorsally. This is the Colles's fracture.

With most injuries to the wrist, the forearm is pronated and the hand is fixed in dorsiflexion. As the victim falls forward, his protecting hand goes out in front of him and to the side. His body weight pronates the forearm and he sustains a Colles's fracture (Fig. 19.4a). Less frequently, the hand

crosses in front of the victim or he falls backwards and the body weight rotates the forearm into supination (Fig. 19.4b). He sustains a Smith's I fracture. As the pronation injury is more frequent, Colles's fracture is more frequent than the Smith's I fracture.

Radiographs

The radiographic appearance of the Smith's I fracture often demonstrates the rotatory nature of the injury in addition to the angulation (Fig. 19.5). By definition, the distal fragment will be displaced volarly with both dorsal angulation (i.e. convex dorsally) and impaction. A careful comparison of the width of the radius just proximal and just distal to the fracture may reveal a significant discrepancy. This is due to rotation of the fracture such that the radial shaft is seen in the oblique plane and the hand and distal fragment in the antero-posterior plane. Often the volar cortex is comminuted. The ulnar styloid may or may not be fractured.

Treatment

The Smith's type I fracture is impacted, dorsally angulated and pronated. Therefore the key to treatment is traction and palmar-flexion of the wrist to disimpact the fragments, followed by manipulation of the wrist into dorsiflexion and supination to realign the fragments.

Plaster cast. If the Smith's type I fracture is treated relatively early and there has been little comminution, reduction can often be maintained by means of a well-moulded plaster cast. We would prefer a long arm-cast or a Munster above-elbow cast that holds the wrist in mild dorsiflexion, applies even support to the volar side of the wrist and forearm and maintains the wrist and forearm in full supination. The cast can be open in the AP plane above the elbow to permit flexion–extension without forearm rotation. Six weeks' immobilization is required. If satisfactory reduction cannot be achieved or if the deformity recurs with plaster immobilization, external or internal fixation is advisable.

External fixation. For external fixation we place two pins transversely through the second and third metacarpals and two pins at the midshaft of the

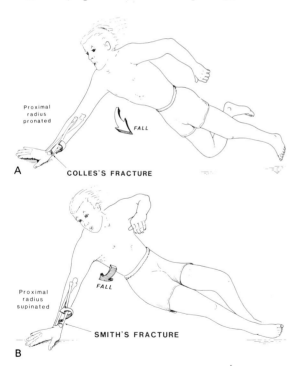

Fig. 19.4 (A) Colles's fracture is produced by a fall forward on the outstretched hand, resulting in pronation of the proximal radius and dorsal displacement of the distal fragment. (B) Smith's fracture is also produced by a fall on the outstretched hand. However, when falling backwards, the body weight supinates the proximal fragment and the distal fragment is volarly displaced

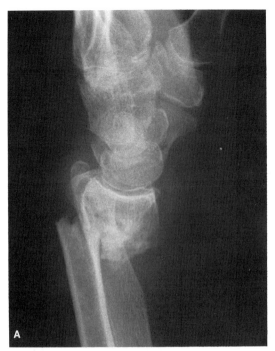 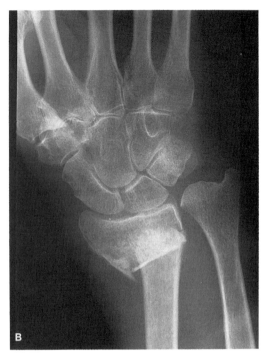

Fig. 19.5 (A) Lateral radiograph of a Type I Smith's fracture demonstrating the characteristic volar displacement of the distal fragment. (B) Anteroposterior radiograph demonstrating the discrepancy in width of the radius proximal and distal to the fracture. Because of rotation at the fracture site, the radial shaft is seen in the oblique plane and the hand and distal fragment in the antero-posterior plane

radius. An external fixation device is attached to the pins, both to reduce the fracture and to hold the reduction during healing. The surgeon should be certain that the rotatory deformity of the fracture has been corrected. Eight weeks of immobilization are usually necessary to assure consolidation of the fracture.

Internal fixation. Open reduction and internal fixation is advised for those Smith's I fractures that cannot be reduced and held by closed treatment or which also have displaced fragments that enter the radio-ulnar or radiocarpal joints. A volar angled T-plate with additional screw fixation of any large comminuted fracture fragments will hold the reduction (Fig. 19.6). Ellis (1965) has advised the use of a small buttress plate that supports the distal fragments without screw fixation distally. This plate is preferred for the treatment of a grossly comminuted Smith's I fracture. One must take care that the plate does not extend past the distal end of the radius. Plates that project distally have caused rupture of the flexor tendons that lie superficial to it (Fuller 1973).

Smith's type II fracture

This is synonomous with the anterior (or volar) 'Barton's II fracture.' It is a fracture of the volar lip of the distal radius, with volar and proximal dislocation of the carpus and of the fracture fragment. The fracture is more frequent in younger patients who do not have osteoporosis and is more common in men than in women. This type of fracture will be discussed under the section on 'Barton's fractures.'

Smith's type III fracture

As classified by Thomas (1957), a Smith's III fracture is of the lower end of the radius within 1 inch (25 mm) of the wrist-joint. It is transverse on anterior-posterior view and slightly oblique on the lateral view. The fracture fragment is displaced and tilted anteriorly. This fracture is often associated with fractures of the metacarpals and is reported to occur almost exclusively in motorcyclists (Paterson 1966, Bhattacharyya & Srivastava 1972). Thomas believed this type of fracture to be due to a forceful blow on the knuckles as the hand grips the motorcycle handlebar.

Mechanisms of injury

The mechanism of injury of the Smith's III fracture appears to be quite different from that of the Smith's I fracture (Fig. 19.7). Whereas the volar displacement of the distal fragment in the Smith's I fracture is due to rotatory and compressive forces, with the Smith's III fracture the main deformity is compressive and angulatory. The hand of the motorcyclist is clenched about the handlebar and is palmar-flexed at the moment of impact. The force of impact is transmitted through the second and third metacarpals and through the tightly gripped handlebar to compress the volar cortex of the distal radius. This results in a shear of the dorsal cortex and volar displacement of the distal fragment. Often, the second or third metacarpal is fractured at the same time.

The mechanism of injury producing this fracture is quite specific and unusual and accounts for the relative infrequency of the Smith's III fracture. In order to understand the mechanism of injury, it is useful to consider fractures that would result in slightly altered circumstances.

1. If the same force of impact were to be inflicted on the fourth and fifth metacarpal heads, much of the force might be dissipated by these metacarpals before it were transmitted to the radius. The mobile fourth and fifth metacarpals would first flex, and then would fracture and dislocate before transmitting the force more proximally.
2. If sudden force were exerted on the second or third metacarpal heads and the hand were not tightly gripping a firm handlebar (or if the wrist were not otherwise stabilized in this position), a partially volar flexed wrist would flex further before transmitting its force more proximally. Under these circumstances, or in cases in which the wrist were acutely palmar-flexed at the moment of injury, a volar lip fracture of the radius (Smith's II or Barton's II fracture) would probably result.
3. If impact occurred with the wrist in neutral position, one would expect a dye-punch fracture of the distal radius. If the impact were to occur

with the wrist in dorsiflexion, there would be injury to the dorsum of the proximal interphalangeal joints and dorsal displacement of the radial fragment.

Treatment

Unlike the Smith's I fracture, reduction of the Smith's III fracture does not require rotation of the fracture fragments. This is an angulatory and compressive fracture and should be reduced by traction and dorsal displacement and tilting of the distal fragment. For closed reduction, the elbow is flexed and the proximal forearm supported by an assistant. The fragments are disengaged by traction and palmar-flexion and then reduced in dorsiflexion. A volar splint or below-elbow circular cast holding the wrist in moderate dorsiflexion should maintain the reduction if the fracture is not badly comminuted. Six weeks of immobilization would appear adequate. If reduction is incomplete or unstable, external fixation with pins in the second and third metacarpals and in the midshaft of the radius, or a volar angled T-plate as described with the treatment of the Smith's I fracture should readily hold the reduced fragments until the fracture has consolidated.

Smith's type IV fracture

Thomas also mentioned a fourth type of fracture which occurs almost exclusively in adolescents and children. It is a 'forward fracture-separation of the lower radial epiphysis or a greenstick fracture of the radius within 2 inches (5 cm) of its lower end.'

In many cases these fractures may be considered as similar to Smith's I fracture in the adolescent. However, there does not appear to be a rotatory component. Descriptions of these fractures by Thomas (1957) and by Paterson (1966) are brief and neither report gives clinical histories nor describes methods of treatment. If the angulation is mild, one need only immobilize the limb below the elbow and protect it until healing occurs. With metaphyseal fractures, any rotatory component should be corrected, if it exists, as rotatory deformities will not remodel with growth. The fracture fragments should be disengaged and the wrist supinated. If there is little rotatory compo-

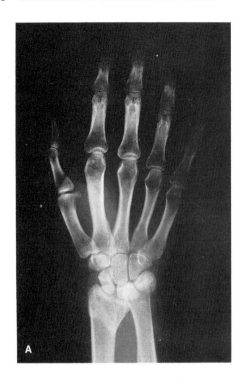

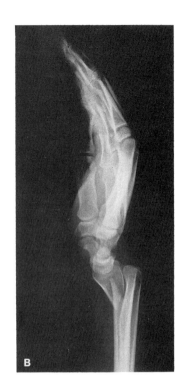

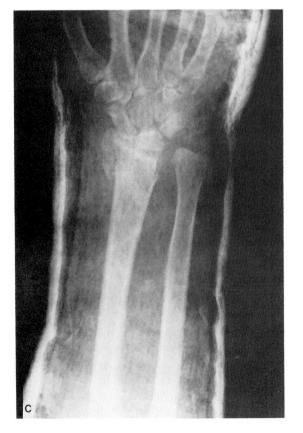

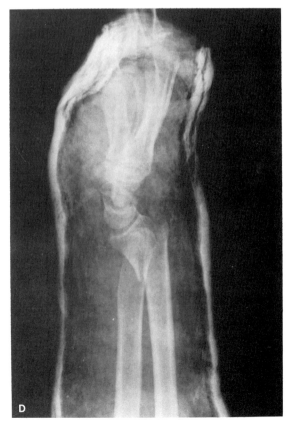

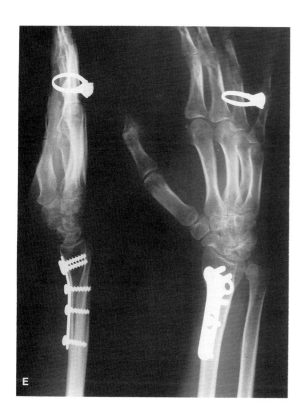

Fig. 19.6 A 50-year-old woman fell and injured her right wrist. (A & B) Antero-posterior and lateral radiographs demonstrated a Smith's type I fracture. (C & D) Acceptable reduction was not achieved by closed treatment. (E) Open reduction and internal fixation with an angled T-plate resulted in anatomical reduction and excellent function

nent and only mild angulation, we need have little clinical concern as remodelling will probably restore normal bone architecture. In these cases, the limb needs to be splinted for four to six weeks and excellent function should result.

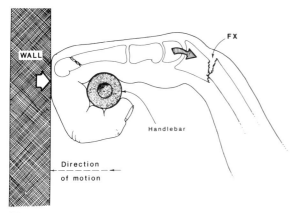

Fig. 19.7 Type III Smith's fracture occurs almost exclusively in motorcyclists. The hand of the motorcyclist is clenched about the handlebar and is palmar-flexed at the moment of impact, producing a shear of the dorsal cortex and volar displacement of the distal fragment. There is often an associated fracture of the second or third metacarpal shaft

BARTON'S FRACTURES

Fractures of the dorsal or volar lip of the distal articular surface of the radius are relatively infrequent. They are unstable and are often associated with carpal dislocation. For these reasons, the results of closed treatment have been poor. Barton was well aware of the instability of this fracture-dislocation and noted that, after reduction of the deformity, 'the moment the extension and counter-extension are relaxed ... the deformity [will] reappear as conspicuously as before; and as often as the effort is renewed and discontinued will the deformity disappear and reappear.' Unlike Barton, most authors have found that the volar fracture is more common than the dorsal fracture (Mills 1957, Flandreau et al 1962, Aufranc et al 1966, Paterson 1966).

Types of fracture and mechanism of injury

Both the dorsal lip fracture–dislocation (Barton's I fracture) and the volar lip fracture–dislocation (Barton's II fracture) of the distal radius are caused by severe angulation of the dorsiflexed or palmar-flexed hand with little rotatory component (Woodyard 1969, De Oliveira 1973, King 1975). When one falls on the palm of the hand, the scaphoid and lunate are wedged in their respective facets at the distal radius. If the volar radiocarpal ligaments remain intact, the carpus may strike the dorsal lip of the radius causing a dorsal lip fracture, or the carpus may be wedged against the volar lip of the radius causing a volar lip fracture (Fig. 19.8). Theoretically, the same injury could avulse the volar lip of the radius by traction on the volar radiocarpal ligaments. Such an injury, however, would probably cause a small cortical fracture. Thus, injury to the fully dorsiflexed hand can either cause a dorsal compression fracture (Barton's type I) or volar compression fracture (Barton's type II) or a small avulsion volar lip fracture. Similarly, a fall on the dorsum of the palmar-flexed hand can cause an avulsion (Barton's I fracture) or impaction (Barton's II fracture). The mechanism of the latter is shown in Figure 19.9. In either case, the carpus is no longer fully stabilized by the distal radius, and will displace with the fracture fragment.

As a rule, the radiocarpal ligaments act as a lever forcing the radiocarpal impaction fracture at either side of the joint. King (1975) notes that at the time of fracture, the ligaments between the lunate and radius may rupture on the side of the joint opposite the fracture, causing even greater carpal instability.

Treatment of Barton's fractures

The treatment of the Barton's fractures has proved difficult due to two factors:

1. The fracture is intrinsically unstable; and
2. Malunion of intra-articular fractures is more disabling than that of extra-articular fractures because of pain.

To understand the reasons why Barton's fractures are unstable, one must consider both the forces and the structures that affect radiocarpal stability. The distal articular surface of the radius is a shallow concavity which, at any moment, articulates with a relatively small area of the convex proximal articular surface of the scaphoid and lunate. During palmar-flexion and dorsiflexion of the wrist, the distal radius articulates with different

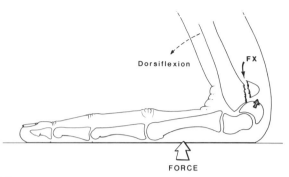

Fig. 19.8 Dorsiflexion injury more commonly causes the volar intra-articular fracture shown. A similar injury may wedge the lunate against the dorsum of the radius causing a dorsal Barton's fracture, or may avulse a small volar bony fragment—Volar Barton's Fracture. The volar lip fracture is most unstable in dorsiflexion

portions of the scaphoid and lunate as they roll forward and back. Because of the shallowness of the distal radius, the articulation is quite unstable unless it is reinforced by the firm bands of volar and dorsal ligaments that support the proximal carpal bones. If either the volar or dorsal lip of the radius is fractured and displaced, the entire carpus becomes unstable and will dislocate proximally, bringing the fragment of the radius with it. With a dorsal lip fracture, instability is greater in palmar-flexion, for in this position the compressive forces

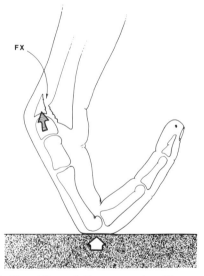

Fig. 19.9 Dorsal Barton's Fracture—a dorsal intra-articular fracture of the distal radius may be produced by impaction or avulsion of the dorsal lip. In either case, the carpus will displace with the fracture fragment in the direction shown. Instability is greater in palmar flexion

act principally upon the dorsum of the distal radius (see Fig. 19.9). With the wrist dorsiflexed, compressive loading shifts to the volar side of the distal radius and therefore in this position the volar lip fractures will be most unstable and tend to displace.

Now consider the means by which we reduce the fracture. Closed reduction of a volar lip fracture requires dorsiflexion of the wrist so that the volar radiocarpal ligaments are made taut and pull the fragment distally. Note that this is precisely the position which puts compressive load on the fracture fragment and forces it to dislocate (Fig. 19.10). If we are to reduce a dorsal lip fracture, we will bring it distally by palmar flexing the wrist.

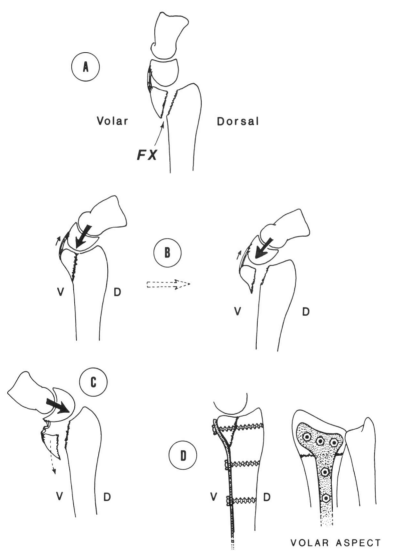

Fig. 19.10 (A) Fracture–dislocations of the distal radius are intrinsically unstable. The carpus is no longer stabilized by the distal radius, and will displace with the fracture fragment. (B) Closed reduction of a volar lip fracture requires wrist dorsiflexion so that the volar radiocarpal ligaments are made taut and pull the fragment distally. However, this position places compressive load on the fracture fragment and permits the wrist to dislocate. (C) Palmar flexion relieves the displacing force on the volar fragment. However, the radiocarpal ligaments are loosened and the fragment may displace. (D) Open reduction and rigid internal fixation have solved the paradox of Barton's fracture

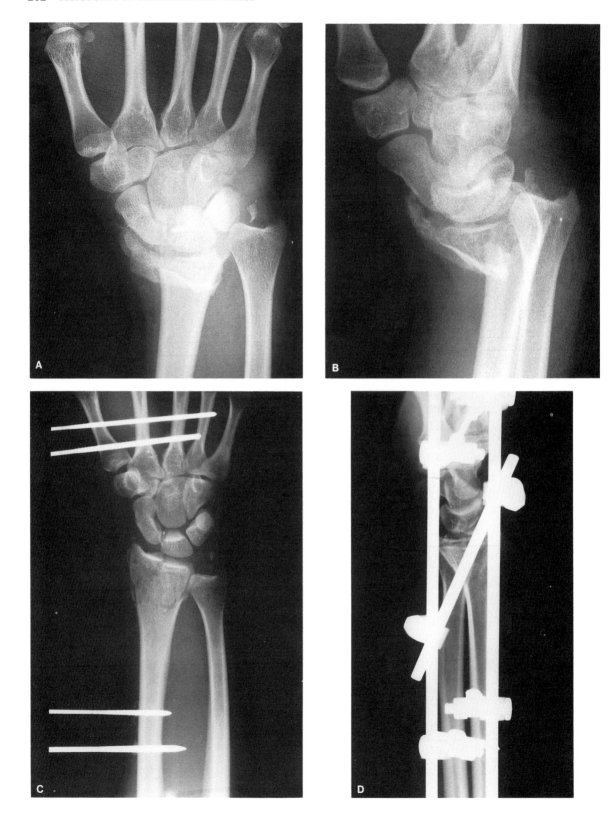

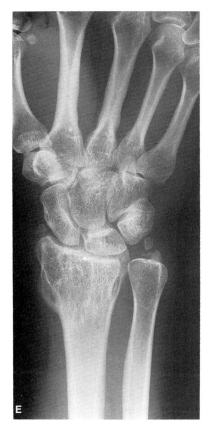
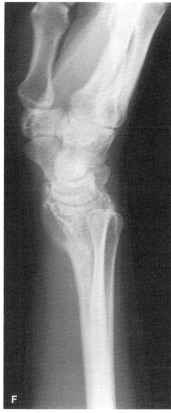

Fig. 19.11 (A & B) A 25-year-old man fell from his bicycle and sustained a right wrist injury. Antero-posterior and lateral radiographs demonstrate a volar fracture–dislocation of the wrist. (C & D) The patient underwent closed reduction of the fracture and application of an external fixation device. (E & F) Eight years after his injury, the patient has a painless wrist. Radiographs demonstrate minimal post-traumatic arthritis

The dorsal radiocarpal ligaments will pull the displaced dorsal fragment into position. Yet, palmar flexion places a compressive load on the dorsal lip of the radius and will thus tend to displace it again.

Thus we have an inherent paradox in the treatment of both dorsal and volar Barton's fractures; the wrist position that will reduce the fracture (by tightening the radiocarpal ligament) is the same position which will displace the fracture (by compressive loading on the fracture fragment). For this reason, Barton's frustration in treating these fracture–dislocations has been shared by many surgeons. Considering the unhappy results of a poorly reduced intra-articular fracture of the distal radius, one can readily appreciate the dissatisfaction and lack of success with closed reduction and plaster immobilization of these injuries.

The integrity of the triangular fibrocartilage that lies between the radius and ulna and supports the triquetrum and lunate has not been studied relative to Barton's fractures. It would appear, however, that this ligament offers little if any stabilization to the central or radial columns of the carpus with volar or dorsal lip fractures of the distal radius.

Although closed reduction and plaster immobilization are usually unsatisfactory in treating the Barton's fractures, there are two other methods: external fixation, and internal fixation.

External fixation

External fixation with pins through the second and third metacarpals distally and through the midshaft of the radius proximally, can be used to reduce the volar or dorsal lip fractures and can maintain position of the wrist while the fracture consolidates (Fig. 19.11). Since external fixation with traction can overcome the compressive force of the carpus against the radius, the wrist should be positioned in the fixator so that the radiocarpal ligaments on the fractured side are made taut. Thus, with

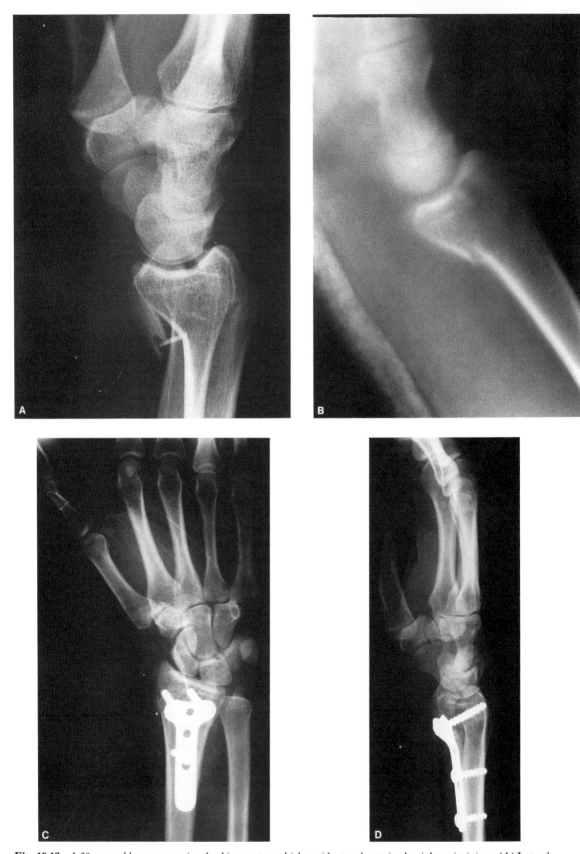

Fig. 19.12 A 20-year-old woman was involved in a motor vehicle accident and sustained a right wrist injury. (A) Lateral radiographs demonstrate a volar lip fracture of the distal radius articular surface. (B) Lateral tomograms confirmed the diagnosis. (C & D) Open reduction and internal fixation resulted in an anatomical position of the fracture fragment and allowed early mobilization of the wrist

Barton's I (dorsal) fractures, the external fixator should immobilize the wrist in palmar-flexion. With Barton's II (volar) fracture, the fixator should be applied with the wrist in neutral or mild dorsiflexion. We would advise serial tomograms in the lateral planes to be assured that the reduction is satisfactory. If the fragment retains a 'stepoff' then internal fixation is required.

Internal fixation

We believe that most Barton's fracture–dislocations are best treated by open reduction and internal fixation. With a Barton's I (dorsal) fracture, we will explore the wrist dorsally through an incision between the third and fourth dorsal compartments, exposing the distal radius and the wrist joint. The fracture is reduced and temporarily held with a Kirschner wire while an angled T-plate is applied. Cancellous screws may be used to hold the distal fragment in place and any dorsal ligament tears are repaired. The patient is permitted controlled active range-of-motion exercises after three weeks. With a Barton's II (Smith's II) volar lip fracture, our surgical approach is to the volar side of the distal forearm and wrist. Finger flexors are retracted ulnarly, FCR and FPL are retracted radially and the insertion of the pronator quadratus often must be elevated to visualize the joint. The wrist joint is opened to assist in accurate reduction of the fracture fragment. As with the Barton's I fracture, an angled T-plate is usually used. Whether or not we use a distal screw depends on the amount of comminution of the distal fragment (Fig. 19.12). The wrist is supported for three weeks and then active controlled range-of-motion exercises are begun.

Our ability to treat the Barton's fractures by open reduction and rigid internal fixation has solved the paradox. Of all fractures about the wrist, it is the Barton's fractures for which internal fixation has proved most useful.

CONCLUSIONS

To obtain a painless, mobile wrist is the goal of any surgeon treating fractures of the distal end of the radius. Unfortunately this goal is not always achieved. Although the Colles's fracture is most frequent in this area, disability caused by malunion and instability following the Smith's fractures and the Barton's fractures are often severe. Each of these fractures requires accurate diagnosis and interpretation in order for the surgeon to be able to render appropriate treatment.

Unfortunately there has been confusion and errors regarding the terminology, the cause and the treatment of these injuries. Perhaps some of this confusion and misunderstanding may be lessened if future authors will identify the fractures by simple anatomical terms in addition to the eponyms. We should clearly define and distinguish the following fractures:

1. Colles's fracture: dorsally displaced, supinated epiphyseal fracture of the distal radius 2–4 cm from its distal articular margin;
2. Smith's I fracture (or reversed Colles's fracture): volarly displaced, pronated epiphyseal fracture of the distal radius 2–4 cm from its distal articular margin;
3. Smith's II fracture (better known as a Barton's II fracture): volar articular lip fracture of distal radius;
4. Smith's III fracture: volarly displaced metaphyseal fracture of distal radius without rotatory deformity;
5. Smith's IV fracture: volarly displaced greenstick or metaphyseal fracture of the distal radius in adolescents;
6. Barton's I fracture: dorsal articular lip fracture–dislocation of the distal radius;
7. Barton's II (or Smith's II) fracture: volar articular lip distal radius fracture–dislocation (*see definition no. 3*).

Many of these fractures can be treated satisfactorily with closed reduction and plaster immobilization. The method of reduction differs depending upon the type of fracture. Some fractures do best with the use of external fixators. Some require open reduction and internal fixation.

It has been said that 'given an eponym, one may be sure that: (1) the man so honoured was not the first to describe the disease ...; or (2) he misunderstood the situation; or (3) he is generally misquoted; or (4) 1, 2 and 3 are all simultaneously true.' (Ravitch 1979).

It would appear that 'Smith's fractures' and 'Barton's fractures' fall into category 4 of this rule of eponyms, as:

1. neither Smith nor Barton were the first to describe the fractures that bear their names;
2. neither Smith nor Barton fully understood the mechanism of injury of the fractures they described; and

3. both Smith and Barton are generally misquoted.

Yet, considering that these great surgeons so vividly and accurately described these fractures over 150 years ago, unaided by radiographs, strain gauges or operative exploration, we are pleased to honour them; even if it must be with inappropriate eponyms.

REFERENCES

Aufranc O E, Jones W N, Turner R H 1966 Anterior marginal articular fracture of the distal radius. Journal of the American Medical Association 196:788–791

Barton J R 1838 Views and treatment of an important injury of the wrist. Philadelphia Medical Examiner 1:365–368

Bhattacharyya A N, Srivastava K K 1972 Smith's fractures. Australian and New Zealand Journal of Surgery 42:141–144

Colles A 1814 On the fracture of the carpal extremity of the radius. Edinburgh Medical and Surgical Journal 10:182–186

De Oliveira J C 1973 Barton's fractures. Journal of Bone and Joint Surgery 55A:586–594

Dupuytren G 1832 Leçons Orales de Clinique Chirurgical Faites a l'Hotel Dieu de Paris par M. Le Baron Dupuytren recueillies et publiées par une Société de Médecine, Germer Baillière, Paris

Ellis J 1965 Smith's and Barton's fractures—a method of treatment. Journal of Bone and Joint Surgery 47B:724–727

Flandreau R H, Sweeney R M, O'Sullivan W 1962 Clinical experience with a series of Smith's fractures. Archives of Surgery 84:288–291

Frykman G 1967 Fracture of the distal radius including sequelae—shoulder-hand-finger syndrome, disturbances in the distal radio-ulnar joint and impairment of the nerve function: a clinical and experimental study. Acta Orthopaedica Scandinavica 108(Suppl):1–155

Fuller D J 1973 The Ellis plate operation for Smith's fracture. Journal of Bone and Joint Surgery 55B:173–178

Goyrand G 1832 Memoirs sur les fractures de l'extrémité

inférieure du radius, qui simulent les luxations du poignet. Gazette de Médecine 3:664–667

Goyrand G 1836 De la fracture par contre-coup de l'extrémité inférieure du radius. Journal Hebdomadaire 1:161–163

King R E 1975 Barton's fracture–dislocation of the wrist. Current practice in orthopaedic surgery 6:133–144

Mills T J 1957 Smith's fracture and anterior marginal fracture of the radius. British Medical Journal 2:603–604

Paterson D C 1966 Smith's fracture—a review. Australian and New Zealand Journal of Surgery 36:145–152

Pouteau C 1783 Oeuvres posthumes de M. Pouteau: Memoire, contenant quelques reflexions sur quelques fractures de l'avant-bras, sur les luxations incomplettes du poignet et sur le diastasis. Ph-D. Pierres, Paris

Ravitch M 1979 Dupuytren's invention of the Mikulicz enterotome with a note on eponyms. Perspectives in biology and medicine 22:170

Roberts J B 1897 A clinical, pathological, and experimental study of fracture of the lower end of the radius with displacement of the carpal fragment toward the flexor or anterior surface of the wrist. Blakiston, Philadelphia

Smith R W 1847 A treatise on fractures in the vicinity of joints and on certain forms of accidental and congenital dislocations. Hodges and Smith, Dublin

Thomas F B 1957 Reduction of Smith's fractures. Journal of Bone and Joint Surgery 39B:436–470

Woodyard J E 1969 A review of Smith's fractures. Journal of Bone and Joint Surgery 51B:324–329

F. D. Burke

20 Colles's fractures: conservative treatment

Colles's fractures account for approximately 10% of fracture attendances at hospital. Because of its relative frequency, the fracture is usually managed by inexperienced junior medical staff. It is often assumed that the management of common injuries is straightforward, but the concept is without logic and, in the case of Colles's fractures, fallacious. Many patients are left with functional difficulties and persistent cosmetic deformity is common. Lidstrom noted that only 41% of Colles's fractures at review had a perfect cosmetic and functional result. There was some functional loss in 20%, and in half of these the loss was significant. There is still a lack of agreement as to the optimal methods of anaesthesia and reduction. The maintenance of the reduction by external splintage during the healing phase remains unsatisfactory, with redisplacement rates quoted from $18–42\%$.

DEFORMING FORCE AND CONSEQUENT LOCAL INJURY

The injury is usually produced by a fall on the outstretched hand. Classically the fracture is extra-articular, one to two inches proximal to the wrist joint. The dorsal cortex buckles, with crushing of a dorsally based cortico-cancellous wedge. The distal end of the radius, which usually faces 20 degrees volarly, is tilted dorsally. If the deforming force continues, a dorsal and radial displacement of the distal fragment occurs associated with proximal migration. The displacement at the fracture can be quantified radiologically in terms of dorsal tilt, radial angulation and shortening (Fig. 20.1). The foreshortening of the radius may produce disruption of the distal radioulnar joint

with impingement of the ulnar styloid against the proximal carpal row, or apparent volar displacement of the distal ulna due to the dorsal displacement of the distal radial fragment and carpus (Fig. 20.2). The disruption may be at the level of the ulnar collateral ligament of the wrist, the styloid, triangular cartilage or more proximally. Intra-articular fractures add the further complication of a disrupted radial articular surface. The dorsal tilt increases tensile loading of volar structures.

MANIPULATION OF THE FRACTURE

Minimally displaced fractures, where the tilt to the radial articulation is less than $20°$ (i.e. the radius still faces volarly), do not require manipulation, and the ultimate anatomical position is rarely significantly worse than that of the original radiograph.

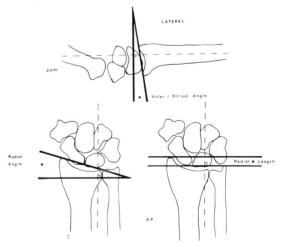

Fig. 20.1 The three measurements of deformity of a Colles's fracture

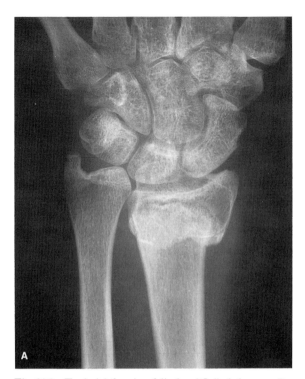 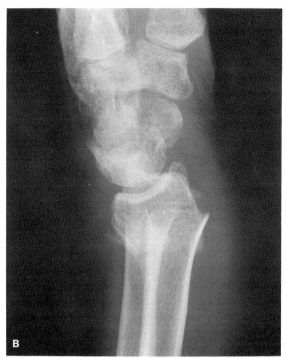

Fig. 20.2 Typical deformity of displaced Colles's fracture. Postero-anterior view shows the radial shortening (A). In this case the radial angle is partly preserved. Lateral view shows that the volar angle has been converted into a dorsal angle (B)

Is manipulation of a more displaced Colles's fracture of benefit? Although slippage following manipulation occurs frequently, we have satisfied ourselves in a local study (Stewart et al 1985a) that a full reduction did benefit the ultimate anatomical result. The well-reduced fractures did lose more position than those less well-reduced, but the final position was considerably better than the initial deformity. Anatomical reduction is therefore advocated for all patients except those with minimally displaced fractures. This ensures the best chance of a good anatomical result, which in turn gives a better chance of a good early functional result. Our survey did not find a direct correlation between the anatomical result and the late functional assessment. The degree of deformity is but one factor which affects the result and the variation in requirements between patients probably plays a more important role in the assessment of an unsatisfactory late result. Major slippage in the first two weeks does merit remanipulation. The majority of such cases in our series obtained lasting anatomical improvement after remanipulation.

Anaesthesia

There is little debate on the timing of manipulation. Most authors advocate reduction at the earliest convenient occasion. The method of anaesthesia, however, is more contentious.

Local anaesthetic direct to the fracture site

The anaesthetic solution is delivered into the haematoma between the bone ends, with additional infiltration to the structures surrounding the distal radioulnar joint. The latter is essential if adequate anaesthesia is to be achieved. The possibility, albeit remote, of introducing infection to the fracture site has concerned some surgeons, while others have found the level of anaesthesia obtained unsatisfactory and questioned the quality of reduction when manipulation is performed with normal tone in the forearm muscles.

The Bier's block

This remains one of the most popular forms of anaesthetic for Colles's fracture reduction. There is the added advantage of relaxation of the forearm muscles. However, the level of anaesthesia is not always satisfactory and the technique offers only limited time for manipulation, application of cast and check radiograph. Increasing discomfort is experienced at the level of the tourniquet, even if a double cuff is used, and it is rarely possible to continue this form of anaesthesia beyond half an hour. If a check radiograph reveals that remanipulation is required, the patient may experience a very unsatisfactory level of anaesthesia. Facilities for swift radiological assessment are essential if this technique is employed. Bier's blocks should only be employed in areas where general anaesthetic facilities are also available. The procedure should be performed by experienced personnel with anaesthetic support in case of cuff rupture which may cause convulsions with respiratory or cardiac arrest. This complication is more likely if cuff failure occurs shortly after the local anaesthetic has been injected into the forearm veins, prior to bonding to local tissues. Long-acting anaesthetics (e.g. Marcaine) are inappropriate for Bier's blocks; they are slower to produce effective anaesthesia and give rise to protracted complications if the cuff should fail. Prilocaine (Citanest) is the preferred agent, having a rapid action with a reduced cardiotoxic effect.

Regional block

Regional block at axillary or supraclavicular level. The commonest complication is patchy inadequate anaesthesia and, infrequently, local haematoma or pneumothorax (in the case of the supraclavicular block).

Lidstrom observed that almost one-quarter of patients manipulated under local anaesthetic had discomfort during the procedure.

General anaesthesia

If the anaesthetic facilities and the patient's general health permit, there is much to recommend reduction under general anaesthesia. This provides relaxation of the surrounding tissues and ample time should remanipulation be required. It seems likely that the accuracy of reduction will relate in part to the adequacy of anaesthesia.

Manipulative technique

There are two main techniques of reduction. The most popular is that described by Robert Jones: the wrist is hyperextended to disimpact the fracture. Longitudinal traction is then applied to the fingers and carpus with one hand, while the surgeon's other thumb presses the dorsal aspect of the distal radial fragment in a volar direction. The fragment may be held reduced by thumb pressure while the adequacy of reduction is assessed clinically. The volar tilt of the lower end of the radius will be revealed by the arc of motion at the wrist. If the range of wrist flexion appears normal, the volar tilt is usually satisfactory. The wrist is then immobilized in a cast and a check radiograph performed.

Böhler described a manual traction technique which required extensive ancillary support. This has been superseded by the use of a variety of traction machines, of which the Chinese finger traps have been the most successful. The technique has much to recommend it, in particular in situations where ancillary support is minimal. After satisfactory anaesthesia, the finger traps are applied to the fingers and thumb (Fig. 20.3). Tilt of the carpus can be controlled by the choice of fingers to which the traction is applied; the use of thumb, index and middle finger produces mild ulnar deviation at the wrist. The arm is then attached to a drip pole at such a level that the elbow lies flexed to 90° with the upper arm free over the edge of the couch. A sling and 5 lb (2.27 kg) of traction is applied to the upper arm (see Fig. 20.3). The fracture is usually reduced by the traction alone if anaesthesia is adequate. The distal fragment is manipulated into satisfactory alignment. Clinical assessment of volar tilt can be performed as previously described without removing the traction. The surgeon has both hands free and can apply a well moulded cast in traction with little chance of losing reduction. A check radiograph in the cast should be performed before anaesthesia is discontinued.

METHODS OF RETAINING REDUCTION

Colles advocated dorsal and volar wooden splints to control the fracture in the healing phase.

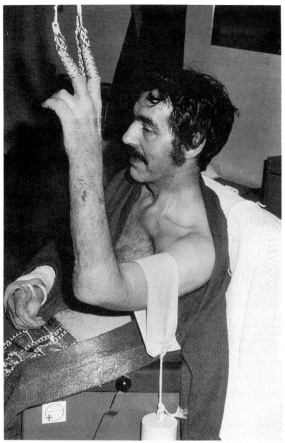

Fig. 20.3 Chinese finger-traps being used to maintain reduction of a Colles's fracture during a plaster change at 10 days

Preformed dorsal and volar metal splints are still used in some centres, but the most popular methods are the use of a below-elbow plaster of Paris cast, a forearm cast brace, or one with a sugar tong extension at the elbow to control pronation/supination. Functional cast-bracing of fractures of the tibia and femur to permit active joint movement during healing have been shown to reduce later stiffness and osteoporosis (Sarmiento 1970, 1972) and an analogous method of treatment for Colles's fractures has been developed by Sarmiento with improved early results in displaced cases (1975). He developed a supinated brace on the theoretical ground that the brachio-radialis muscle is a major deforming force on the fracture fragments and is relaxed in supination (1965), and went on to show in 93 displaced fractures better anatomical end results were achieved in those patients treated in

supination as opposed to pronation (1980). However, there appeared to be no difference in the early functional results between the two treatments.

Our local study (Stewart et al 1984) compared the efficacy of the Colles's forearm plaster cast, the forearm cast-brace and the supinated cast-brace. The three groups (243 patients) were well matched in terms of age and sex. Three radiographic measurements were made at each stage of treatment and the final anatomical result determined using the criteria employed previously by Sarmiento (1975). Of the study group, 193 fractures were felt to merit manipulation. All were initially placed in a plaster backslab in mild wrist flexion and ulnar deviation. At an average interval of nine days, the wrist was transferred to the chosen form of immobilization. Eleven fractures required remanipulation at this stage. Function was assessed in detail at three and six months using Sarmiento's modification (1975) of Gartland and Werley's system (1951). The ultimate anatomical result was not related to the form of immobilization but was related to the efficacy of reduction. Loss of position in the braces was no greater than those in plaster casts. The functional result at three months was likewise not related to the form of immobilization, and hence not influenced by early wrist or finger motion, but was related to the severity of initial displacement of the fracture and to a lesser degree to the anatomical result. This latter effect was lost at six months. Early hand function and supination in the treatment of displaced Colles's fractures as advocated by Sarmiento was found to confer no anatomical or functional advantage. The study concluded that there was no indication to change from the use of conventional plaster casts in routine cases. A below-elbow cast-brace would be indicated if preferred by the patient or in situations where stiffness of the fingers was judged to be a likely complication (e.g. rheumatoid arthritis). Patients with symptoms or previous history suggestive of sympathetic dystrophy might benefit from the increased finger mobility and wrist flexion obtained by the cast-brace.

It was interesting to observe in this series that the increased wrist mobility in the cast-brace did not appear to improve the results in intra-articular fractures, nor did the position of immobilization affect the ultimate position. In most cases the wrist was held in mild flexion and ulnar deviation, but those splinted in neutral dorsipalmar flexion did not have a less satisfactory ultimate anatomical result. The Cotton Loder position (see p. 322) (extreme wrist flexion) would therefore seem unnecessary, particularly as the position may precipitate median nerve compression. The fracture position should be reviewed radiologically at one week and if significant loss of position is found remanipulation is required. In this series the improvement obtained at remanipulation was usually maintained.

ROLE OF HAND THERAPY IN COLLES'S FRACTURES

All patients attending with a Colles's fracture should be interviewed at an early stage by the therapist and advice given on retaining mobility of the shoulder and elbow. In the longer term, only a small number of patients will require therapy to regain shoulder or wrist mobility following Colles's fracture. All such patients should be monitored by the doctor and, if evidence of shoulder stiffness, sympathetic dystrophy or, at a later stage, marked wrist stiffness becomes apparent, swift referral for intensive therapy is required. Hand therapy should be regarded in the same way as an antibiotic— prescribed for specific indications, for a limited period, and at a sufficiently high dosage to be effective. Low-dose maintenance therapy squanders resources and is of doubtful benefit.

COMPLICATIONS OF COLLES'S FRACTURES

Stiffness

Shoulder stiffness is a complication which can largely be avoided by constant vigilance and early referral to therapy. Prompt intervention is particularly important in these cases for the condition, once established, is extremely slow to reverse. If shoulder pain is a prominent feature, intra-articular steroid injection is often of benefit. Reduced mobility at the wrist is a frequent sequel to Colles's fracture, particularly in the elderly. Although a reduced range of dorsal and palmar flexion may be observed on clinical examination,

elderly patients rarely regard the wrist as stiff. Thirty degrees of dorsal and palmar flexion will allow an almost full range of activities to the elderly. However, younger patients will complain of difficulties if engaged in occupations or activities which require full upper limb dexterity (e.g., tool setters or car mechanics). Disruption of the distal radioulnar joint may reduce pronation/supination range with a profound reduction in upper limb function at any age. Loss of pronation is the more disabling of the two. Darrach or Baldwin procedures, coupled with intensive postoperative hand therapy, may improve pronation–supination range and, to a lesser degree, dorsipalmar flexion.

Finger stiffness may be caused by post-traumatic oedema or follow sympathetic dystrophy. Fibrin is laid down in the soft tissues by the oedematous exudate and may restrict subsequent tendon or joint motion. This is most commonly seen around the metacarpophalangeal and interphalangeal joints. If oedema is allowed to diffuse around the collateral ligaments in a lax position, the effect of subsequent fibrin deposits will be to shorten them. This is particularly important at the metacarpophalangeal joints where the ligaments are lax in extension and tighten progressively when flexed. Ideally, when oedema is anticipated, the hand should be splinted with the joints in such a position that the collateral ligaments are under tension. This reduces the chances of subsequent stiffness of the hand with fore-shortening of the collateral ligaments. Clinical experience and anatomical dissection indicate that the most favourable position in which the fingers may be placed is $90°$ of flexion at the metacarpophalangeal joints, and virtually full extension of the interphalangeal joints. The thumb is held extended at the metacarpophalangeal and interphalangeal joints and abducted from the palm to avoid a first web space contracture. The metacarpophalangeal joints of the fingers are the most difficult to maintain in optimum position. Palmar oedema tends to force them into an unfavourable semi-extended position. The position of metacarpophalangeal joint flexion and interphalangeal joint extension is perhaps best maintained with the use of a volar splint with the wrist held in extension. However, this form of splintage is difficult to maintain in the presence of a mildly flexed wrist and is generally regarded as unsatisfactory in the management of Colles's fractures. The digits are left free, the surgeon relying on early mobilisation of the fingers to avoid joint contracture and tendon adhesion. Nevertheless, some restriction in joint mobility or tendon excursion may follow Colles's fracture, particularly in elderly patients. If oedema is associated with disproportionately severe pain, a diagnosis of sympathetic dystrophy should be considered. Guanethidine blocks, coupled with intensive hand therapy, are most effective if employed before the condition becomes fully established.

Dupuytren's disease

The effect of local trauma on the appearance or progression of Dupuytren's disease is of interest.

The incidence of the disease in manual workers is no higher than the incidence in clerks (Early 1962). The disease is evenly distributed between dominant and non-dominant hands. For these and other reasons discussed by Fisk (1974), it is generally accepted that chronic minor trauma does not play a role in the causation of Dupuytren's disease.

However, one occasionally sees a patient with pre-existing Dupuytren's disease which appears to have been exacerbated by an episode of trauma to the involved limb, a correlation supported by Clarkson (1961) after a survey of numerous authorities. Hueston (1968) has postulated that injury may exacerbate Dupuytren's disease by an alteration in the pattern of blood flow to the hand. In our series, the incidence of Dupuytren's disease was 4% at three months and 11% (23% patients) at six months. Two patients had noticed palmar nodules prior to the fracture. Sixteen patients were noted to develop the condition between three and six months. All cases were mild, taking the form of palmar nodules in 13 patients out of the 23, palmar bands in nine patients and a digital nodule in one patient. Twenty-one patients were seen between 15 and 27 months after fracture (mean 20.7 months) and the disease process had not progressed significantly in any patient. Minor progression was seen in two patients; two patients felt that the nodules were definitely less prominent, and the remainder were unchanged. Only two patients had contractures at final review: both involved the proximal interphalangeal joint and were limited to 15 and 20° respectively.

Using the incidences of the disease for each decade of age in both sexes quoted by Early (1962), the predicted incidence in our group is 4.2%, which is statistically significantly lower than the actual incidence at six months of 11% (0.05 > P > 0.01). This increase in incidence of Dupuytren's disease following Colles's fracture has not previously been noted. Bacorn and Kurtzke (1953), in a study of 2100 cases of Colles's fractures, noted only four cases (0.2%); neither Lidstrom (1959) nor Frykman (1967) in their detailed reviews noted any cases, and Colles's fracture as a predisposing factor is not mentioned in the monograph on Dupuytren's disease edited by Hueston and Tubiana (1974).

It seems likely that an episode of limb trauma exacerbates a pre-existing tendency to develop Dupuytren's disease and that Colles's fracture accelerates the Dupuytren process, although this is only temporary, and rapid development of contractures is unlikely to occur.

Pain

Pain over the lower end of the radius usually settles over the first three or four months after injury. However, disruption of the distal radioulnar joint may cause persistent discomfort around the lower end of the ulna. This may be caused by degenerative changes between radius and ulna (where the discomfort is often greatest during rotatory movements of the forearm). The relative shortening of the radius can disrupt the triangular cartilage or produce impingement between ulna and the proximal carpal row. Either condition may cause prolonged wrist pain, most commonly on dorsiflexion. The Darrach or Baldwin procedures may both be effective in obtaining pain relief.

Median nerve compression

We found (Stewart et al 1985b) an incidence of carpal tunnel syndrome of 17% at three months: this is much higher than those of previous reports, which vary from 0% (Lidstrom, 1959) to a maximum of 5.4% (Pool, 1973). This reflects specific clinical searching by a hand surgeon. The incidence had settled to 12% by six months. There was a subsequent operation rate of 3.4% of the whole group (eight patients) for persistent troublesome symptoms. At operation, seven patients had definite median nerve compression in the carpal tunnel (Fig. 20.4) and afterwards their symptoms resolved. There is a tendency to underestimate the frequency of this condition after Colles's fracture.

Both Lynch and Lipscomb (1963) and Sponsel and Palm (1965), in their papers on carpal tunnel syndrome following Colles's fractures, observed that symptoms came on soon after reduction in the majority of cases, and usually before three months. They considered that the main aetiological factors were the position of immobilization of the wrist, and oedema and haematoma in the carpal tunnel, especially following fractures with intra-articular extension. In our local series there was only one acute case, due to immobilization in extreme palmar flexion, which settled completely after correct splintage. There were, however, ten new cases at six months, with two of these subsequently requiring decompression. The reason for this difference is that none of our patients, except the one mentioned, were immobilized in significant wrist palmar flexion. In Lynch and Lipscomb's paper, of the 15 extremities in which the position of immobilization was known, 12 had the Cotton Loder position of full flexion and ulnar deviation. In Sponsel and Palm's paper, 3 of 19 patients had their wrists in the Cotton Loder position. Carpal tunnel syndrome after Colles's fracture appears to be common if looked for.

There was a specific correlation of the incidence of this delayed Carpal Tunnel Syndrome with the mean residual dorsal angle of the associated fractures, median nerve compression being more frequent in cases with a high residual dorsal tilt (Fig. 20.4). In addition, there was an increased incidence in the elderly. The aetiology would appear to be due to the effect of the changed anatomy acting over several weeks in older patients, whose nerve tissue tolerates the effect of trauma and pressure relatively poorly. Tenosynovitis of the flexor tendons, suggested by Lynch and Lipscomb (1963) as a possible cause of compression, may be a consequence of this altered anatomy.

The view that these fractures are not worth

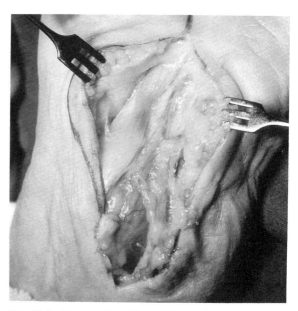

Fig. 20.4 Compression of the median nerve resulting from a Colles's fracture

reducing in the elderly should therefore be challenged because it is accepted that the final anatomical result is related to the completeness of reduction (Green & Gay 1956, Lidstrom 1959, Pool 1973, Van der Linden & Ericson 1981, Stewart et al 1985).

The clinical success rate of seven out of eight following classical carpal tunnel decompression tends to refute the suggestion of Lewis (1978) that treatment of this syndrome following Colles's fractures produces poor results.

Ulnar nerve compression

Ulnar nerve compression at the wrist is uncommon following Colles's fracture. Only two patients in our series developed ulnar sensory symptoms: one case was mild and settled by six months, but the other was troublesome and was decompressed at six months following positive electromyographic tests. The patient was a woman of 56 with malunion and marked radial deviation.

Radial nerve compression

Mild irritation of the terminal branches of the radial nerve is a frequent complication following the application of an Orthoplast cast-brace, despite considerable care in the moulding. In our series, 11 patients developed this complication (all in the cast-brace group). All but one settled in six months.

Tendon rupture

Extensor pollicis longus rupture remains an uncommon complication following Colles's fracture. There was one patient in our series, and Frykman notes an incidence of 0.7% in his review. The complication usually arises in the minimally displaced Colles's fracture, perhaps because the intact overlying retinaculum holds the tendon against the displaced edge of bone. An attrition rupture occurs several weeks after the fracture. More widely displaced fractures may disrupt the retinaculum and allow the tendon to stand free from the fracture margin. The attrition rupture damages a length of the tendon and tendon transfer (EIP to EPL) is indicated for those who remain significantly incapacitated. The degree of incapacity is not always large and relates in part to the patient's requirements and extensor pollicis brevis function.

Weak grip

This symptom may be caused by a variety of factors. Limited wrist extension or finger stiffness may be responsible. Pain around the inferior radioulnar joint may limit the ability to grasp firmly.

Cosmetic deformity

This remains one of the most frequent and distressing features of the injury. Colles observed that 'the deformity will remain undiminished through life'. Frykman noted that 50% of the patients in his series had significant ulnar prominence of the distal end of the ulna, radial deviation or dorsal angulation. Ulnar prominence may be reduced by fairly simple surgery. Corrective osteotomy of the distal radius is a more major procedure and is reserved for gross residual angulation. A dorsal wedge (opening) osteotomy is required, for a volar closing wedge will simply increase the disparity between length of radius and ulna.

CONCLUSION

Colles's fracture remains a difficult problem to manage satisfactorily. Our survey indicated that only 69% of patients had achieved an excellent or good rating six months later.

Anatomical reduction is advocated for all patients except those with minimally displaced fractures. This ensures the best chance of a good anatomical and early functional result, and also a good cosmetic result which is important to the patient. In addition, a good anatomical result lowers the risk of the patient developing carpal tunnel syndrome; this 'protection' applies particularly to the elderly patient.

Maintenance of reduction remains a problem, with no method of external splintage providing adequate control. Would accurate reduction and internal fixation with Kirschner wires improve cosmetic and functional results? The literature does not offer firm guidance on this matter. The role of hand therapists is to provide advice for all Colles patients, but to reserve intensive treatment for those in need.

REFERENCES

Bacorn R W, Kurtske J F 1953 Colles's fracture. A study of two thousand cases from the New York State Workmans Compensation Board. Journal of Bone and Joint Surgery 35A:643–658
Bohler L 1842 The treatment of fractures, 4th edn. William Wood, Baltimore
Clarkson P 1961 The aetiology of Dupuytren's contracture. Guy's Hospital Reports 110:52–62
Colles A 1814 On the fracture of the carpal extremity of the radius. Edinburgh Medical and Surgical Journal 10:182
Early P F 1962 Population studies in Dupuytren contracture. Journal of Bone and Joint Surgery 44B:602–613

Fisk G 1974 The relationship of trauma to Dupuytren's contracture. In: Hueston J T, Tubiana R (eds) Dupuytren's Disease (1st edn). Churchill Livingstone, Edinburgh, 43–44
Frykman G 1967 Fracture of the distal radius including sequelae—shoulder–hand–finger Syndrome. Disturbance in the distal radio-ulnar joint and impairment of nerve function. A clinical and experimental study. Acta Orthopaedica Scandinavica Supplement 108
Gartland J J, Werley C W 1951 Evaluation of healed Colles's fractures. Journal of Bone and Joint Surgery 33A:895–907
Green J T, Gay F H 1956 Colles's fracture residual disability. American Journal of Surgery 91:636–642

Hueston J T 1968 Dupuytren's contracture and specific injury. Medical Journal of Australia 1 : 1084–1085

Hueston J T, Tubiana R (eds) 1974 Dupuytren's disease (1st edn). Churchill Livingstone, Edinburgh

Lewis M H 1978 Median nerve compression after Colles's fracture. Journal of Bone and Joint Surgery 60B : 195–196

Lidstrom A 1959 Fractures of the distal end of the radius. A clinical and statistical study of end results. Acta Orthopaedica Scandinavica Supplement 41

Lynch A C, Lipscomb P R 1963 The Carpal Tunnel Syndrome and Colles's fracture. Journal of the American Medical Association 185 : 363–366

Pool C 1973 Colles's fracture. A prospective study of treatment. Journal of Bone and Joint Surgery 55B : 540–544

Sarmiento A 1965 The brachioradialis as a deforming force in Colles's fractures. Clinical Orthopaedics 38 : 86–92

Sarmiento A 1970 A functional below the knee brace for tibial fractures. Journal of Bone and Joint Surgery 52A : 295–311

Sarmiento A 1972 Functional bracing of tibial and femoral shaft fracture. Clinical Orthopaedics 82 : 2–13

Sarmiento A, Pratt G W, Berry N C, Sinclair W F 1975 Colles's fractures—functional bracing in supination. Journal of Bone and Joint Surgery 57A : 311–317

Sarmiento A, Zagorski J B, Sinclair W F 1980 Functional bracing of Colles's fractures—a prospective study of immobilisation in supination versus pronation. Clinical Orthopaedics 146 : 175–183

Sponsel K H, Palm E T 1965 Carpal Tunnel Syndrome following Colles's fracture. Surgery, Gynaecology and Obstetrics 121 : 1252–1256

Stewart H D, Innes A R, Burke F D, 1984 Functional cast bracing for Colles's fracture. A comparison between orthoplast cast bracing and conventional plaster cast. Journal of Bone and Joint Surgery 66B : 749–753

Stewart H D, Innes A R, Burke F D 1985 Factors affecting the outcome of Colles's fracture. An anatomical and functional study. Injury 16 : 289–295

Stewart H D, Innes A R, Burke F D 1985 Hand complication in Colles's fracture. Journal of Hand Surgery 10B(1) : 103–107

Van der Linden W, Ericson R 1981 Colles's fracture. How should its displacement be measured and how should it be immobilised? Journal of Bone and Joint Surgery 63A : 1285–1288

21 Colles's fractures: combined internal and external fixation

The management of fractures of the distal radius still poses important problems although, in the last decade, considerable improvement has been achieved, especially regarding new and sophisticated techniques of external fixation (Cooney 1983, Firica et al 1981, Forgon & Mammel 1981).

Evidence accumulated throughout the literature (Bacorn & Kurtzke 1953, De Palma 1952, Castaing 1964, Cole & Obletz 1966, Dobyns & Linscheid 1975, Dowling & Sawyer 1961, Frykman 1967, Gartland & Werley 1951, Rauis et al 1979), indicates a strong correlation between restoration of bone anatomy and recovery of function. At present, the most efficient and innocuous method of reduction is by gentle, prolonged (Böhler 1942, Cooney et al 1979) longitudinal traction applied to the relaxed upper limb after adequate anaesthesia. The crucial problem remains how to stabilize these unfortunately ubiquitous fractures until they become well united. Morbidity, costs and ability to use the limb throughout treatment may also be important factors (Cagnol 1975, Cooney et al 1980, Lee-Osterman & Bora 1980). The purpose of this chapter is to describe a method for the stabilization of extension-compression fractures of the distal radius, by a combined system of internal and external fixation (Fig. 21.1).

INDICATIONS

The present method is designed for the percutaneous intra-medullary osteosynthesis and external fixation of Pouteau-Colles's fractures which are basically unstable and require reduction, re-reduction or have overt comminution. Although

the primary indications are for handling extension-compression fractures, in some selected cases of the flexion-compression type (Smith's fractures) the same basic principles hold true.

This procedure is especially helpful in bilateral fractures and in those where concomitant soft-tissue injuries require a quick, stable and easy method for stabilizing fractures which allows access to the skin. Soft-tissue injuries can thus be adequately treated at both the initial and subsequent changes of dressings, skin graft inspection, burns and the like. On several occasions, the procedure has been used to relieve an acute carpal tunnel syndrome, caused by a Colles's fracture reduction and immobilization in the potentially aggressive Cotton-Loder position (Lee-Osterman & Bora 1980). In these patients, the nerve may be released following stabilization of the fracture.

CONTRAINDICATIONS

These include severely contaminated wounds, or unreliable patients like alcoholics, psychotics and unmotivated, depressed individuals.

OPERATIVE TECHNIQUE

In this method, the sterile phase includes both percutaneous intramedullary osteosynthesis and application of an external mini-fixator, followed by another phase in which either a plaster or thermoplastic forearm and wrist support is added.

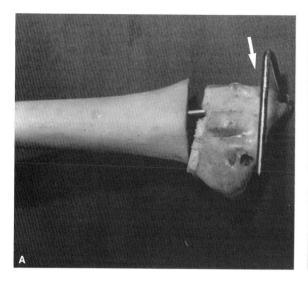
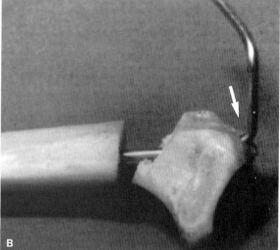
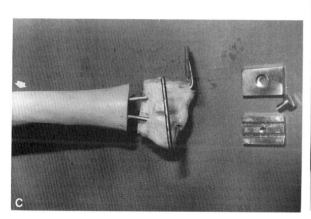
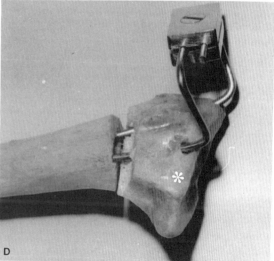

Fig. 21.1 Experimental demonstration in which the radial wire tends to correct the radial deviation of the distal fragment through the steel wire's elastic force (A). Similarly the dorsal wire tends to keep the dorsal tilt of the distal fragment corrected (B). Both wires in place, gripped by the narrowest part of the medullary canal (arrow). Their divergent distal parts will support the distal radial fragment. Here, it is separated from the proximal fragment for demonstration purposes. Once adequately bent, the protruding wires will be clamped together by the external mini-fixator (C). This experimental model of the distal radius was dorsally wedged to imitate an extension–compression extra-articular fracture. It was then stabilized with the combined technique of external and internal fixation. The ideal site of penetration for the dorsal wire should always be medial (ulnar) to Lister's tubercle, preferably transfixing the pyramid-shaped dorso-medial area of the bone marked by the asterisk (D)

Sterile phase

For the sterile phase—always to be performed in the operative theatre and under general or regional anaesthesia—we have designed a set of instruments (Fig. 21.2) comprising a wiredriver, an external mini-fixator ('Mini-U-Fix', pat. pend.) and an Allen-type screwdriver. Either thick Kirschner wires or thin Steinmann pins can be used, provided they measure 30 cm in length and 2 mm in diameter. These wires are first bent with the slotted wiredriver which also serves as a modular wirebender. Thus, the blunt end of the wire is pushed

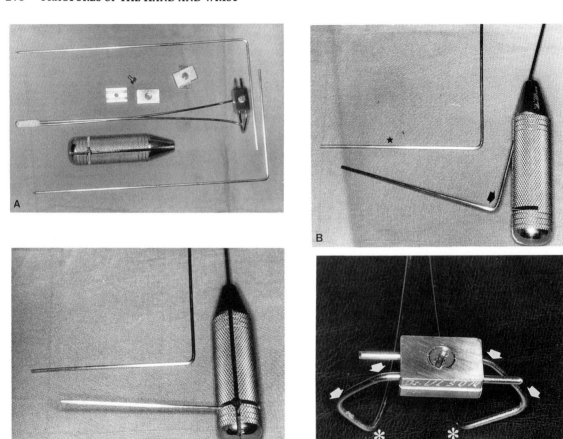

Fig. 21.2 (A) Set of wires, wiredriver and mini-fixator employed in the combined method of internal and external fixation. (B) The star indicates the outer segment of the wire which is the same length as the wiredriver (10 cm), used to bend the wire. (C) Once bent, the wire is fitted into the longitudinal slot of the wire-driver and turned into the locked position, either in the right or left transverse slot. (D) The Eiffel-tower shape of the wires united by the mini-fixator; asterisks indicate the pre-bent angles and the arrows show the two subsequent bendings performed externally on the protruding portions of the wires

down the slot until it stand flush with the bottom end of the wiredriver. By flexing the protruding 20 cm extension of the wire, it is bent to a 90° angle. The now angulated wire is introduced at the slotted crossing and locked into either the right or left position, depending on the surgeon's hand dominance.

Reduction is usually performed manually, that is to say without any special apparatus (Böhler 1942, Frykman 1967, Lidström 1959). Whilst the assistant applies countertraction on the flexed elbow, the surgeon gently but firmly exerts a longitudinal distraction of the fracture by holding the thumb in one hand and the middle and long fingers in the other (Fig. 21.3a). Reconstitution of

the full length of the radius by persistent traction is essential (Castaing 1964, Cooney et al 1980). For reduction of the dorsally displaced distal fragments the volar cortex, usually broken in a simple transverse line, may be used as a fulcrum (Cooney et al 1979). A radiographic control may now be obtained. The flexion and ulnar deviation of the wrist are kept by the surgeon whilst the assistant, with both hands, holds the patient's forearm which in turn is supported by a stack of sterile towels. The surgeon's free hand then performs the percutaneous fixation.

The entry point for this is found by palpating the radial styloid process, just dorsal to the tendons of the first extensor compartment. The skin and

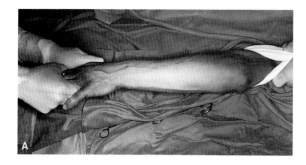
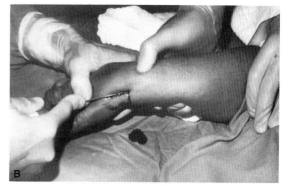
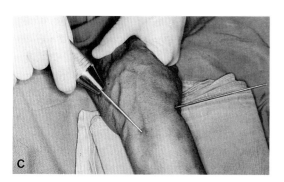
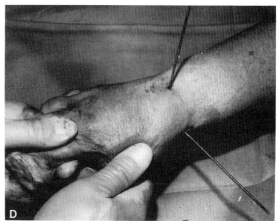

Fig. 21.3 (A) The fracture is manually reduced by Böhler's technique after complete sterile preparation and draping of the upper limb. (B) An assistant holds the proximal forearm and the surgeon inserts the radial wire first. Its direction is changed as soon as the cortex is engaged so as to enter the medullary canal. (C) The dorsal wire is introduced second. (D) Check radiographs can be obtained after the first wire is in place, but this is usually done when the second one has also been inserted. (An image intensifier is useful for monitoring the introduction of the wires.) The external parts of the wires are almost perpendicular to the arm because of the pre-bent angle of 90°, now just beneath the skin

subcutaneous tissues are penetrated with the wire at almost a right angle to the surface.

As soon as the outer cortex is pierced, the penetrating wire must change direction: it is now placed at an acute angle to the longitudinal axis of the radius (Fig. 21.3b). By rotating the wiredriver alternately clockwise and counterclockwise and exerting continuous moderate pressure, the cancellous area of the styloid is entered and the fracture site is quickly traversed by the point of the wire until it reaches the medullary canal of the proximal fragment. If the angle is not right the progressive sliding of the wire may be slowed down when it encroaches on the inner surface. In this case, a little back-up manoeuvre and another attempt to penetrate the medullary canal will be required. Here, the use of sledpointed wires (like a Rush

nail) are especially helpful (Rush 1954). Quick progress of the wire and a telltale friction of its tip against the inner surface of the radius indicates that it is accurately placed. Another radioscopic control can now be taken provided an image intensifier is at hand.

The need for manual introduction can best be appreciated when a long wire is mounted on the handle, because its flexibility enables the surgeon to 'feel' penetration into the medullary canal.

When the tip of the wiredriver approaches the skin, the handle is dislodged laterally and removed from the partly introduced wire which is then pushed manually further into the canal by a direct grasp on the bent segment or tail. Once the radial wire has been fully introduced up to its pre-bent angle, a similar procedure is used for the dorsal wire.

For this, the point of penetration should be on the dorsoulnar aspect of the radial epiphysis (Fig. 21.3c) so as to transfix the often present die-punch fragment (Scheck 1962) through its ulnar-most side. Again, the wire is at first introduced perpendicular to the bone surface but its direction should then become quite oblique, in order to reach the medullary canal after the tip of the wire has been deflected against the inner surface of the radial and volar side of the bone. In the adult radius, whether in a man or woman, there is enough room for two 2 mm diameter Kirschner wires at the narrowest part of the medullary canal (Sage 1959). Again, the wire is introduced right up to its angle (Fig. 21.3d). A radiographic control is taken in two projections, at right-angles to each other. When correctly placed, the wires form an isosceles triangle, the apex of which lies in the medullary canal proximal to the middle one-third of the bone, whereas its basis faces the radiocarpal joint (Fig. 21.4).

The tails of both wires are then bent in opposite directions to contour the dorsum of the wrist, at a distance of about 1.2–1.5 cm, which is the clearance required for changing dressings under the external fixator. Before bending the radial wire vertically, the best possible wire position is estimated to avoid either tension or compression of the skin between both penetration sites.

With the aid of a pair of long-nosed pliers, the radial wire is held 1.5 cm from the skin whilst the wiredriver flexes it ulnarly. The dorsal wire is bent in a similar fashion (Fig. 21.4c). A distance of 3–4 mm should separate both horizontal segments of the wires.

The external fixator is mounted, starting with the lower plate which has two parallel slots for lodging the wires. The dorsal or upper plate is also fitted with slots and a central screw. Once tightened, the tail ends of the Kirschner wires are cut off (Fig. 21.4d). In some cases, where more severe comminution calls for additional compression from side to side, an approximation of the wires before finally tightening the central screw can produce the desired effect.

A double layer of gauze soaked in betadine is placed around the wires and on the skin under the fixator, after which a layer of sterile stockinette is applied up to the mid-arm level. The sterile phase has now been concluded.

Unsterile phase

Care should be taken not to enclose either of the wires when applying the forearm and wrist support: a well-padded plaster gutter splint on the volar and ulnar sides (Fig. 21.5). The redundant stockinette is rolled off distally over the splint for a final finish. It is important to keep all the fingers and the thumb absolutely free.

AFTER-CARE

Care while apparatus is in place

During the first 24 hours, the hand is well-elevated on pillows and, upon being discharged from hospital, the patient's arm should be kept in continuous sling elevation (Rauis et al 1979) for the first 3 days. Frequent shoulder exercises and use of the hand are encouraged as early as possible (Dobyns & Linscheid 1975).

Although analgesics are prescribed, antibiotics are not routinely given. The sling is discontinued after the first postoperative week. Shoulder and finger exercises are checked and the site of skin penetration is cleansed and again dressed with betadine.

Similar clinical controls are performed once weekly; there is little need for radiographic control, although in special cases where fixation proves to be less stable, a check radiograph can be obtained during the second or third postoperative week.

Removal of wires

After 6 weeks the external fixator is released by loosening the central screw and the intramedullary wires are removed under local anaesthesia (Castaing 1964, Sevitt 1971). When both penetration sites and the radiocarpal and radioulnar joints have been infiltrated, first the dorsal wire is removed and then the radial one. The skin just distal to both wires should be depressed to facilitate exposure of their subcutaneous angulation. A simple pull on the wire may result in soft tissue

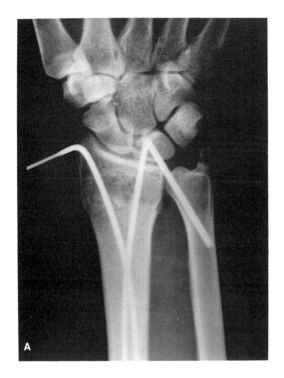

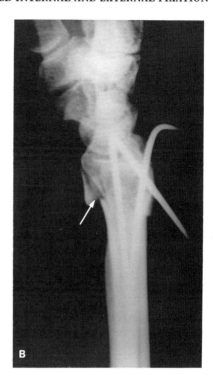

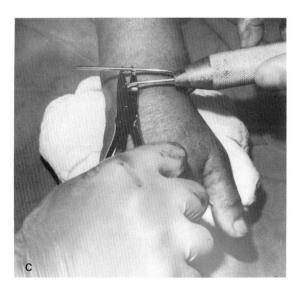

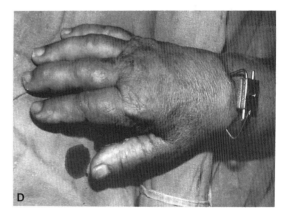

Fig. 21.4 (A) Postero-anterior picture discloses a good longitudinal correction of the radial length with restoration of the radial angle and articular surface. An inverted Eiffel-tower silhouette is formed by the intramedullary wires. (B) On the lateral film the distal ends of the wires also diverge. The correction of the dorsal deviation or tilt is best obtained when the volar cortex is in apposition and can be used as a fulcrum for the reduction, as indicated by the arrow. (C) Both wire tails are bent externally, leaving enough room for oedema and dressings of the penetration site. Before bending each wire twice in opposite directions so that they lie parallel, the best position is found in order to avoid excessive skin tension: the wire tails should be sufficiently separated to prevent skin pressure. (D) The wires are bent and firmly fixed by the external mini-fixator, after which the excessive wire tails are cut off

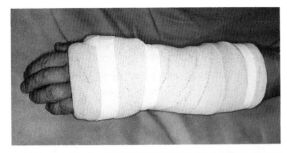

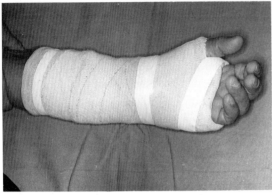

Fig. 21.5 A well-padded volar-ulnar plaster gutter or heat-moulded plastic splint is applied. It must permit full motion of the fingers and thumb. The forearm is placed in $30°$ or $40°$ supination, leaving the elbow free. The redundant stockinette is rolled off distally to cover the bandages

damage. The wire is therefore grasped with a pair of pliers and, whilst the skin is depressed at the site of penetration, the wire is pulled out and up. A plaster splint is maintained during the week that follows.

Rehabilitation

As most patients start using their hands early in the healing phase, a formal rehabilitation programme may not be required. The patients are checked every week for shoulder or finger stiffness and, when these are present, they are submitted to a closely supervised physical and occupational therapy programme. Emotionally unstable patients require special attention to prevent shoulder-hand-finger dystrophy (Dobyns & Linscheid 1975).

RESULTS

From April 1979 to April 1982, a prospective and consecutive series of 120 patients with extension–compression fractures was studied. No attempt

was made to select these patients for treatment and twelve trained surgeons were responsible for fixation of the fractures. There were 88 female and 32 male patients, whose median ages were respectively 57 (18–87) and 43 (18–84) years.

All the fractures considered recent were treated within 21 days after the accident. At the time of fixation the fractures were, on average, 5 days old. In the present study, the distribution of such fractures according to Frykman's classification was as follows:

Type   I = 0.5%;
Type   II = 9.16%;
Type III = 4.16%;
Type   IV = 7.5%;
Type   V = 7.5%;
Type   VI = 7.5%;
Type VII = 14.18%;
Type VIII = 45.0%.

The less severe classes (I–IV) corresponded to 27%, whereas the more severe ones (V–VIII) to 73% of the fractures.

To study the degree of stabilization in the proposed method, standardized radiographic controls were obtained with posteroanterior and lateral views at four stages of treatment (plus, of course, the original films before reduction).

Radiograph   I = final intraoperative control
Radiograph   II = at the fifth or sixth postoperative week, before wire removal
Radiograph III = at the fifth or sixth week, after wire removal
Radiograph IV = 6 months after operation

All films were marked by one person according to two linear and two angular parameters (Fig. 21.6). The former included the radial angle and dorsal-volar angulation, or volar angle, whereas the latter included the radial length and the distal radioulnar difference.

Anatomical results

A study of the anatomical results was made by comparing the four radiographic parameters in the four stages of treatment. The opposite radius was used as a normal control whenever possible. Table 21.1 shows the average values in the different stages of treatment.

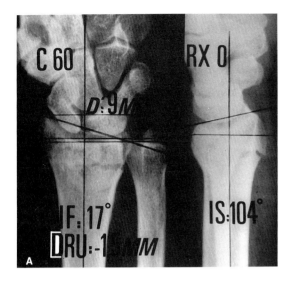
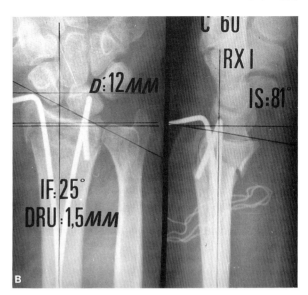
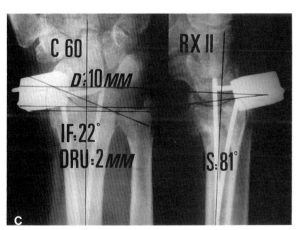
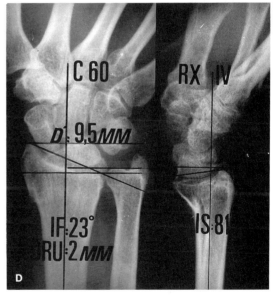

Fig. 21.6 Case 60: (A) in the initial radiographs, the parameters were: IF (radial angle) = 17°; DRU (distal radioulnar difference − 1.5 mm; D′ (radial length) = 9 mm and IS (volar angle) = 104°. (B) The films taken at operation showed improved radial length and good correction of the dorsal tilt, from 24 (or 104°) to 9° (or 8°) of volar angle. (C) Six weeks later, just before removing the combined fixation, the radial length (D′) was only 2 mm shorter than that on the radiograph immediately after fixation. (D) This shortening remained unaltered until the final control at six months (RX-$_{IV}$). The same applies to the volar angle

Table 21.1 Anatomical results

Stages	Parameter			
	RA°$\pm$s	VA°$\pm$s	RUD$^{mm}\pm$s	D′$^{mm}\pm$s
XR$_I$	25.1 $\pm$ 3.2	84.9 $\pm$ 6.6	0.55 $\pm$ 1.6	11.0 $\pm$ 2.3
XR$_{II}$	24.8 $\pm$ 3.8	84.1 $\pm$ 5.8	1.44 $\pm$ 1.6	9.7 $\pm$ 2.7
XR$_{III}$	24.3 $\pm$ 3.8	84.3 $\pm$ 6.1	1.67 $\pm$ 1.6	9.4 $\pm$ 2.7
XR$_{IV}$	24.4 $\pm$ 4.1	84.0 $\pm$ 6.6	1.64 $\pm$ 1.7	9.3 $\pm$ 2.6

In the statistical analysis of results, the most significant data relate to the volar angle and to the radial length.

Volar angle

No significant differences were found in the serial radiographic control average values (radiograph I to radiograph IV). However, as compared to the opposite, normal side, the angles after reduction were higher, indicating a slightly incomplete reduction of the dorsal angulation at the time of fracture fixation. The volar angle (VA_I) with the fixator in place averaged $84°.9 \pm 6°.6$, as compared to the normal volar angle (VA_N) of $80°.8 \pm 2°.4\star$.

Radial length

The average reduction value (D'_I) was close to the normal one (D'_N) and both were significantly higher than the subsequent control values:

$$D'_N \text{ and } D'_I > D'_{II} D'_{III} D'_{IV} \dagger$$

The anatomical results were expressed as proposed by Lidström (1959) and Frykman (1967) and Table 21.2 shows how our results compare with theirs.

Correlation between the patient's age and anatomical results

A study of the anatomical results according to the four parameters adopted at the four different stages of treatment and for the age groups ranging from the third to the seventh decades, showed: (1) the age factor had no influence on the anatomical results; (2) the loss of reduction is not influenced by age with the present method of fracture stabilization.

Functional results

A functional evaluation using the point system proposed by McBride (1948) and adopted by

$\star$ TUKEY'S TEST: F calc = 10.0; F crit = 2.85; Critic value = 2.12.

$\dagger$ $XD'_N = 11.30$ mm ± 2.05 mm   TUKEY'S TEST:
  $XD'_I = 10.99$ mm ± 2.31 mm   F crit = 2.47
  $XD'_{II} = 9.67$ mm ± 2.73 mm   F calc = 33.04
  $XD'_{III} = 9.37$ mm ± 2.70 mm   Critic value = 0.68.
  $XD'_{IV} = 9.30$ mm ± 2.61 mm

several authors (Cooney et al 1979, Dowling & Sawyer 1961, Forgon & Mammel 1981, Gartland & Werley 1951) was routinely carried out at the final radiographic control during the sixth postoperative month (Figs 21.7A–D). The results were: 'excellent' 29.5%, 'good' 53%, 'satisfactory' 11.1% and 'poor' 5.7%. The average follow-up period was 10 months.

Loss of grip strength

At the final functional evaluation the bilateral grip strength was measured as 'loss' or 'reduction' of strength in relation to the normal side. The results showed the following average values: 'excellent' 21.1%, 'good' 23.6%, 'satisfactory' 39.2% and 'poor' 31.0%.

The study of reduction in grip strength was not included in the McBride (1948) evaluation of functional results. A definite loss of strength, as measured by the Jamar dynamometer, was observed in all groups at the sixth postoperative month. Such loss was less pronounced in the functionally gratifying results ('excellent' and 'good') which showed a 23% reduction as compared with the undesirable results ('satisfactory' and 'poor'), where a more pronounced reduction of 37% was statistically significant.

Cosmetic results

The cosmetic results, evaluated according to Frykman's criteria (1967) at the sixth postoperative month, were: 'normal or near normal appearance as compared to the normal side' 51%; 'caput ulnae more prominent' 46%; 'mild to moderate radial deviation' 3%; 'dinner-fork deformity' 0%.

As demonstrated by several authors (Bacorn & Kurtzke 1953, Castaing 1964, Cooney et al 1979, Gartland & Werley 1951), there was a strong

Table 21.2 Anatomical results of united fractures (N = 100)

Deformity	Volar angle (φ)		Shorten-ing (mm)	Lidström (1959)%	Frykman (1967)%	Present series (1983)%
Absent	90	or	3	24%	25%	66%
Mild	91–100	and/or	3–6	39%	42%	33%
Moderate	101–114	and/or	7–11	32%	38%	1%
Severe	115	and/or	12+	5%	5%	0%

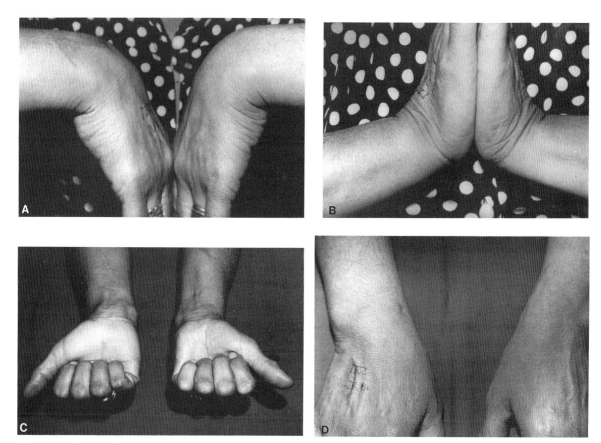

Fig. 21.7   Case number 60: ranges of movement and cosmetic result at the time of final evaluation, six months after fixation

correlation between the anatomical and functional results. The 'excellent' and 'good' results in Table 21.3 correspond to 82.35% of 'absent' and 'mild' anatomical deformities. 'Poor' results nevertheless occurred with normal or near normal anatomy, in two patients with dystrophic reactions.

In Table 21.4, the relationship between fracture type and functional results demonstrates a high rate of 'excellent' and 'good' results in both the subgroups of less severe (I–IV) and more severe (V–VIII) fractures, respectively corresponding to 92.8% and 79.6%. All 'poor' results occurred in the more severe subgroups.

The rate of 'excellent' and 'good' results is shown in this table, although the 13.2% difference between subgroups I to IV (less severe) and V to VIII (more severe) may be statistically insignificant.

Table 21.3 Relationship between functional and anatomical results

Functional criteria	Anatomical criteria				
	Absent	Mild	Moderate	Severe	Total (%)
Excellent	17	3	0	0	20 (29.5)
Good	19	17	0	0	36 (53.0)
Satisfactory	6	1	1	0	8 (11.8)
Poor	2	2	0	0	4 (5.7)
Total	44	23	1	0	68 (100.0)

Table 21.4 Rate of excellent and good results for different fracture types

Fracture type	Functional rating			
	Excellent (+Good)	Satisfactory (+Poor)	Total	Excellent +Good(%)
I–IV	13	1	14	(92.8)
V–VIII	43	11	54	(79.6)
Total	56	12	68	(82.3)

Complications

The major complications observed during treatment were: sympathetic reflex dystrophy (4%); finger stiffness (14%); superficial pin-tract infection (5%); cosmetic deformity (3%).

No complications were noted in approximately 74% of the cases, whereas in 26%, at least one of the above listed was present.

Of the cases presented, 4% had median nerve involvement due to an initial plaster cast immobilization with a flexed wrist or oedema. In all patients, the occurrence was classified as a transient neurapraxia that disappeared after fixation of the fracture and immobilization of the wrist in a straight position.

All superficial infection cleared promptly with local povidone-iodine pin-site cleansing and antibiotic treatment. In all cases, the wires were kept in place until the proposed period of treatment had been concluded.

Sympathetic dystrophy was by far the most difficult complication, since it affected the functional end-results. All cases of sympathetic dystrophy developed finger stiffness.

CONCLUSION

The present method for stabilizing Colles's fractures derives from two long-established and accepted methods of fracture fixation: (1) the three-point elastic intramedullary osteosynthesis proposed by Rush (Rush 1954, Fusi 1959); and (2) the external fixation of fractures by means of rigid frames mounted on threaded pins transfixing the bone fragments (Brooker et al 1983, Cooney 1983, Forgon & Mammel 1981, Jakob 1983).

In the distal radius, three anatomical landmarks are especially resistant to fracturing due to their pyramidal bone processes and cortical bone content: the radial styloid, the dorso-medial part of the ulnar notch of the radius and the volar-medial part of the ulnar notch. Such resistant areas are

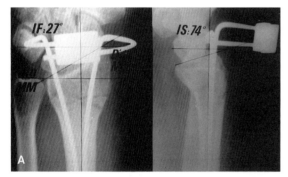

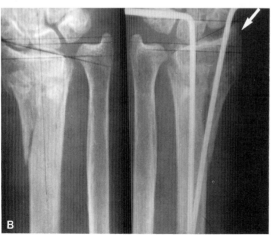

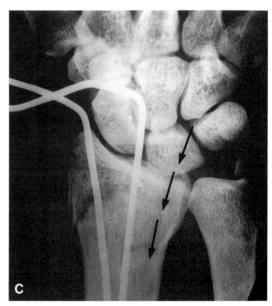

Fig. 21.8 (A) Example of an ideally reduced and fixed Colles's fracture, in which the wires form an inverted isosceles triangle. (B) In this case, the radial wire was misplaced and both the radial angle and the radial shortening lacked reduction. The white arrow shows the ideal point of entry. (C) Another example of wire misplacement. The black arrows point to the correct direction. These wires will only partially stabilize the fracture, because they form a right-angled triangle and not an isosceles one

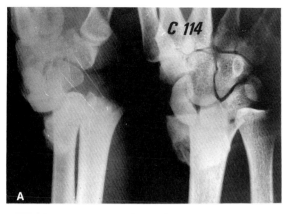
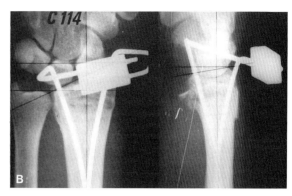
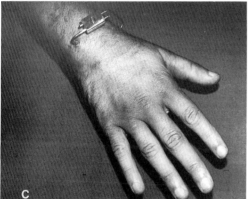
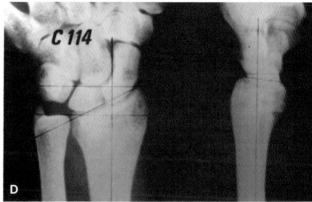

Fig. 21.9 (A) Case number 114: initial radiographs of a severely displaced Colles's fracture which was compound anteriorly. There was compression of the median nerve. (B) Radiographs of same wrist taken at the time of the closed reduction and percutaneous intramedullary osteosynthesis with external fixation. (C) Appearance of the hand and wrist at six weeks, just before removal of the wires. The patient had good recovery of the median nerve. (D) Final radiograph at six months

almost invariably present, even in severely comminuted fractures, and can be used to advantage when performing the fixation proposed in this chapter. Thus, the radial wire should penetrate the styloid, whilst the dorsal one is aimed at the dorsomedial 'pyramid' or 'dye-punch fragment'.

When the radial wire is introduced, the elastic force at play acts against the distal radial fragment and pushes it ulnarly (Fusi 1959, Rush 1954), correcting the radial deviation and preventing the recurrence of this component. Upon introducing the dorsoulnar wire, its elastic force tends to keep the dorsal tilt of the fracture in the corrected position. Once adequately applied, both wires should form an isosceles triangle (Fig. 21.8). The sides of this triangle are slightly parabolic since the wires are under elastic deformation (Ulson 1983, Zinghi & Lanfranchi 1980). Upon being clamped

together, the wires form a semi-rigid triangular frame, anchored in the funnelled tubular bone. Such mechanical characteristics prevent proximal migration of the frame, which is gripped by the medullary canal at the junction of the middle and distal thirds of the radius. The elliptical cross-section of the medullary canal not only contributes to the rotational stabilization of the semi-rigid frame, but it is also large enough to accept wires of 2 mm at its narrowest point.

The distal fragments of a typical comminuted Colles's fracture are kept from collapsing by the crossing and converging direction of the wires (Fig. 21.9) much in the same way that hay is kept high in a manger. Kapandji (1976) described intrafocal fixation for Colles's fractures which resembles the present technique in that both systems avoid proximal collapse or shortening, with the crossed wires forming a support for the distal fragments.

The external fixator is a mechanically crucial component as it not only keeps the wires steady, preventing their independent movement, but also largely eliminates rotational stress on the fragments caused by pronation and supination. When compression is desirable for the approximation of distal fragments in the frontal plane, both wires are compressed before the central screw is tightened. The present external fixator design compares favourably to other models in terms of bulk and simplicity, allowing the hand to be used throughout treatment without interfering with the clothes worn by the patient, an especially desirable feature in cold climates.

As previously mentioned, the wires will be gripped at the narrowest point of the middle third of the bone canal, where they support the fractured radius, neutralizing the flexion-extension forces acting on the sagittal plane. Although minimal motion can occur at the fracture site as in any semi-rigid system, primary bone healing may be stimulated as suggested by Firica et al (1981).

The periarticular soft tissues, i.e. the capsular, ligamentous and teno-retinacular structures enveloping the distal fragments, help to keep them in the reduced position. Such soft-tissue support provided by the transfixing angulations of the wires are also important points for stabilizing the fracture.

The skin and the extensor retinaculum must be depressed to facilitate exposure of the right-angle in the wire at the time of its removal.

Editor's note: The equipment described in this chapter can be purchased from IMPOL-Instrumental e Implantes Ltda., Al. Itupiranga 86, 04294 São Paulo, Brazil

REFERENCES

Bacorn R W, Kurtzke J F 1953 Colles's fracture. A study of two thousand cases from the New York State Workman's Compensation Board. Journal of Bone and Joint Surgery 35A:643–658

Böhler L 1942 The treatment of fractures (4th edn). William Wood, Baltimore

Brooker A F, Cooney W P, Chao E Y (eds) 1983 Principles of external fixation. Williams & Wilkins, Baltimore, ch 8, p 103

Cagnoli, H 1975 Acta Ort. Latinoamericana 3:281

Castaing J 1964 Les fractures récentes de l'extrémité inférieure du radius chez l'adulte. Revue de Chirurgie Orthopédique et Réparatrice de L'Appareil Moteur 5:41–696

Cole J M, Obletz B E 1966 Comminuted fractures of the distal end of the radius treated by skeletal transfixion in plaster cast: an end-result study of thirty-three cases. Journal of Bone and Joint Surgery 48A:931–945

Cooney W P 1983 External fixation of distal radius fractures. Clinical Orthopaedics and Related Research 180:44–49

Cooney W P, Linscheid R L, Dobyns J H 1979 External pin fixation of unstable Colles's fractures. Journal of Bone and Joint Surgery 61A:840

Cooney W P, Dobyns H H, Linschield R L 1980 Complications of Colles's fractures. Journal of Bone and Joint Surgery 62A:613–619

DePalma A 1952 Comminuted fractures of the distal end of the radius treated by ulnar pinning. Journal of Bone and Joint Surgery 34A:651–662

Dobyns J H, Linscheid R L 1975 Fractures and dislocations of the wrist. In: Rockwood CA and Green DP (eds) Fractures, Vol 1, J B Lippincott, Philadelphia, ch 7, p 345

Dowling J J, Sawyer B J 1961 Comminuted Colles's fractures. Journal of Bone and Joint Surgery 43A:657–668

Firica et al 1981 L'osteosynthèse stable élastique, nouveau concept biomécanique. Étude expérimentale. Revue de Chirurgie Orthopédique et Réparatrice de L'Appareil Moteur. Suppl. II 67:82–91

Forgon M, Mammel E 1981 The external fixator in the management of unstable Colles's fracture. International Orthopaedics (SICOT) 5:9–14

Frykman G 1967 Fractures of the distal radius including sequelae—shoulder-hand-finger syndrome, disturbance of the distal radioulnar joint and impairment of nerve function. A clinical and experimental study. Acta Orthopaedica Scandinavica 108 (suppl):30

Fusi F 1959 Indicazioni e limiti dell'osteosintesi endomedollare transtiloidea nel trattamento delle frature dell'estremo inferiore del radio. Minerva Ortopedica 10:95–105

Gartland J J, Werley C W 1951 Evaluation of healed Colles's fractures. Journal of Bone and Joint Surgery 33A:895–907

Jakob R P 1983 The small external fixator. AO Bulletin p 1–51, Swiss Association for the Study of Internal Fixation, Bern

Kapandji A 1976 L'Osteosyntèse par double embrochage intra-focal. Annales de Chirurgie 30:903–908

Lidström A 1959 Fractures of the distal end of the radius. Acta Orthopaedica Scandinavica Suppl. 41:1–118

Lee-Osterman A, Bora F W Jr 1980 Injuries of the wrist. In: Heppenstal R B (ed) Fracture treatment and healing. W B Saunders, Philadelphia, ch 19, p 513

McBride E D 1948 Disability evaluation. Principles of treatment of compensable injuries. J B Lippincott, Philadelphia

Rauis A, Ledoux A, Thiebaut H, Van der Ghinst M 1979 Bipolar fixation of fractures of the distal end of the radius. International Orthopaedics (SICOT) 3:89–96

Rush L V 1954 Closed medullary pinning of Colles's fracture, Clinical Orthopaedics and Related Research 3:152–162

Sage F P 1959 Medullary fixation of fractures of the forearm. A study of the medullary canal and a report of fifty fractures of the radius treated with a prebent triangular nail. Journal of Bone and Joint Surgery 41A:1489–1516

Scheck M D 1962 Long-term follow-up of treatment of comminuted fractures of the distal end of the radius by transfixation with Kirschner wires and cast. Journal of Bone and Joint Surgery 44A:337–351

Sevitt S 1971 The healing of fractures of the lower end of the radius. Journal of Bone and Joint Surgery 53B:520–531

Ulson H J R 1983 Pouteau-Colles's fracture. Stabilization with percutaneous intramedullary osteosynthesis and external fixation. In: Book of Abstracts, 2nd Congress of the International Federation of Societies for Surgery of the Hand, Boston, pp 81–82

Zinghi G F, Lanfranchi R 1980 Osteosynthesis with Rush's double nail by the 'Eiffel-Tower' method in pseudarthrosis impacted in good position and retarded union. Italian Journal of Orthopaedics and Traumatology VI (1):85–95

William P. Cooney

22 Distal radial fractures: external fixation

Colles's account in 1814 of the fracture which bears his name (Fig. 22.1) still provides the classic description:

'This fracture takes place at about an inch and a half above the carpal extremity of the radius. If the surgeon lock his hand in that of the patient's, and make extension, he restores the limb to its natural form, but the distortion of the limb instantly returns on the extension being removed. Should the facility with which a moderate extension restores the limb to its form induce the practitioner to treat this as a case of sprain, he will find, after a lapse of time sufficient for the removal of similar swellings, the deformity undiminished. Or, should he mistake the case for a dislocation of the wrist, and attempt to retain the parts in situ by tight bandages and splints ... he will find, at the expiration of a few weeks, that the deformity still exists in its fullest extent and that it is now no longer to be removed by making such extension of the limb. By such mistakes, the patient is doomed to endure for many months considerable lameness and stiffness of the limb, accompanied by severe pains on attempting to bend the fingers and the hand.'

This description by Colles is more than of historical interest; it relates the unfortunate story of problems associated with the treatment of fractures of the distal radius. We are reminded by Colles that failure to achieve proper reduction and inability to maintain fracture reduction remain the most serious problem in the treatment of this common injury. However, he continues 'One consolation only remains, that the limb will at some remote period again enjoy perfect freedom in all its motions and be completely free of pain: the deformity, however, will remain undiminished through life'. Unfortunately most surgeons find that this satisfactory functional outcome is not always achieved and that persistent problems are frequent after Colles's fracture, to the considerable dissatisfaction of the patient (Cassebaum 1950, Bacorn & Kurtzke 1953, Lidström 1959, Dowling & Sawyer 1961, Scheck 1962).

Modern concepts in the treatment of fractures of the distal radius require a clear definition of the different types of fractures and a classification such as that of Frykman (1967) to provide a basis for improved treatment. Fractures that are outside the main articular region of the wrist (extra-articular fractures—Frykman I and II) should be separated from those that involve the main articular area of the wrist (intra-articular fractures—Frykman III-VIII): see Table 22.1. Each requires a different method or approach to treatment. Similarly, fractures with dorsal displacement of the distal radius should be distinguished from those that have volar displacement and factors of comminution, angulation, shortening and displacement should be assessed since they may alter the treatment and change the concepts upon which treatment is usually based (Cooney et al 1979).

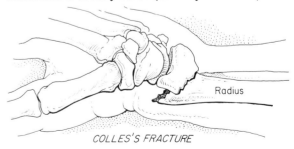

COLLES'S FRACTURE

Fig. 22.1 Colles's fracture—metaphyseal

Table 22.1 Frykman classification

Type	Distal ulnar fracture	
	No	Yes
Extra-articular	I	II
Intra-articular		
radiocarpal	III	IV
radioulnar	V	VI
radiocarpal and radioulnar	VII	VIII

In this chapter, we will concentrate on the treatment of displaced and unstable fractures of the distal radius, especially those fractures that are intra-articular, involving both the distal radius and distal ulna and that involve subluxation or dislocation of the distal radioulnar joint. Colles's fracture and Smith's fracture are generic terms that do not describe the entire story of distal radial fractures. Straightforward extra-articular Colles's and Smith's fractures can usually be treated satisfactorily by simple cast immobilization. The types of fracture considered in this chapter are those which are intra-articular and comminuted and, as a result, are unstable fractures and should therefore be considered for more aggressive treatment such as external skeletal fixation.

PRINCIPLES

There are three main principles which apply in the treatment of fractures of the distal radius. The main principle in treatment that applies to all complex distal radius fractures is that stated by Böhler (1937): *'maintain reduction of the fracture by fixed traction.'* This principle has been restated in scientific terms by Adrey (1970) and Vidal et al (1979) who have termed this technique 'ligamentotaxis'. This implies maintaining reduction by fixed traction through the ligaments attached to the distal radius. By maintaining longitudinal traction, loss of reduction can be prevented, and anatomical alignment can be maintained. In applying this principle of treatment (DePalma 1952, Blechert-Toft & Kaalund-Jensen 1971, Marsh & Teal 1972, Augustine 1974), previous methods which use hyperflexion and hyperextension manoeuvres would be disruptive and should be avoided. A method of sustained traction followed by gentle manipulative reduction using direct pressure on the fracture fragments is preferred. Once obtained, the reduction is then maintained by fixed traction, following the principle set forth by Böhler.

The second principle of treatment is to obtain *anatomical reduction of the fracture by aligning the volar cortex.* With dorsal comminution, the volar cortex provides the fulcrum to prevent dorsal angulation and shortening (Cooney et al 1979). A volar buttress to lock the distal radial fracture fragments in a reduced position is essential to maintain reduction; dorsal alignment, though desirable to achieve an anatomical reduction, is of only secondary importance to fracture stability (Frykman 1967). The mechanical realignment which results from accurate reduction of the volar cortex prevents secondary carpal instability, diminishes malalignment of the distal radioulnar joint, limits shortening of musculo-tendinous units and improves the position of intra-articular fracture fragments which, if they remained displaced, would lead to cartilage degeneration. We have been impressed that, with restoration of normal anatomy, the wrist can regain almost 90% of normal motion and strength and that functional achievements previously unobtainable with the 'conventional' methods of treatment can be obtained.

The third principle in treatment is *accurate reduction of the distal radioulnar joint* (Brady 1963, Sarmiento et al 1975). In previous descriptions, fractures of the distal ulna, which are often associated with tearing of the ligamentous support of the distal radioulnar joint were usually ignored. Frykman (1967) made an important contribution to our understanding of distal radial fractures by describing the complications associated with an unreduced distal ulna. He provided a classification of fractures of the distal radius that took into account the presence or absence of a fracture of the ulna (Table 22.1). Reduction of the distal radioulnar joint by placing the forearm in a supinated position restores the articular cartilage contact areas and stabilizes the triangular fibrocartilage ligament system in correct anatomical position. With an unstable distal ulna, 'the surgeon will find that the end of the ulna admits of being readily moved backwards and forwards' (Colles 1814). Reduction and immobilization of the bone and ligament support of the distal radio-ulnar joint is therefore an important principle that contributes to the best treatment of fractures of the distal radius.

INDICATIONS FOR EXTERNAL FIXATION

1. *Unstable distal radial fractures* of the Frykman types III–VIII. Unstable fractures have by definition more than 25° of dorsal angulation and 10 mm of radial shortening. Comminution and intra-articular fracture fragments will commonly add to the inherent instability.
2. *Loss of reduction* after closed reduction and application of a plaster cast. When there is loss of reduction, after cast immobilization, of more than 10° of dorsal angulation, alone or in combination with radial shortening of 10 mm, then further loss of reduction can be expected and this implies an unstable distal radial fracture.
3. *Bilateral fractures* of the distal radius.
4. *Open injuries* with unstable fractures of the distal radius and/or ulna.

To help further in deciding the need for primary external fixation, the Frykman classification has been very reliable in our experience and correlates well with the anticipated results. The majority of fractures treated with external fixation are Frykman types III–VIII. Even more importantly, fractures that are very unstable (intra-articular Frykman types VII and VIII) are absolute indications and have responded well to external fixation.

Contra-indications

External fixation is not required in the majority of uncomplicated and stable fractures of the distal radius. Closed reduction and immobilization in a plaster cast or sugar-tong splint is performed in over 80% of these fractures that we are called upon to treat (Brindley 1972). Conservative measures are particularly preferred in the elderly patient (over the age of 75), patients with underlying osteoporosis and young patients with an open growth plate. In the young adult with a significantly displaced and intra-articular fracture of the distal radius, open reduction and internal fixation with supplemental bone graft has become our treatment of choice.

Other contra-indications include patients with upper limb paralysis, additional fractures in the hand, wrist or forearm that preclude pin placement and psychological rejection by the patient of an external frame with pins.

The presence of burns, open wounds, or segmental extremity injuries has not precluded use of external fixators which in fact have made the management of such patients easier.

TYPES OF FIXATORS

There is a variety of external fixation techniques which can be applied to accomplish the desired goal. We will describe four methods of external fixation that we believe have advantages over pins and plaster and other methods of treatment and which currently are in use at the Mayo Clinic. Each of these external fixation techniques involves placement of pins into the hand, most commonly the second and third metacarpals, and proximal pins into the distal radius.

Our first experience involved the *Roger Anderson frame* (Fig. 22.2) which has separate units, holder clamps, side bars and cross pins (Anderson & O'Neil 1944). This frame is quite adjustable to any

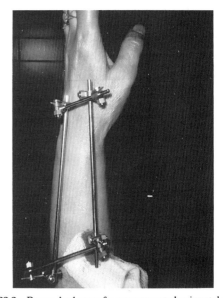

Fig. 22.2 Roger Anderson frame: separate horizontal and vertical side bars attach to universal joints, through which smooth or Crowe pins are placed into the hand metacarpals and distal radius

clinical situation, easy to apply by junior house staff or resident and can be readjusted if desired during treatment (Grana & Kopta 1979).

The second frame in common use is the *Hoffman* C-series (Fig. 22.3). This is a unilateral frame with a sliding compression–distraction central bar (Hoffman 1954). In contrast to the Roger Anderson frame, it provides stability primarily in one plane

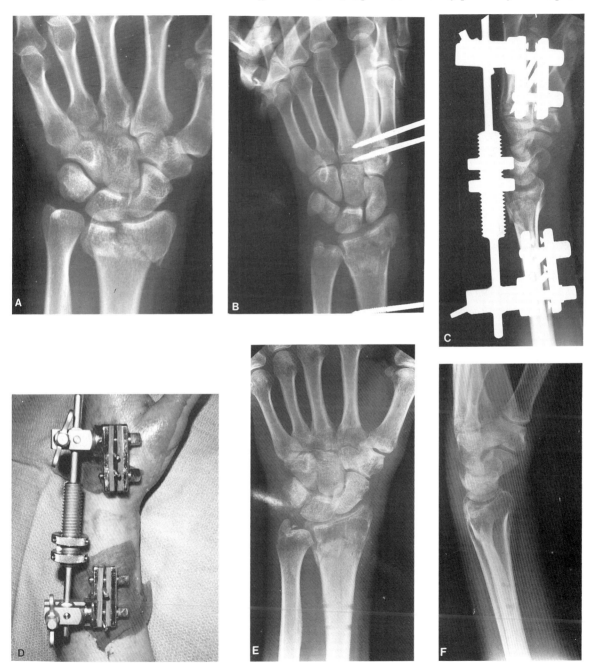

Fig. 22.3 Hoffman C-Series: (A) distal radial fracture, entering radio-carpal joint; Frykman type IV. (B & C) AP and lateral radiographs with frame applied after distraction, reduction and transverse pin insertion. *Note* older type of pins without complete threads to the pin tip. (D) Fixator applied laterally. Distraction or compression can be obtained through sliding C-bar. (E & F) AP and lateral 2 weeks after removal of frame; anatomical reduction of the fracture has been maintained

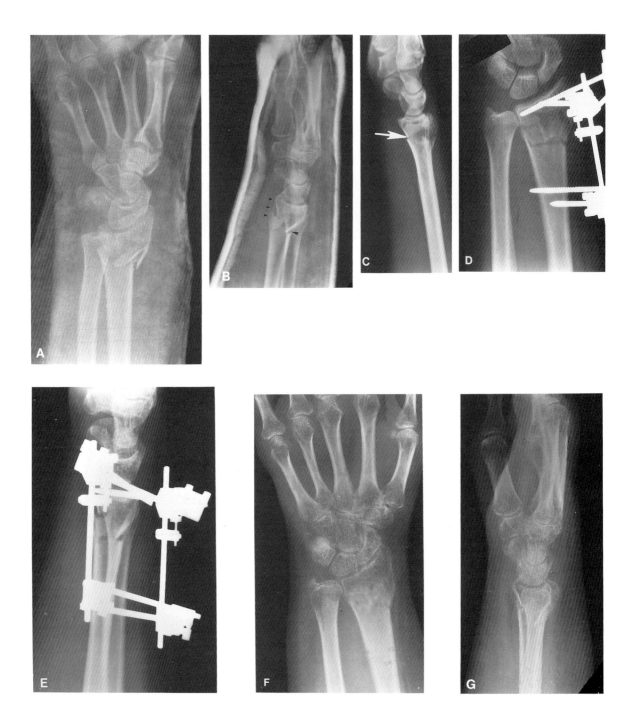

Fig. 22.4   Mini-Frame (Jacquet): (A & B) comminuted distal radial fracture after closed reduction and cast application. Arrows show dorsal displacement of distal fracture fragments. (C) Lateral demonstrating alignment of volar proximal and distal cortices which is necessary to secure reduction and prevent dorsal displacement. (D & E) AP and lateral of the distal radius showing anatomical reduction of the intra-articular part of the fracture. (F & G) Lateral two months after original fracture. Reduction of distal radius and ulna maintained : *note* osteopenia

while maintaining distraction. It is usually applied to the lateral side of the wrist, with pins transversely placed in the metacarpals and distal radius (Adrey 1970).

A third frame, popular in Europe, is the *mini-exoskeleton fixator of Jacquet* (Fig. 22.4) which was developed for soft-tissue and skeletal support of severe hand injuries (Asche & Burney 1982). It has

been applied with minor modifications to fractures of the distal radius (Forgon & Mammel 1981, Riggs & Cooney 1983). It has the advantage of small size for use in elderly patients, especially women, and the second advantage that the pins are placed in the distal radius so that the carpus may be free to move in an effort to prevent wrist stiffness. It cannot be used when distraction of

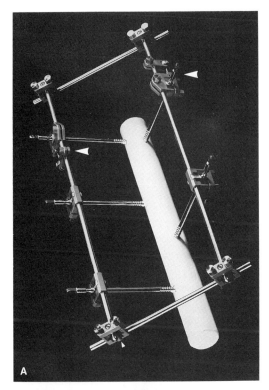

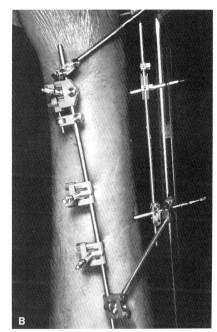

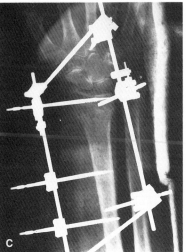

Fig. 22.5 Jacquet mini-frame extended across distal radio-carpal joint (A) model. Hoffman pins (3 mm) fit within sliding clamps (small arrow) after removing central C-crimp. Compression and distraction can be applied through the sliding swivel clamps (large arrows). (B) Mini-frame applied across wrist-joint. Radiological appearance. (C) After 3–4 weeks the metacarpal pin can be removed to initiate wrist motion, but the fracture remains immobilized by the proximal frame and radial pins

highly unstable fractures is desired, unless it is further modified to have a bar across the wrist into the hand metacarpals (Fig. 22.5).

The fourth frame consists of the pre-set *Ace-Colles quadrilateral frame* (Fig. 22.6A), which is placed dorsally over the distal radius (Cooney 1983). Pins are inserted through the frame which acts as a pin-guide for accurate placement. Universal couple joints allow for minor adjustment in pin position and both compression and distraction can be applied after the fracture has been reduced and the frame applied. The main advantage of this frame is the use of a pre-drilling and tapping system that allows for insertion of threaded pins. Recent studies of the mechanics and biology of external fixation have shown that the pin-bone interface is the weakest link in the external fixation system. These studies (Chao and Pope 1983) stress the importance of improved pin fixation systems which the Ace-Colles fixator provides. The disadvantages of the Ace-Colles quadrilateral frame are the lack of adjustability and improper pin place-

ment when used in the hands of an inexperienced surgeon.

TECHNIQUE

The technique which we have employed over the past 10 years for treatment of fractures of the distal radius is based on the principle of first obtaining anatomical reduction of the fracture by traction and gentle manipulation and, second, maintaining that reduction with fixed traction by external skeletal fixation (Fig. 22.7). To obtain reduction:

1. Place the extremity in finger-trap traction with 3–5 kg of counter-traction, once adequate Bier block or axillary block anaesthesia has been obtained;
2. Reduce the fracture by direct pressure on the distal fragments, avoiding hyperflexion or hyperextension manoeuvres;
3. Confirm adequate reduction by AP and lateral X-rays of the wrist. On the lateral view, the

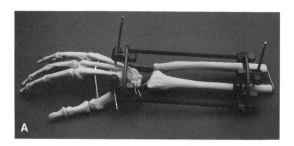
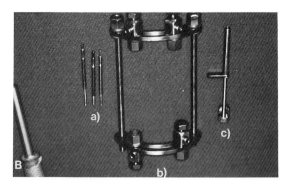
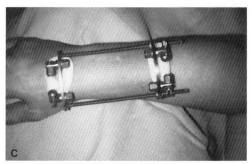

Fig. 22.6 Ace–Colles fixation frame. (A) Model applied to skeleton of forearm and hand. Pins are placed in the metaphyses of the second and third metacarpals and non-parallel pins in the radius. (B) Equipment for insertion of pre-drilled pins with (a) threaded pins of sizes 2.0, 2.5 and 3.0 mm (b) pre-drilling frame (c) pin/drill guide. By removing central collet in the pin-holding clamps, drill-guide is inserted through the frame and accurate pin placement obtained. (C) Frame *in situ*. It has a low profile and can be worn with Ace bandage, or with plaster support

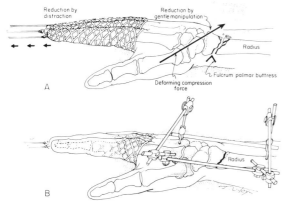

Fig. 22.7 Technique of fracture reduction and immobilization: (A) reduction obtained by distraction and gentle manipulation with effort made to align palmar cortex which can be used as a fulcrum to sustain the reduction. (B) External fixation with a quadrilateral frame (Roger Anderson type)

volar cortex should be perfectly reduced, i.e. the proximal volar cortex overlapping the distal volar cortex (*see* Fig. 22.4C);

4. Maintain the forearm in neutral rotation or supination to reduce the distal radioulnar joint;

5. Apply the external fixation frame with fixed traction (3–5 kg) being maintained. With the Roger Anderson or Hoffman frames, place the fixation pins free-hand into the *base* of the second and third metacarpals, with parallel pins in the distal third of the radius. With the Ace-Colles frame (Fig. 22.8), the frame is placed directly over the distal forearm in line with the third metacarpal. Using the frame as the pin guide, self-drilling, self-tapping pins are inserted into the third metacarpal and a second

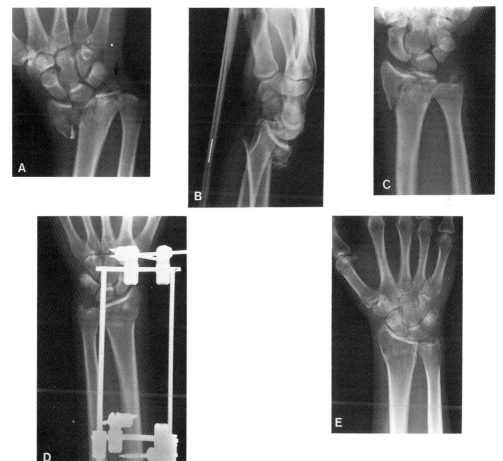

Fig. 22.8 (A & B) Comminuted Frykman type IV fracture of distal radius. *Note* displaced ulnar styloid (arrow) and severe radiocarpal joint injury. (C) Reduction of intra-articular fracture by traction. (D) External fixation with Ace–Colles fixator for anatomical alignment of radiocarpal joint. (E) Final AP radiograph five months after initial fracture

pin placed in the transverse plane into the second metacarpal. The position of the frame is adjusted with alignment on the forearm. With the newer Ace-Colles system, the frame has a drill guide that allows pre-drilling of the bone and then the insertion of self-tapping pins that have a firm hold in bone. The heat of bone drilling and potential for pin loosening appears to be less utilizing the latter technique (Green C. A. & Matthews 1981);

6. Pin fixation of the distal ulna to the distal radius with a 0.035 inch (0.9 mm) Kirschner-wire can be performed if the distal ulna is unstable.

Pitfalls

With the above technique, a number of pitfalls should be avoided. First, the external frame should not be used to obtain the fracture reduction or manipulated to correct a loss of reduction. To do this puts undue stress on the pin–bone interface and leads to loosening of the pins. Secondly, during the insertion of pins, soft tissues such as tendons, nerves and vascular structures should be avoided. The base of the second metacarpal is relatively free of soft-tissue attachment, but on the dorsum of the hand the extensor tendons over the second and third metacarpals must be separated for atraumatic insertion. For the third metacarpal, we prefer a small incision and either spreading the nerves and tendons with a haemostat or, with the pre-drilled system, using a drill-guide placed directly on the base of the shaft of the third metacarpal. For the insertion of pins into the distal forearm, dorsal and radial longitudinal incisions are made, the soft tissues are spread with a haemostat and the drill-guide is inserted. Finally, proper placement of the pins requires that the distal two pins are placed in the metaphysis of the second and third metacarpals, while the proximal pins are placed into the diaphysis of the radius but not at the same level. A low-speed, high-torque drill can be used but ideally a pre-drilled system is best, with the pins inserted using a hand chuck as described for the Ace-Colles's fixator.

After the pins are fully inserted and the external fixator applied, final AP and lateral radiographs are obtained to check for fracture reduction and the position of the pins. Minor corrections are made at this time.

After-care

A sterile dressing with betadine ointment is applied to the pinholes and the wound is left undisturbed to reduce skin motion and provide a seal at the skin–pin interface. A plaster splint may be added for soft tissue support and when there is an associated injury of distal radioulnar joint. Otherwise, no plaster support is needed.

Following external fixation, we encourage patients to resume the activities of daily living using the injured extremity. It is important to emphasize finger extensions early, to prevent adhesions along the extensor tendons. Local anaesthesia injected around the distal pins can assist in obtaining extensor tendon function. By applying rigid fracture fixation, gliding tendons and mobile finger joints can be maintained while the fracture heals.

External fixation is continued for 7–8 weeks, with radiographs and clinical examinations at one, two and six weeks. If a significant loss of reduction occurs within the first two weeks, reduction is repeated under an axillary block and additional pin fixation is applied. The pins can be removed as an out-patient procedure, after which an orthoplast or neoprene wrist cock-up splint is worn for two weeks as forearm and hand strength returns.

RESULTS

From our experience with over 200 unstable fractures of the distal radius, we have been able to analyse the advantages of external fixation techniques. We have reported (1979) the results for the first 60 consecutive cases using exclusively the Roger Anderson system; 54 of the 60 (90%) had good or excellent results.

More recently (1983), we reviewed 100 additional patients who were treated with the four external fixation frame systems described earlier (Roger Anderson, Hoffman, Mini-frame Jaquet; Ace-Colles): there were 22 excellent, 64 good, 10 fair and 4 poor results; 86% good or excellent results. The individual results from the four fixator systems are shown in Table 22.2. Only the C-series

Table 22.2 Results from 100 consecutive distal radius fractures treated with external fixation

	Fixators			
	Roger Anderson	Ace Colles	Mini-Fixator (Jacquet)	C-Hoffman
Number of patients	60	15	15	10
Results				
Excellent or good	54 (90%)	14 (93%)	12 (80%)	6 (60%)
Fair	4	1	3	2
Poor	2	0	0	2
Complications (%)	30	26	33	30

Hoffman did less well than anticipated (62% good or excellent results). The other frame systems had 86–92% satisfactory results. The four poor results were related to upper limb dystrophy, with median neuropathy in two and a painful fixator in the other two. The results from primary external fixation and secondary external fixation are quite similar. The fracture types were Frykman types III–VIII, over half of the cases being types VII and VIII; 90% of the fractures were intra-articular and 85% had moderate to severe comminution.

The attitude of the patient is always in question when a new technique is applied to an old problem. From our studies, we have found that patient satisfaction was extremely high, with over 90% reporting acceptance of the apparatus and pleasure with the result; 85% of patients had returned to all activities of daily living and 95% were completely pain-free. Only 12% had clinical deformity and 3% were dissatisfied with their result. Grip strength averaged 60% of the uninjured side and flexion–extension motion was 70% of the uninjured extremity. There was excellent return of pronation–supination (90% of normal). Few patients have required a subsequent Darrach resection of the distal ulna (5% of the original 60 patients). Many of the wrists have restoration of normal anatomy with little evidence, on X-ray, of the previous distal radial fracture.

Complications of external fixation

Complications continue to be the main problem in treatment of unstable distal radial fractures (Green, S. A. 1981). External fixation has without question reduced the number of serious complications but unfortunately has added several of its own (Table. 22.2). From our previous studies, we have found that complications can occur in up to 30% of the patients treated for distal radial fractures (Cooney et al 1980). Carpal tunnel syndrome, radiocarpal and radioulnar arthrosis, and loss of fracture reduction were in the past the most common (accounting for 66% of all complications). With external fixation, the majority of these problems have been reduced: in our most recent series there was an 8.3% incidence of serious complications (Cooney 1983).

With external fixation, pin-tract problems have developed as potential difficulties (Fig. 22.9). Loosening of the pins is the most frequent of these. In the Roger Anderson series, smooth pins were used and loosening occurred in 12%; 1.2% of these developed pin-tract osteomyelitis. Loss of reduction accompanied some cases of pin loosening. With the newer techniques of inserting the pins and attention to the details of this process, problems of pin-tract loosening have become fewer, and more serious complications, such as carpal tunnel syndrome, upper limb dystrophy, loss of fracture reduction and post-traumatic arthrosis, also appeared to be much less common. Our preference for external fixation is related to the fact that the complications associated with external fixation are decidedly less than those found with pins and plaster (Green, D. P. 1975, Chapman et al 1982): 40% vs. 16% pin-tract problems. With the Roger Anderson system, pins and methacrylate or pins-in-plaster systems, smooth pins continue to be used but with an increased incidence of pin loosening. Both Hoffman and Fisher threaded pins have decreased pin problems (from 12% to 4%), and the best results are from the pre-drilled pin system of the Ace-Colles unit.

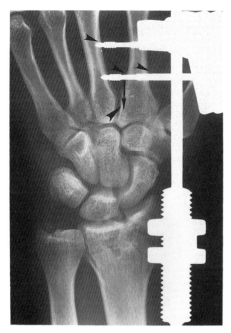

Fig. 22.9 Errors in pin placement: continuously threaded pins are preferred, which should be placed through cancellous bone in the metaphysis or through both cortices of the diaphysis. The pins shown are too distal, improperly inserted and of the wrong type

The greatest concern in using external fixation, that of tendon and peripheral nerve damage, has not been a serious problem, despite our initial use of closed techniques. Open insertion of the pins should always be considered in the forearm where neurovascular structures are in jeopardy but semi-open insertion appears to be a safe procedure provided anatomical factors are considered and proper pin placement is used as recommended by S. A. Green (1981).

CONCLUSION

External fixation has been applied in approximately 30% of fractures of the distal radius that we have treated since our first use of the technique in 1973. Remarkable improvement in fixator design, the development of accurate and safe techniques for insertion of the pins and the definition of specific indications for use have greatly improved the results compared with the unsatisfactory earlier

reports of this procedure and that of 'pins and plaster' (Cole & Obletz 1966, DePalma 1952, Green, D. P. 1975). Research efforts have further helped to establish the optimum number of pins, the preferred site of pin placement, the indications for half-frame versus full quadrilateral frames and the weak link of the system: the pin–bone interface (Chao & Pope 1983).

It is most important to point out that external fixation of distal radius fractures is not meant to replace traditional methods of closed reduction and cast immobilization but to supplement it as a method of treatment for the more unstable fractures. We have found, however, increased applications for this procedure as our experience grows. We would recommend it for selected Colles's, Smith's and Barton's fractures as the clinical situation indicates. Open fractures, segmental fractures and highly comminuted fractures of the distal radius, irrespective of the specific type, respond well to external fixation and there is no reason to fear lack of bone union due to the distraction component of the technique. Mobilization of joints proximal and distal to the fracture site is more readily obtained with this technique than by immobilization in a long-arm cast. Distraction across the wrist joint and immobilization of joints has not resulted in functionally significant loss of motion. To date, we have not found it necessary to incorporate hinge or universal joints as part of the external fixation unit (Cooney et al 1980). Future improvements in external fixators will no doubt occur. Both lighter weight and plastic, radiolucent frames will be developed and improved pins and techniques for introducing them, similar to those used for internal fixation, will emerge. The benefits of controlled radiographs such as image intensification, already in use in our clinical practice, will increase the accuracy of fracture reduction and pin placement. Longitudinal traction across a hand table may replace overhead traction, providing the surgeon with an easier approach for insertion of pins.

The final acceptance of external fixation for fractures of the distal radius awaits the critical comparison by colleagues less familiar with its use and by those who have always preferred simpler methods of treatment. In comparing current results with historical standards described by Gartland

and Werley (1951), it appears that the high level of success, both clinically and radiographically, obtained by external fixation cannot be duplicated by classic casting or splinting methods. When correctly applied, external skeletal fixation provides rigid immobilization of the fracture fragments, prevents redisplacement and assures the best cosmetic and functional result for the patient.

REFERENCES

Adrey J 1970 Le fixateur externe Hoffman couple en cadre étude bioméchanique dans les fractures. Gead, Paris

Anderson R, O'Neil G 1944 Comminuted fractures of the distal end of the radius. Surgery, Gynecology and Obstetrics 78:434–440

Asche G, Burney R 1982 Indikation fur die anwendunz des mini fixateur externa. Aktuel Traumatology 12:103

Augustine R W 1974 Stabilizing the Colles's fracture. Michigan Medicine 73:319–320

Bacorn R W, Kurtzke J F 1953 Colles's fracture: a study of two thousand cases from the New York State Workmen's Compensation Board. Journal of Bone and Joint Surgery 35A:643–658

Barton J R 1838 Views and treatment of an important injury of the wrist. Medical Examiners 1:365

Blechert-Toft M, Kaalund-Jensen H 1971 Colles's fracture treated with modified Böhler technique. Acta Orthopaedica Scandinavica 42:45–57

Böhler L 1937 Die technik der knochenbruch behandlung, Maudrich, Vienna

Brady L P 1963 Double pin fixation of severely comminuted fractures of the distal radius and ulna. Southern Medical Journal 56:307–311

Brindley H N 1972 Wrist injuries. Clinical Orthopaedics 83:17–23

Cassebaum W H 1950 Colles's fracture: a study of end results. Journal of American Medical Association 143:963–965

Chao E Y S, Pope M 1983 The mechanical basis of external fixation. In: Seligson D, Pope M (eds) Concepts in External Fixation. Grune and Stratton, New York

Chapman D B, Bennett J B, Bryan W J, Tullos H S 1982 Complications of distal radius fractures: pins and plaster treatment. Journal of Hand Surgery 7:509

Cole J M, Obletz B E 1966 Comminuted fractures of the distal end of the radius treated by skeletal transfixion in plaster cast. An end result study of thirty-three cases. Journal of Bone and Joint Surgery 48A:931–945

Colles A 1814 On the fracture of the carpal extremity of the radius. Edinburgh Medical Surgical Journal 10:182–186

Cooney W P, Linscheid R L, Dobyns J H 1979 External pin fixation for unstable Colles's fractures. Journal of Bone and Joint Surgery 61A:840–845

Cooney W P, Dobyns J H, Linscheid R L 1980 Complications of Colles's fractures. Journal of Bone and Joint Surgery 62A:613–619

Cooney W P 1983 External fixation of distal radius fractures. Clinical Orthopedics 180:44–49

DePalma A F 1952 Comminuted fractures of the distal end of the radius treated by ulnar pinning. Journal of Bone and Joint Surgery 34A:651–662

Dowling J J, Sawyer B Jr 1961 Comminuted Colles's fractures: evaluation of a method of treatment. Journal of Bone and Joint Surgery 43A:657–668

Forgon M, Mammel E 1981 The external fixator in the management of unstable Colles's fracture. International Orthopaedics (SICOT) 5:9–14

Frykman G 1967 Fracture of the distal radius including sequelae: shoulder-hand-finger syndrome, disturbance in the distal radioulnar joint and impairment of nerve function. A clinical and experimental study. Acta Orthopaedica Scandinavica Supplement 108

Gartland J J Jr, Werley C W 1951 Evaluation of healed Colles's fractures. Journal of Bone and Joint Surgery 33A:895–907

Grana W A, Kopta J A 1979 The Roger Anderson device in the treatment of fractures of the distal end of the radius. Journal of Bone and Joint Surgery 61A:1234–1238

Green S A 1981 Complications of external skeletal fixation. Charles C Thomas, Springfield (Illinois)

Green C A, Matthews L S 1981 The thermal effects of skeletal fixation pin placement in human bone. Orthopedic Transactions 5:261

Green D P 1975 Pins and plaster treatment of comminuted fractures of the distal end of the radius. Journal of Bone and Joint Surgery 57A:304–310

Hoffman R 1954 Osteosynthése externe par fisches et rotates. Acta Chirurgica Scandinavica 107:72–88

Lidström A 1959 Fractures of the distal end of the radius. A clinical and statistical study of end results. Acta Orthopaedica Scandinavica Supplement 41

Marsh H O, Teal S W 1972 Treatment of comminuted fractures of the distal radius with self-contained skeletal traction. American Journal of Surgery 124:715–719

Riggs S A, Cooney W 1983 External fixation of complex hand and wrist fractures. Journal of Trauma 23:332

Sarmiento A, Pratt G W, Berry N C 1975 Colles's fractures: functional bracing in supination. Journal of Bone and Joint Surgery 57A:311–317

Scheck M 1962 Long-term follow-up of treatment of comminuted fractures of the distal end of the radius by transfixation with Kirschner wires and cast. Journal of Bone and Joint Surgery 44A:337–351

Vidal J, Buscayret C, Connes H 1979 Treatment of articular fractures by 'ligamentotaxis' with external fixation. In: Brooker A, Edwards C C (eds) External Fixation. The Current State of the Art. Williams and Wilkins, Baltimore

What happens afterwards?

3

R. H. C. Robins

23 Rehabilitation

PRINCIPLES

Rehabilitation after fracture is inseparable from its treatment. This principle applies just as much to the hand as it does to the hip. When an elderly woman breaks her neck of femur, an operation must be performed which will enable her to bear weight on the leg and walk within a few days of injury. In this way, the pattern of activity is preserved and rehabilitation commences as soon as the patient comes under treatment. One of the fundamental contributions made by Sir Reginald Watson-Jones to the management of fractures was to emphasize the importance of activating all those parts which it was not necessary to immobilize in order to achieve union. Prolonged immobilization by external methods is no longer considered advisable and alternative techniques are available, but the principle remains: rehabilitation does not await healing of the fracture. It *accompanies* its definitive treatment.

What then is meant by rehabilitation in this context?

1. It is the preservation of function in uninjured parts of the hand. This seemingly simple concept embraces several requirements: the avoidance of unnecessary immobilization of digits not involved in the injury, care in the positioning of the fingers, prevention of oedema, and active exercises.
2. The restoration of active motion in the fractured fingers, the recovery of strength of grasp and pinch, improvement in sensibility and the quality of the soft tissues.
3. Progress needs to be measured. Unless the range

of motion in injured digits is recorded, the effect of treatment cannot be evaluated. Moreover, nothing encourages a patient more than the evidence that his efforts are being rewarded by a steady increase in movement and strength. In the more serious cases a detailed functional assessment is required, whereby his performance is measured in the context of the activities of daily living.
4. The patient's return to work, or, if necessary his retraining and resettlement in an alternative occupation. Until this point has been reached, rehabilitation cannot be said to be complete.

How is rehabilitation to be related to treatment and what are its aims? One of the objects of treatment should be to make rehabilitation easy for the patient. If this is not considered and inappropriate methods are followed, a fractured finger can lead to a stiff hand (Fig. 23.1), even if only a single finger is broken. The main object of physical therapy is to make it possible for the patient to do it for himself. The purpose of this chapter is to discuss first, how preventive and remedial measures should be put into practice in the context of the well managed case and second, to consider what can be done for the neglected hand when the factors of prolonged immobilization, persistent oedema, or delayed wound healing have resulted in severe joint stiffness. But first, who is to be responsible for this treatment and how is progress to be measured?

Hand therapy

Standard practice in the UK implies that the patient with a fracture in the hand will attend a

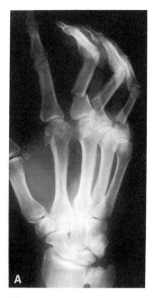
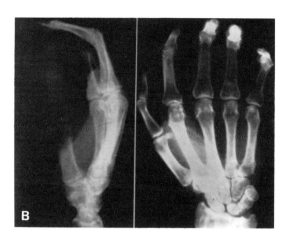
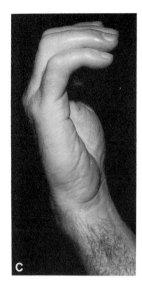

Fig. 23.1 Fractures of the proximal phalanges. Initial appearance (A). Union in perfect position after immobilization in plaster for two months (B). The result: atrophy of the fingers with complete stiffness at all joints (C). Prolonged immobilization is the commonest error in the treatment of finger fractures

fracture clinic or hand clinic, after initial treatment in the accident and emergency department. The more severe cases will be admitted under the care of the orthopaedic, plastic or hand surgeon. The supervision of the after-care is the responsibility of the surgeon concerned, but the actual day-to-day treatment is normally carried out by the physiotherapist, often later joined by the occupational therapist. Traditionally the physiotherapist employs various exercise and mobilization techniques, whereas the occupational therapist relates these to the activities of daily living and the requirements of the patient's job and may also design and make splints to encourage recovery of function. In practice these roles may overlap to a great extent, a situation which has led to the development of the discipline of hand therapy. This is already established in North America with its own society, many of whose members devote the whole of their professional time to rehabilitation of the hand. In Britain a group has recently been formed of occupational and physiotherapists who have a prime interest in this field. One of the requirements is the efficient assessment and recording of disability and the response to treatment.

Hand assessment charts

Over the years many attempts have been made to design charts for recording hand function, but most have failed because they were too elaborate in concept and too time-consuming to complete. A successful chart should be attractive in its lay-out and quick to fill in, saving time in the hospital records and not creating extra work.

Charts recently promoted by the British Orthopaedic Association comprise a series covering recent injuries, sensory function, range of motion and functional assessment. In the context of rehabilitation after fracture, the latter two are relevant and are reproduced by permission of the British Orthopaedic Association (Fig. 23.2).*

Range of motion

Three ways of recording range of motion, active or passive, are provided. First, is the actual measurement by goniometer of the *arc of motion* for each individual joint, and second the *overall*

* These charts are available from The Pilgrims Press, Caxton House, Ongar, Essex CM 5 9RB, England, U.K.

Hand range of motion chart

Hospital

Injured hand: left/right
Dominant hand: left/right
Method of recording joint ranges:

Number
Name
Address

Dorsal

Palmar

Diagnosis ....
....

Date of birth　　　　　　　Age　　　　　　　　　M/F
Occupation

		P	A	P	A	P	A	P	A	P	A	Normal ranges
Date of injury	Details											
Dates of operations												
Examination dates												
Passive/Active		P	A	P	A	P	A	P	A	P	A	Normal ranges
Thumb	MCP											
	IP											
	Pulp to base of little (cm) **Flexion**											
Index	MCP											
	PIP											
	DIP											
	Pulp to crease (cm)											
	Nail to table (cm)											
Middle	MCP											
	PIP											
	DIP											
	Pulp to crease (cm)											
	Nail to table (cm)											
Ring	MCP											
	PIP											
	DIP											
	Pulp to crease (cm)											
	Nail to table (cm)											
Little	MCP											
	PIP											
	DIP											
	Pulp to crease (cm)											
	Nail to table (cm)											
Span	Thumb index (cm)											
Span	Index little (cm)											
Grip strength												
Pinch strength												

Fig. 23.2(A) Range of motion chart. Space on the back is allowed for Odstock tracings (see opposite)

Odstock Tracings
Solder wire & catheter tubing

State:	E.g. Ring finger, active	Colour code	Date
Active/Passive			
Flexion/Extension			
Identify digit			
Mark joints			

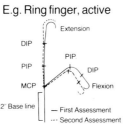

range recorded as the distance in centimetres by which the finger-tip fails to reach the distal palmar crease on flexion or the finger nail fails to reach the horizontal plane on extension (*see* Fig. 23.2a). Space is provided in which consecutive measurements can be tabulated over a period of time. Some clinicians and therapists find that a diagrammatic record gives a clearer picture as to progress , and certainly this may be more convincing to the patient. Accordingly the back of the chart is left largely blank in order to accommodate *Odstock tracings* (*see* Fig. 23.2b). This simple method employs a malleable material, such as solder wire passed through thin rubber tubing, applied closely to the back of the finger and a tracing made in maximal flexion and extension. The positions of the joints are then marked on the diagram. Serial tracings are made at intervals of time and colour-coded, which give a pictorial record of progress in mobilization.

Additional information which can be written on the front of the chart includes measurements of the span between the thumb and index finger and that between the index and little fingers. Strength of pinch and strength of grip may be recorded by any technique which the examiner favours. A number of spring gadgets have been devised for this purpose; a pneumatic cuff inflated to a standard pressure provides a good measure of power grip. A column is included for normal range of movement for those patients who may have hypermobile joints of alternatively relatively stiff ones. The vitally important matter of sensory assessment is recorded on a separate chart, but this is not relevant to an uncomplicated fracture and outside the scope of this chapter.

Functional assessment

The functional assessment chart (*see* Fig. 23.2c) is applicable to all patients with permanent disability, including those with joint stiffness, pain, weakness, or instability attributable to fractures. On the reverse of the form is tabulated in serial manner the patient's performance in response to certain activities designed to test specific aspects of hand function (*see* Fig. 23.2d). This is the evidence on which the therapist bases the conclusions summarized on the front of the form. The disability in the hand is placed in the context of physical handicap in the rest of the upper limb and elsewhere in the body and relates it to difficulties experienced at work or at home. This assessment of disability by the patient may be contrasted with the comments of the therapist and the view taken by the patient towards his or her handicap and to any proposals about surgery to alleviate it. This sort of evaluation finds its widest application in rheumatoid arthritis, but it is equally relevant to a crushed hand with multiple fractures.

MANAGEMENT OF RECENT FRACTURES

Fracture healing and joint mobility

The causes of finger stiffness after fracture of the metacarpals or phalanges are either involvement of

Hand functional assessment chart

Hospital

Consultant

Affected hand: left/right
Dominant hand: left/right

Number
Name
Address

Diagnosis .... Date of birth   Age   M/F
.... Occupation

Main problems	Pre-op	Post-op
Hand		
Upper limb		
Lower limb		
Spine		
Severity of pain and relevant drugs		
Difficulties at home		
O T Home assessment yes/no		
Difficulties at work		
Work assessment yes/no		
Attitude to disability		
Attitude to surgery		

Functional assessment   Recommend grade 0-5

		Pre-op date	Post-op date
Light pinch	Pick up pencil		
	Write name		
	Pick up pin		
Heavy pinch	Use tweezers with pin		
	Strike match		
	Do up zip		
Tripod pinch	Small screwdriver **unscrew plug**		
	Open safety pin		
	Lid off saucepan		
Grasp	Hold tumbler		
	Lift full teapot (2 pints)		
	Lift full kettle (2 pints)		
Opposition	Scissors cut paper		
	Do up buttons		
	Wind watch		
Pronation Supination	Screw jam jar		
	Wring cloth		
	Turn yale key in lock		
Miscellaneous	Handle money		
	Pick up telephone		
	Dial telephone		
	Manage walking aids and type of aids used		
	Release grip		
Comment			

Manual dexterity		Time in Seconds					
		Pre-op date		Post-op date			
	Pick up 24 marbles using	Left	Right	Left	Right	Left	Right
	Thumb/Index						
	Thumb/Middle						
	Thumb/Ring						
	Thumb/Little						
	Between 2/3 fingers						

Examiner ....

Fig. 23.2 (C & D)   Functional assessment chart. The conclusions are summarized on the front

the joint in the injury or the effects of immobility, whether this be due to immobilization of the joint for a prolonged period or to reluctance on the part of the patient to keep the fingers moving because they are painful and swollen. If the joint itself is seriously damaged, some degree of disability is inevitable, but when this is not so, the outcome may depend upon the correct choice of treatment. The onset of stiffness in uninjured fingers should always be preventable if these principles are followed: immobilization should be confined to the parts which are fractured, oedema should be countered by elevation of the limb and avoidance of compression dressings and splints, and finger exercises should be commenced at the earliest stage possible.

In order to resolve this conflict between active exercise and passive immobilization, treatment can be considered as falling into three choices: immediate mobilization, immobilization by plaster of Paris, or other material, with or without prior manipulation ('le traitement orthopédique' of the French) or internal fixation after open or closed reduction ('le traitement chirurgicale'). The exact indications for these different methods are discussed elsewhere in this book, but the principle behind them all forms the basis for rehabilitation after fracture: to achieve and maintain a stable reduction of the fracture and permit mobilization of the joints at the earliest opportunity. These treatment policies will now be examined as they apply to various fractures in the hand.

Since the time in the last century when Lucas-Championère advocated massage and movement in the treatment of fractures, rebelling against the contemporary ideas of prolonged immobility, to the present-day conflict (apparent rather than real) between the rigid surgical fixation as exemplified by the AO group in Switzerland and the functional bracing advocated by those who follow the teaching of Sarmiento (Sarmiento & Latta 1981), there has been confusion about the relative merits of what might seem to be irreconcilable views about how fractures should be treated. Originally this was doubtless true, because immobilization could be equated with dis-use and its attendant complications of muscle wasting, joint stiffness and osteoporosis. Nowadays, selection of methods of treatment is based on the knowledge of the stability

of the fracture and the acceptability of the position of the fragments. Thus the treatment of stable fractures of the digits should be based on early joint movements. Certain fractures in unacceptable position may be corrected by manipulation and afterwards be stable and thus suitable for protected movement. A good example is fracture of the fifth metacarpal neck. The great majority of these fractures need no reduction, but if the head of the metacarpal is prominent in the palm, reduction can be effected by a force directed backwards along the line of the fully flexed proximal phalanx of the little finger. The fracture is then treated by active exercises, because once reduced it is stable. A rare type of fracture in this area is oblique and unstable; in such instances, an open reduction and stabilization by screw is needed in order to allow unrestricted movement.

Fractures of the fingers requiring immobilization by external means are usually treated with moulded plaster of Paris slabs or with strips of metal padded with foam. Unless there is some special reason to the contrary, these are applied to the volar surface and are retained by open-wove bandages or strips of adhesive plaster. Great care must be taken to avoid constriction to the circulation which may cause swelling or, worse, ischaemia. Fractures with displacement require prior manipulative reduction. The position of the fingers and the time during which they are immobilized are both vitally important factors if stiffness is to be prevented. The safe position of immobilization has been emphasized by James (1970). The metacarpophalangeal joints should be flexed about 70° and the proximal interphalangeal joints 20°, in which positions the collateral ligaments are stretched and not therefore prone to develop irreversible contractures. All rules may sometimes be bent and there will be occasions when the surgeon may decide that ankylosis of a severely damaged joint may be inevitable, in which case the position of function should be used, about 40°.

How long is safe? Similar arguments apply here as to the use of a tourniquet. All surgeons become uneasy at the application of a pneumatic cuff beyond 90 min; this period is frequently exceeded, but at one's peril in the older patient or one in whom the circulation may already be impaired through injury or disease. Three weeks is the safe period of immobilization, but in favourable conditions this may be extended to four weeks, or longer in the case of the thumb. Unless there is bone loss, non-union of finger fractures (excluding avulsed fragments) is uncommon except for the proximal phalanx of the thumb, the bone distal to the wrist most likely to need grafting. Policy decisions should therefore be made on clinical examination rather than radiographic appearances. It is vital to mobilize finger fractures within 3–4 weeks of injury, by which time sufficient stability should have been restored. A major error is constantly being made when the programme of treatment is halted because of an unpromising radiograph or a misleading radiological report. If the objective of mobilizing the fingers within the expected period of time cannot be achieved, internal fixation should be used and this decision should be made as soon as possible after injury. The indications for internal fixation of finger fractures are quite clear (Robins 1961) and, while techniques may change, principles do not. There are a number of indications for internal fixation as follows:

1. Shaft fractures after failure of closed treatment or where it is considered essential to avoid immobilization: e.g. where there is pre-existing chronic arthritis
2. Fractures with displacement close to, or involving, the joint, excluding tiny fragments
3. In certain instances, to afford stability after major hand injuries, especially where there is vascular damage

Since it is the soft tissues which determine oedema and stiffness, it is important not to add unnecessary surgical trauma to the wound of injury. For this reason the relatively non-invasive Kirschner wires have much to recommend them over implant materials, which require wide dissection and stripping of soft tissues for their use. Whether the fractures are isolated or multiple, open or closed, the object of treatment is to relieve pain and to stabilize the skeleton so that active movements may be started early: in short, to immobilize the fracture and mobilize the joints.

Mobilizing techniques

It is one thing to say 'go for early movements' and sometimes quite another to put it into practice. There should be no difficulty in a simple, stable closed fracture but objectives must vary in response to the severity of the injury; for instance, crush injuries with open fractures will usually end up with some permanent disability, the degree of which will depend to some extent on the determination of the patient as well as the quality of the treatment. Even in the simple case, it is insufficient just to tell the patient to move the fingers. All fresh fractures are painful and pain is the chief deterrent to active movement. Sometimes surgical relief of pain is indicated; for example, release of the subungual haematoma with a fracture of terminal phalanx. More usually it is the application of a simple support allowing controlled movement. An adjacent uninjured finger can provide this by being taped to the injured one. This technique has two added advantages: it controls rotation, something easily checked by watching the plane of the finger nails as the digit flexes; and it acts as a lively splint providing active, assisted movements. Another very useful method, in place of strapping, is the Bedford support: a double-barrelled elasticated tube which fits over two fingers. For the metacarpals, an elastic crêpe bandage should be adequate.

If there is significant swelling, a sling is indicated, applied in such a way that the hand is at least level with the opposite shoulder. It should not be worn for longer than necessary, but whether it is worn or not, the shoulder must be exercised regularly.

The patient is encouraged to exercise first the uninjured parts of the hand and then to bring in the fractured digital ray, carrying out slow and deliberate movements and actively holding the digit in flexion and extension with maximal power for a few moments.

Similar considerations apply to mobilizing fractures shortly after internal fixation, but here there will be greater difficulty and more supervision by the therapist will be required. Although the use of Kirschner wires or other implants can free the hand from the need for external splints for treatment of the fracture, damage to and repair of other structures may impede the ability to start active motion, but unless there are overriding considerations, dressings should be minimal and movements started within them. Elevation is important and if exercises are to be effective, the patient must be positioned so that his arm is comfortably supported and free from unnecessary restraint. All this seems very obvious, but it is the neglect of these simple rules which is the commonest avoidable cause of hand stiffness after injury. There are, however, constraints imposed by pain, uniting fractures and perhaps also the presence of dressings.

When the fracture has united or passed the point of no return in this direction, treatment needs to be more aggressive and also more specific. Take, for example, fractures of the proximal or middle phalanges of the fingers. If they are of significant degree, movement at the interphalangeal joints will not return without much hard work on the patient's part. Unless the therapist instructs the patient exactly how to move the finger, all the effort will be wasted on the metacarpophalangeal joint which will probably be no problem. The most effective way is to make a rounded wooden block, one end to be grasped in the palm and the other to fit just short of the relevant digital crease (Fig. 23.3). Not only does this provide support and leverage where it is needed, but by keeping it always handy it is a constant reminder to the patient of what to do. For the metacarpophalangeal joints, where an element of rotation is involved, a lump of plasticine or putty, or a squash ball, according to the tastes of the patient, are all potentially effective. However, this is prohibited in the early stages after fracture, because there is a risk of displacing the fragments. It is also not recommended when the object of treatment is to restore motion to the interphalangeal joints.

Exercises designed to mobilize the wrist and forearm follow the normal methods of physiotherapy, but two points need emphasis. First, the most important arc of movement in the wrist is neither flexion/extension nor radial/ulnar deviation but the oblique plane comprising extension and radial deviation at one extreme and flexion and ulnar deviation at the other. Secondly, the common pattern of wrist/finger movement is wrist extension/finger flexion through to wrist flexion/finger extension. Any exercise programme to increase strength and mobility in the wrist and hand, but

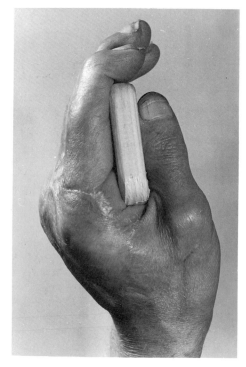

Fig. 23.3 Exercise block for the terminal joints (for the proximal interphalangeal joints it will be correspondingly smaller)

particularly following fractures of the wrist, should make use of these natural patterns of movement, concentrating the patient's attention on the component which is uninjured. Thus with a stiff wrist, encouraging the patient's grasp will enhance the strength and range of wrist extension. This is a principle of occupational therapy which will be referred to later.

In the after-treatment of the more complex finger fractures, the technique of continuous passive motion may have a useful role but at present this has not been evaluated. Another variant combining fracture treatment and rehabilitation is the use of dynamic traction for the early mobilization of fractures of the proximal interphalangeal joint. Azouz and Schenck (1985) have recently reported a series of ten patients with comminuted intra-articular fractures treated by a traction apparatus consisting of a 'hayrake' splint with a rigid arc equidistant from the proximal interphalangeal joint in all positions. Rubber bands were used for traction, attached at one end to a movable component of the arc and at the other to a transosseous wire placed horizontally, distal to the involved joint. Splinting was maintained for an average of seven weeks and the position varied from full flexion to full extension on a timed schedule. At 12 months, the ten patients obtained an average range of motion from 7 to 90°. Such results would seem in this limited series to compare favourably with those expected from open surgical procedures.

The use of splints

The word splint signifies immobilization, but this was not always so. An earlier meaning was the parts of a suit of armour which allowed movement while exerting control, as at the bend of the elbow. This meaning is in keeping with the dynamic splint as understood by hand surgeons today. Splints must be designed to interfere as little as possible with the use of the hand. For this reason, many are of limited value in this context. An exception to this is the arm-chair finger splint conceived and described by Capener about 40 years ago, but designed and made by Suter, the orthotist to the Devonian Orthopaedic Association (Fig. 23.4). In the tradition of other Exeter appliances it embraces the principle of the coiled spring, in this case using piano wire. While velcro straps may have replaced

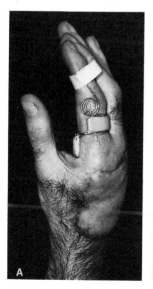
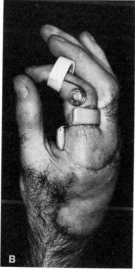

Fig. 23.4 The Capener arm-chair splint provides both assisted extension for stretching a contracture (A) and resisted flexion for developing strength (B)

leather, the basic design remains unchanged and it is the one device with almost universal application in the attempt to restore strength and movement to the stiff finger. It is able to give assisted extension and resisted flexion at the same time. Because finger flexion is so much stronger than extension, and has to be so, the need in rehabilitation is to assist extension by giving a steady stretching force and to resist flexion in order to give the strong flexor muscles something to work against. The arm-chair splint may therefore be used as an exerciser by day, being slipped on and off as necessary, and worn at night as a splint to stretch the finger in extension and oppose the tendency of the finger to contract down during sleep. It should not be used at night until the patient has become accustomed to its use by day, or there will be a risk of provoking dorsal oedema by obstructing the venous return.

THE STIFF HAND AFTER FRACTURE

Discussion so far has been concerned with the restoration of function after fracture when this has been under the control of the surgeon and therapist from the time of injury. While this does not guarantee a successful outcome, at least the worst pitfalls should be avoidable and, if the policy already described is followed, a result should be obtained commensurate with the severity of the injury; where this falls short of what is acceptable, reconstructive or ablative surgery can be decided upon. Severe stiffness in the fingers after injury can have many causes, of which fractures may be one, but often it is the gross damage to the soft tissues and the consequent oedema which is the most important factor, especially in crush injuries. The condition is made worse when the need for early mobilization has not been realised and when tissues of impaired vitality have been preserved, leading to delay in healing or to secondary amputation. The situation is particularly regrettable with closed crushing injuries in which uncontrolled oedema has led to generalized thickening of the soft tissues and adhesions between the mobile parts. Apart from the vascular problems caused by direct trauma, there are also neurovascular problems which may complicate relatively minor fractures, generally of the wrist, and going under the names of Sudeck's atrophy or reflex sympathetic dystrophy. Greater awareness of the cause of this condition and its dissociation from the psychological aura which has previously surrounded the diagnosis has led to more rational treatment. Quite a different therapeutic approach is required in the management of this condition from that needed for the stiff hand following either neglect of simple fractures or severe local trauma. One thing, however, is common to all: the surgeon must explain the nature of the problem, the programme of treatment and the expected outcome. In all instances, progress will be slow and the patient must be told this; also that whatever may be done in the way of treatment, whether this be physical, medical or surgical, the deciding factor is the motivation of the patient to get better. The first duty of the surgeon and the therapist is to restore the confidence of the patient, which is nearly always lacking, and to stimulate the will to recover.

Sudeck's atrophy

Acute atrophy of bone together with swelling, pain and loss of function was first described by Sudeck in 1900. Although the original description was in the foot, it is now recognized as being commoner in the hand and usually complicates relatively trivial trauma such as a minor fracture of the wrist. In the early stages after injury it is characterized by redness, swelling and burning pain, but this gives way to a cold, clammy, pale, stiff hand. In the most severe cases the hand is frozen with neither active or passive movement in the fingers. The similarity between this reflex sympathetic dystrophy and causalgia, the painful sequel of peripheral nerve damage, is so striking that most authorities consider them to be at either end of the same neurological spectrum: pain following partial nerve lesions or major causalgia, and minor causalgia (sympathetic dystrophy) where the damage is to the very fine terminal axons. The treatment of Sudeck's atrophy follows similar lines to causalgia, where hypersensitivity to noradrenaline is an important feature. Barnes (1954) showed that most cases of causalgia from gunshot wounds could be relieved by sympathetic block, or sympathectomy.

The clinical management of these conditions was revolutionized by the introduction of guanethidine blocks by Hannington Kiff (1974). These are easier to perform and longer in their effect than sympathetic blocks. Withrington and Wynn Parry (1984) recommend avoiding sedation so that the patient is encouraged to try and desensitize the hyperpathic skin by stroking and rubbing the skin and exercising in physiotherapy followed by productive activity in occupational therapy. This treatment can be repeated frequently and is more effective when given intensively than spread out over a longer period of time.

Management of the stiff hand

Sudeck's atrophy above, is a special case. The trauma component is slight, the neurovascular one considerable. Their combined effect is often devastating, but with a potential for recovery which may be complete.

The stiff hand after multiple fractures is likely to be less painful but lead to a disability at least partly dependent, not only on the severity of the fractures, but also on the degree of the accompanying soft tissue injury.

Assessment of patient and treatment planning

Faced with this problem on the first consultation, the surgeon needs a plan of management. The first requirement is to establish a base-line by recording the physical examination and a full functional assessment on the lines referred to at the beginning of this chapter. The physical examination takes particular note of associated features, including the quality of the skin cover, the presence of pain, oedema and altered sensibility, as well as the state of union of the fracture and the mobility of the joints.

The next stage is to determine the ultimate aim of treatment based on the physical examination and the functional assessment. While it is generally true that a decision about secondary surgery should await the time of maximal improvement after physical treatment, this is not always so. Firstly, no patient can cooperate fully if the hand is painful or insensitive or if wound or scarring is unsatisfactory. Secondly, a slavish adherence to the principle that everything viable should be saved may lead to the preservation of a useless digit which is holding up the recovery of function in the rest of the hand. It is sometimes necessary to sacrifice a part for the good of the whole. This is a decision which should be taken relatively early before irreversible changes have had time to take place in other parts of the hand injured less seriously or not at all. It is therefore sometimes necessary to carry out an elective amputation prior to commencing intensive physical treatment, just as it may be helpful to revise a scar or to operate on a painful neuroma. However, it is more usual that other forms of conservative treatment such as oil massage for an adherent scar, sympathetic blocks for vascular impairment or transcutaneous nerve stimulation for painful peripheral nerve pain will be indicated and all these methods may be used at the same time as treatment to restore mobility.

Mobilization of stiff fingers

This can be a long and often rather painful process and the patient's confidence must be gained at the outset. The assessment already referred to helps to achieve this, because the patient will appreciate that the problem is understood and being approached in a rational manner. Moreover, the regular recording of the range of movement of each joint will demonstrate improvement. The knowledge that he is getting better is the most valuable incentive to the efforts of the patient.

Treatment should be on a daily basis with each occasion alternate spells of physical treatment and occupational therapy. The former starts with a warming-up period of heat and massage before proceeding to active exercises and passive stretching. Active exercises are designed to restore flexion; here passive movements play only a small part and, even then, are combined with instruction to the patient to flex actively at the same time. The exercise block already described is of great value in this situation and should be the patient's constant companion. By dint of the greater strength of the long flexors over the extensor apparatus, so that there is no extensor function comparable to the power grasp, the regaining of active extension has to be attempted through passive stretching and

serial splintage. The experienced therapist knows how far extension can be pushed by gradual traction on the digits without the risk of provoking a painful reaction. At this point the digit is splinted. In the past, plaster-of-Paris was used for this purpose, but now one of the heat-moulded plastics is more appropriate (Fig. 23.5). This is worn at night as a static splint and by day may be taken on and off. It is vitally important that, in an effort to improve extension, the power and range of flexion should not suffer. If the fingers are stiff in extension, a fabric glove with adjustable tapes to keep the fingers flexed may be worn at night (Fig. 23.6). Static splints can be made to support the whole

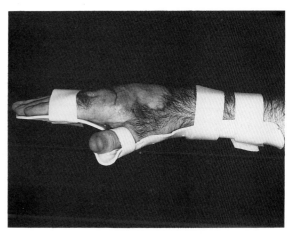

Fig. 23.5 Heat-malleable static night splint to maintain extension

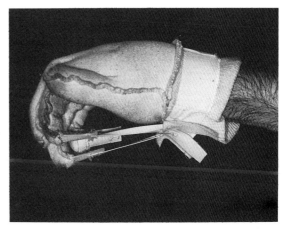

Fig. 23.6 Fabric glove with adjustable tapes secured with velcro to maintain flexion. Fitted with elastic tapes (as shown here) it becomes a dynamic splint

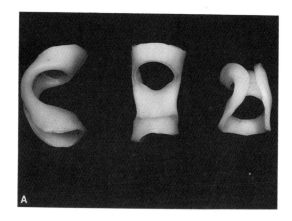

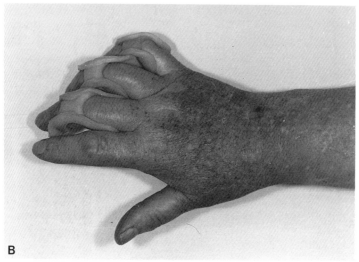

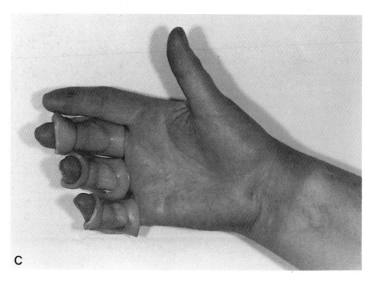

Fig. 23.7 Static thermoplastic splints holding interphalangeal joints in maximal extension, while leaving exposed maximal tactile area (A–C)

hand or can be tailored to an individual joint or joints. Their object is to maintain the range of extension achieved by the therapist, holding it while further improvement is attempted. Dynamic splints in this context, excluding the arm-chair splint for the individual finger, interfere with function. While it may be useful exercise to flex the fingers against traction mediated through elastic bands or spring wire, the hand cannot be used for much when encumbered by an elaborate splint, and it is, above all, use that is essential for recovery. Conscientiously used, an exercise block is more effective.

In the treatment of the stiff hand, physiotherapy may not be fun, but occupational therapy should be. Activities here may take the form of production by working a machine or recreational games in which a spirit of competition may be introduced. Whatever means are adopted, the ends are the same: to grip more and more powerfully objects of decreasing size and to open the hand gradually to grasp objects of increasing diameter. Regular functional assessments are carried out until maximal improvement has been reached. At this point consideration is again given to the possibility of improvement by surgery. This may take the form of operations aimed at improving motion, such as capsulotomy, volar plate release or excision of an adherent superficialis tendon, correcting deformity by oesteotomy, stabilizing a painful interphalangeal joint by arthrodesis or replacing a metacarpophalangeal joint by implant athroplasty. In fact, the commonest operation is amputation of a part or the whole of a finger which is painful, useless or a hindrance to the function of the whole hand.

These processes of rehabilitation must take account of the patient's daily life and resettlement in employment. If it is clear from the nature of the injuries that the previous job will be unattainable, plans for future training should be formulated as soon as possible and be incorporated in the programme of treatment.

CONCLUSION

What then is the conclusion from all this? Advances are made in our understanding of the nature of pain and the means for its relief. Materials used in treatment may change, but the principles do not. In the case of most fractures, joint stiffness can be prevented by prompt attention to active exercises aided by simple splints. In the more serious case, a much more intensive programme is required involving all the resources of remedial therapy. Thrice-weekly sessions in a physiotherapy department are totally inadequate. Treatment means a preliminary warm-up in physiotherapy followed by active work in occupational therapy and then back to physiotherapy. Weekly recording of progress should be made. Between attendances the patient must work at the exercises shown. Above all, the therapists must demonstrate that they are interested in the patient's recovery, and must motivate him or her towards restoration of function by personal effort because in this situation others can only create the conditions favourable to recovery. All these principles were stated by Wynn Parry in 1958 and have been reiterated constantly since that time (Wynn Parry 1981). 'If patients with severe injuries to the hand are to regain maximal function as quickly as possible, intensive treatment for several hours a day is required from a highly skilled therapeutic staff, under the direction of a doctor with specialized knowledge of all aspects of the problem'.

REFERENCES

Azouz D, Schenck R R 1985 Dynamic traction and early mobilization for fractures of the proximal interphalangeal joint. Paper read at Annual Meeting of American Society for Surgery of the Hand, Las Vegas

Barnes R 1954 Causalgia. A review of 48 cases in Peripheral nerve injuries. Report of Medical Research Council p 156–185

Capener N 1956 The hand in surgery. Journal of Bone and Joint Surgery 38B:128–151

Hannington Kiff J 1974 Intravenous regional sympathetic block with guanethidine. Lancet i:1019–1020

James J I P 1970 The assessment and management of the injured hand. The Hand 2:97–105

Lucas-Championnière J 1895 Traitement de fractures par le massage et la mobilisation. Paris

Robins R H C 1961 Injuries and infections of the hand. Edward Arnold, London, ch 10

Sarmiento A, Latta L L 1981 Closed functional treatment of fractures. Springer-Verlag, Berlin

Sudeck P 1900 Uber die akute Entzundliche Knochenatropie: Archiv fur Klinische Chirurgie 62:147

Withrington R H, Wynn Parry C B 1984 Painful disorders of peripheral nerves. Postgraduate Medical Journal 60:869–875

Wynn Parry C B 1981 Rehabilitation of the hand (4th edn). Butterworths, London

N. J. Barton

24 Complications

'Hand fractures can be complicated by deformity from no treatment, stiffness from over-treatment, and both deformity and stiffness from poor treatment.' In this memorable sentence, Swanson (1970a) has summarized the whole problem. Doctors sometimes forget that the natural history of untreated fractures is to unite: this is seen in animals, in primitive and isolated tribes, and in prehistoric skeletons.

There are certain bones, such as the tibia and the scaphoid, with a strong tendency to non-union, but most fractures through most bones (and especially through the cancellous parts of those bones) will unite if left alone: it will, however, be malunion. In most cases the purpose of treatment is not to make the bone join up, but to make it join up in the correct position.

This requires some form of immobilization, whether by splintage or internal fixation, and in the *hand*, the question is whether the game is worth the candle. As Swanson makes clear, it is unfortunately true that many fractures of the hand would have obtained a better result if the patient had never seen a doctor, and this is a terrible condemnation of our attitudes. In some ways, the problem is getting worse because keen young orthopaedic surgeons who have been taught (one might even say indoctrinated) about the advantages of internal fixation and have had some experience in such techniques, are all too keen to apply them to the hand, where the situation is very different in two respects. First, internal fixation of small bones is more difficult and has little or no margin for error: drills tend to slip off the sharply curved surface of the bone and, if a mistake is made, new fracture lines may be created so that fixation becomes

impossible. Second, in no part of the body is the radiological result less important by comparison with the functional result in terms of range of movement, and a greater range of movement may be achieved without operation by simple early mobilization.

In the *wrist*, immobilization is nearly always necessary, to prevent non-union in the carpus and malunion in the distal radius. A large range of movement at the wrist, though desirable, is less necessary than in the hand.

With these thoughts as a background, this chapter will review the complications of fractures of the hand and wrist: how to prevent them, and how to treat them if they do occur. In a sense, this whole book can be considered as being about how to prevent the various complications and some aspects have been very fully covered already, but it may be of value to underline the most important points and fill in a few gaps.

STIFFNESS

This must come first, because it is the most common problem. Indeed, it would not be going too far to say that if a bad result follows any type of hand injury, the problem is likely to be stiffness. The management of the stiff hand is described briefly in Chapter 3 and more fully in Chapter 23, but there are different types and causes of stiffness, most of which are avoidable, and prevention is better than cure. One must, therefore, consider the causes of stiffness.

Incorrect immobilization

This term embraces two errors: the hand may

incorrectly be immobilized when it would have been better to mobilize it straightaway, or it may rightly be immobilized but in the wrong position. Worst of all, both mistakes may be made simultaneously and unfortunately this is not rare.

Unnecessary immobilization

In Chapter 3, Professor James has distinguished between unstable fractures of the phalanges for which some form of immobilization is needed, and stable ones, which are best treated by early active movements. Similarly, in Chapter 10 it is made clear that most metacarpal fractures can be treated very simply.

This may not emerge clearly from the contents of this book. Chapters 3, 4, 5 and 6 describe different methods of immobilizing phalangeal fractures, the methods described in Chapters 4, 5 and 6 being designed to allow as much joint movement as possible while supporting the fracture. Chapters 9, 10 and 11 define indications for operation on metacarpal fractures, and Chapters 13, 14 and 15 discuss operative techniques for certain particularly difficult problems. Thus a large proportion of Part 1 concerns special techniques for the more difficult fractures, because this book is directed to experienced and presumably discriminating surgeons. However, it cannot be over-emphasized that these surgical methods are only indicated in a very small proportion of routine fractures in the hand. Of the hand fractures seen in an ordinary fracture clinic, probably about 50% can be treated by the method sometimes known in Britain as 'supervised neglect' (with the emphasis on the supervised), 35% need immobilization, and 5% need internal or external fixation.

Another possible example of unnecessary immobilization which may be harmful (though not in the sense of causing stiffness) concerns the thumb when treating a scaphoid fracture. The orthodox treatment in Britain is by a below-elbow plaster cast extending to the proximal phalanx of the thumb. 'In this way the trapezium and the trapezoscaphoid joint will be immobilized' says Fisk (1982) in the sixth edition of Watson-Jones' Textbook of Fractures, though it is interesting that Watson-Jones himself, in the third edition (1943) recommends a plaster which includes the first

metacarpal but stops short of the MCP (metacarpophalangeal) joint. Böhler (1935), in his textbook, advises leaving the thumb completely free and specifically says that scaphoid fractures should be treated in the same way as Colles's fractures. London's book (1961) agrees with Böhler. There are both theoretical and practical reasons for leaving the thumb free. Böhler et al (1954) suggest that immobilization of the thumb 'restricts free play of the thumb muscles, thus eliminating the compression-effect on the carpal scaphoid and hindering the union of the fragments'. The plaster extending to the proximal phalanx may also be an example of the phenomenon described by Hicks (1960): external splintage as a cause of movement in fractures, because the patient can, by flexing the distal phalanx of the thumb against the end of the plaster, distract the entire ray. In practice, it is much more inconvenient for the patient to have the thumb in plaster and there is no evidence that it helps: Böhler et al (1954), comparing two groups of 35 patients, found that in those in whom the thumb was immobilized five developed non-union but when the thumb was left free only two failed to unite. Admittedly, these were dorsal plaster splints rather than complete plasters, and the numbers probably do not reach significance. A large prospective randomized trial is needed and this is now under way in Nottingham.

Immobilization in the wrong position

The hand. It is perhaps worth trying to clarify the terminology for positions of the hand. Much confusion has arisen in the past by the use of the term 'position of function'. This term should be abandoned as it has no meaning and is indeed a misconception: the hand functions by moving from one position to another. In particular, this term has often been confused with the *position of rest*, that is to say the position adopted by the hand when the patient is asleep or anaesthetized, with the MCP joints fairly straight and the IP (interphalangeal) joints semi-flexed. This position of rest is unfortunately rather similar to the *position of stiffness* or, even more vividly, 'position of failure' which is the position in which the hand tends to become stiff, as so well described by Koch (1935), with the MCP joints extended, the IP joints flexed, and the thumb adducted.

In a rather different category is the *position of arthrodesis*: that position in which a particular joint should be fixed if it is never going to move again. This position varies from joint to joint and from finger to finger; moreover it is unlikely to apply to more than a few joints in the hand, however badly that hand may have been affected by injury or arthritis.

Last, and most relevant to this chapter, is the *position of immobilization*. The present writer believes that the more widespread use of the position for immobilization of the hand advocated by Professor James of Edinburgh (with the IP joints straight, the MCP joints flexed and the thumb in palmar abduction) has been one of the most important causes of improvement in the results of hand injuries over the last 20 years. This is often called the Edinburgh position or the James position: he himself calls it the 'safe position'. It may be compared with the position in which you park your car if it has a faulty battery and you anticipate difficulty in getting it started: you leave it at the top of the hill so that you can get it running downhill. The position of immobilization is like this because, although it is not the position in which you want to leave the hand permanently, it is the easiest position from which to get it moving again.

Chapter 3 describes the reasons for adopting this position and the method of achieving it. I find it helpful to use a second plaster slab dorsally to maintain the desired position though, as these hands are liable to swelling, one must ensure that the two slabs do not meet at their edges. It is easy to neglect the thumb, which can develop an adduction contracture after a severe injury of the hand even though the thumb itself was not injured: the thumb should either be left free for active exercises, or immobilized in palmar abduction.

The wrist. The position for immobilization of scaphoid fractures is far from universally agreed. Berlin (1929) dissected 60 cadaveric wrists and concluded that the least separation of the fracture fragments occurred when the wrist was in radial deviation and 45% dorsiflexion, a view confirmed more recently by Thomaidis (1973). This position has, on the whole, been accepted as the one in which scaphoid fractures should be immobilized, but some authorities disagree with it: indeed, as Fisk (1982) pointed out, any extreme position will immobilize the carpus.

Squire (1959) recommended dorsiflexion with ulnar deviation, a position supported by cadaveric studies by King et al (1982) but criticized by Fisk (1970) as likely to distract the fragments. When one exposes a scaphoid fracture, it sometimes seems as though palmar flexion is the position which closes the fracture and Broome and Cedell (1964), in a small series of patients, claimed that union took place more quickly when the wrist was in neutral than in a standard cast in dorsiflexion. It seems extraordinary that there should be room for difference of opinion about an apparently simple mechanical problem such as this, but it is interesting that McLaughlin (1954) who operated on many scaphoid fractures found that no one position of the wrist could be relied upon to reduce or immobilize the fracture.

There is also disagreement about the position of the forearm. Cadaveric studies by Verdan (1960) suggested that pronation and supination of the forearm caused movement at the fracture site; for this reason, some surgeons use above-elbow casts, but even here there is disagreement. Squire (1959) and King et al (1982) recommended, in addition to the position of the wrist mentioned above, that the forearm should be immobilized in full supination. However Lindström (1975) having reviewed 373 cases with a follow-up period of more than 7 years, found no difference in the final outcome between patients treated in an above-elbow plaster as recommended by Verdan or a below-elbow Böhler cast. Alho and Kankaanpää (1975) made a prospective comparison between patients randomly allocated to treatment in above- or below-elbow casts, both extending down to the IP joint of the thumb. They found no difference in the speed of union and non-union was actually more common in the above-elbow group (6 out of 41) than in the below-elbow group (2 out of 51). More prospective studies are needed to provide the answer to the simple, important and practical question 'What sort of plaster should we use?' The difficulty, however, is defining the end-point to be measured and, in particular, deciding when union has been achieved.

In treating Colles's fractures, the position of the wrist is dictated by the manoeuvre needed to obtain reduction: since the distal fragment of radius is too small to grasp, it is manipulated indirectly through the ligaments by pulling on the more distal bones.

A position of marked flexion of the wrist was formerly advocated and for many years I, in my English ignorance, imagined that this was called the 'cotton-loader position' after that used by workers in the cotton-fields of the southern states of the USA. In fact it is named after two surgeons called Cotton and Loder, but their names have been applied to this position by oral tradition and they do not seem to have recommended it in writing. Cotton was an eminent surgeon in Boston, Massachusetts, who published a text-book on fractures in the early part of the twentieth century. The identification of Loder is not certain but Dr Roy Meals of Los Angeles has found that an orthopaedic surgeon called H. B. Loder, who graduated from Harvard in 1894, had his office at 512 Commonwealth Avenue, Boston, only a few doors away from Cotton who was at number 520. It therefore seems very likely that he is the man, especially as neither of the other two Doctor Loders practising in the USA in the 1920s was a surgeon.

This very flexed position is not now favoured, and certainly should not be maintained for more than 10 days, partly because it is uncomfortable and partly because it may result in permanent loss of extension at the wrist-joint. In Colles's fractures which are so unstable as to seem to need this position, consideration should be given to external fixation (*see* Chapter 22) or combined internal and external fixation (*see* Chapter 21).

Pronation is an important part of the manoeuvre to reduce a Colles's fracture and it seems logical, in younger patients at any rate, to maintain this by using an above-elbow plaster in that position, but in practice this has been shown to confer no advantage (Pool 1973). Van der Linden and Ericson (1981) found that the position of the wrist did not make much difference either: what affected the outcome was the amount of original displacement and the success of reduction. In contrast, Smith's fractures are reduced by supination (*see* Chapter 19), but it is unwise to keep an elderly patient's arm in supination for more than three weeks or it may never regain a good range of pronation.

Fractures into joints

Prevention of joint stiffness

Here, perhaps, is the greatest opportunity for the surgeon to improve upon the natural history of the untreated injury. Detailed accounts are given in Chapter 7 of the management of articular fractures in the phalanges, in Chapter 9 of fractures of the metacarpal heads, and in Chapter 11 of fractures and dislocations involving carpometacarpal joints (though only that of the thumb has a large range of movement).

The most common articular fractures of the hand are those in which a *small fragment of bone is avulsed* by ligament, capsule or tendon. Opinions differ as to whether these should, in general, be immobilized or not; probably it does not make much difference, though avulsion of the insertion of the ulnar collateral ligament of the MCP joint of the thumb (Stener & Stener 1969) requires open reduction for the same reason as the more common ligamentous injury (Stener 1962). Occasionally this ligament avulses two fragments of bone, one of which is much displaced while the other is not (Fig. 24.1): operation is indicated because the displaced fragment usually carries most of the ligament and is displaced superficial to the adductor aponeurosis in the typical way.

If the fracture is accompanied by *subluxation* of the joint, it is essential that the subluxation be reduced and kept reduced until the fracture and periarticular structures have healed. This is most commonly seen in Bennett's fracture and at the PIP (proximal interphalangeal) joint: both are rare injuries on which a surprisingly large number of papers have been published. Their treatment is discussed in Chapters 7 and 11 of this book. The important thing is to reduce the subluxation and hold it reduced: if this is done, the fracture will look after itself.

Displaced fractures carrying a *large proportion of articular surface* provide, in general, one of the strongest indications for fixation. Methods of fixation of fractures of the lower end of the radius have been described in Chapters 19, 21 and 22. In the fingers such fractures, which are not common, are most often seen in the head of the proximal phalanx (*see* Chapter 7). At this site the result of conservative treatment is almost always poor, with

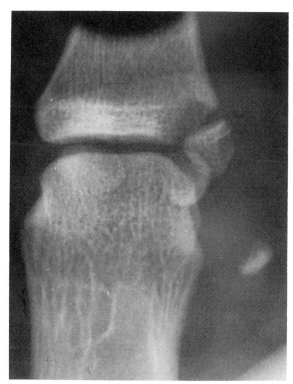

Fig. 24.1 In fractures of the ulnar corner of the base of the proximal phalanx of the thumb, there are occasionally two bony fragments, one displaced and one not. The ulnar collateral ligament may be attached to the displaced one, which is displaced superficial to the adductor expansion as described by Stener

a finger that is painful, stiff and crooked, whereas McCue et al (1970) have shown that excellent results can be obtained by open reduction and internal fixation; Barton (1984a) has described a technique for doing this. Both fracture-subluxations and fractures with large fragments should be treated in such a way as to allow early mobilization, whether in an extension-block splint or after internal fixation. Certain methods of external fixation may also permit early movement (*see* Chapter 13).

With severe comminuted fractures involving a joint, a decision must be made at the outset as to whether there is a realistic prospect of restoring useful movement or not. If not, the joint may be arthrodesed straight away. This author considers that a single stiff PIP joint is a considerable disability and would, if at all possible, always prefer reconstruction by internal fixation or even replacement arthroplasty. At the DIP (distal interpha-

langeal) joints, in the thumb or in the wrist, arthrodesis is acceptable and may be the best solution.

Treatment of joint stiffness

The methods of mobilization of stiff joints have been admirably described by Robins in Chapter 23. If these fail, can anything further be done by the surgeon?

The obvious treatment would appear to be manipulation under anaesthetic, but in the post-traumatic stiff hand this is more likely to do harm than good.

Arthrolysis alone is seldom helpful, but, combined with division of contracted periarticular structures, can give good results in the MCP joints or PIP joints. Watson's (1979) approach to the PIP joint has proved particularly rewarding.

Where a fracture into a joint has united in a displaced position, it is possible to do operations to correct the deformity and restore a smooth joint surface (Fig. 24.2). These are difficult procedures and unlikely to be successful unless the reduced bony fragment, which may be very small, can be internally fixed well enough to allow early movement.

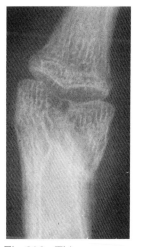
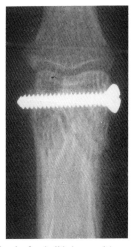

Fig. 24.2 This young man sustained a football injury to his index finger which caused an oblique fracture of one condyle of the head of the proximal phalanx, which was not properly treated and was allowed to unite with proximal displacement of the fragment causing pain, deformity and limitation of flexion to a range between 15 and 65°. After osteotomy, realignment of the joint surface and screw fixation the lateral deformity was corrected and the range increased to from 0 to 80°

A much simpler procedure will allow a gratifying increase in movement in those cases where a long oblique or spiral fracture, whose distal end reaches into the side of the head of the phalanx, has united in a shortened position. Although the articular surface on the end of the bone (that which looks transverse on a PA X-ray film) has not been breached, the whole distal fragment has settled back so that the long spike of bone forming the distal end of the proximal fragment is obstructing flexion, either by directly blocking the base of the middle phalanx or by obstructing the normal forward movement of the collateral ligament in flexion (Fig. 24.3). Provided the alignment of the finger as a whole remains satisfactory, all one need

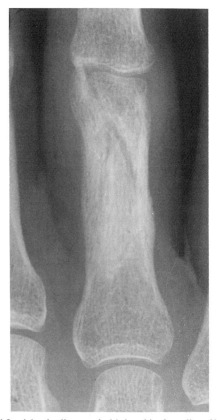

Fig. 24.3 A bookseller caught his hand in the collar of his horse and sustained a spiral fracture of the distal part of the proximal phalanx. The distal fragment displaced proximally, was not reduced and the fracture united in this position, with a spike of bone (consisting of the distal end of the proximal fragment) limiting flexion of the PIP joint to 60°. Later, the spike was removed and within a week he could flex the joint to 90°

do is to *trim off the bony spike* until full movements are possible (*see also* Fig. 9.6).

Adherence of tendons

Prevention

An important advantage of early mobilization of stable fractures, or fractures which have been made stable by internal fixation, is that the tendons are prevented from sticking down.

In the finger, Lamphier (1957) has pointed out that the front of the proximal phalanx is the floor of the tunnel for the flexor tendon. During a review of 148 fractures of the shafts of the phalanges, Barton (1979) analysed 53 displaced fractures of the mid-shaft and found that, of those which were reduced, 15 had excellent or good results with 22 fair or poor but, of those which were not reduced, none were excellent, only 3 good, and 11 fair or poor. It is clear that reduction is much more likely to be followed by a good result; moreover if the result is not good, due to tendon adherence (but joint movement has been maintained) it can be made good by tenolysis.

Stiffness of the wrist after fractures of the distal radius which did not enter the joint may be due in part to adherence of the tendons at the fracture site, and Dias et al (1987) found that patients with Colles's fractures treated by early mobilization (undisplaced fractures in a crepe bandage and displaced fractures in a plaster restricting extension but allowing free flexion of the wrist and fingers) regained movements of the wrist and fingers more quickly than those treated in a conventional cast, without suffering more pain or developing more deformity.

Treatment

Tenolysis is an accepted procedure after tendon injuries, but it is not as well-known as it should be that it is equally useful, indeed more useful, after fractures, especially in the phalanges where the tendons are very closely applied to the bone and the normal excursion is considerable (McGrouther & Ahmed 1981). Figures 24.4a and b show a fracture which resulted in a finger with a good range of passive movement but very limited active range. Figure 24.4c shows how the active flexion

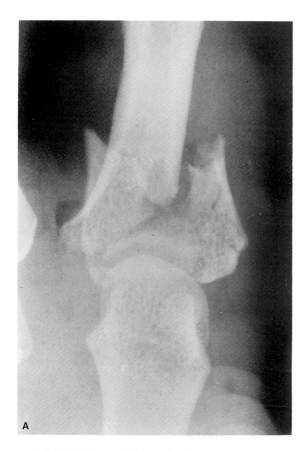

A

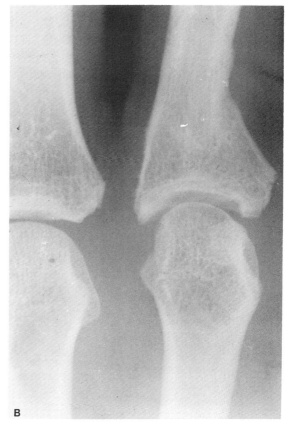

B

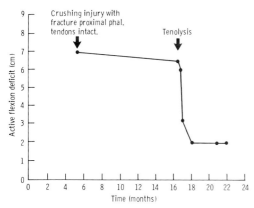

P. McN. Aged 21 years. LEFT INDEX FINGER

Graph: Active flexion deficit (cm) vs Time (months). Annotations: "Crushing injury with fracture proximal phal. tendons intact." and "Tenolysis".

Fig. 24.4 Comminuted fracture of the base of a proximal phalanx, treated by early mobilization (A). After union. Almost full passive movement of the joint but active flexion very restricted, due to adherence of the flexor tendon (B). After flexor tenolysis, he could flex the tip of the finger to within 2 cm of the proximal palmar crease (C)

deficit (the distance by which the fingertip fell short of the distal palmar crease) was improved by tenolysis, and this benefit was lasting. Coonrad and Pohlman (1969) have shown the value of tenolysis of the extensor tendons after fractures of the base of the proximal phalanx; this procedure may be combined with corrective osteotomy.

Occasionally comminuted fractures of the distal end of the radius are complicated by adherence of the long tendons of the fingers: this is seen most often after unsatisfactory internal fixation, usually for Smith's fractures. The finger joints will rapidly stiffen, but if they can be mobilized by physiotherapy and the patient is well motivated, then tenolysis can be very worthwhile, converting a disgruntled patient into a satisfied one. (I should stress the word *unsatisfactory* in relation to internal fixation: good internal fixation of a Smith's or Barton's fracture allows early movement and this helps to prevent adherence of tendons.)

NON-UNION

This complication is common in the scaphoid, rare in the hand, and almost unknown after fractures through the cancellous bone of the distal radius.

Carpal bones

Fractures of the hook of the hamate are notoriously prone to non-union; in fact the fracture is seldom diagnosed until non-union is established. The capitate is also subject to non-union. Both these are mentioned in Chapter 18.

However the bone in the upper limb where non-union is a real problem is the *scaphoid*, and this demands special consideration.

Non-union of the scaphoid

Prevention. Since most of the effort put into diagnosing and treating scaphoid fractures is directed to preventing non-union, there is little to add to the accounts given in Chapters 16 and 17 of the management of recent scaphoid fractures by conservative and operative means.

There are, however, important points to be made about the incidence and diagnosis of non-union, and, especially, treatment. Attitudes are changing with the realization that established methods are not entirely satisfactory, and the exploration of many new techniques. Although some of these have been mentioned in Chapter 17, a review of the different methods of management of non-union seems appropriate.

Incidence. One of the few things we know for certain about scaphoid fractures is that there are many people walking around sublimely unaware that they have an ununited scaphoid fracture, or even that they have ever fractured their scaphoid, until some new injury happens to bring it to light. We therefore simply do not know how common scaphoid fractures are, or what is the true incidence

of non-union. If an injury so minor as to be ignored or forgotten by the patient can cause a scaphoid fracture which fails to unite, it seems likely that similar injuries cause scaphoid fractures which do unite. However, untreated scaphoid fractures are more likely to proceed to non-union than treated ones: out of 46 patients operated on and reviewed by the author for non-union of the scaphoid, only nine had been adequately treated for the original injury, usually because the patient never attended hospital or failed to co-operate in treatment. Once the fracture has been diagnosed and treated, it should be easy to establish the rate of non-union, but the observant reader will have detected a difference of opinion between the authors of Chapters 16 and 17 about this.

Diagnosis. The truth is, and this has not received nearly enough attention in the past, that it is very difficult to tell when or whether a scaphoid fracture has united. Obviously such a short bone cannot be stressed manually like a tibia, so the only way of telling clinically whether the fracture has united is by tenderness. However, tenderness is, at the best of times, a subjective matter and in this case it is elicited by pressure in the anatomical snuffbox which is always tender if one presses hard enough, because one is pressing on the terminal sensory branches of the radial nerve.

The answer should lie in radiological examination, but how does one decide that the films indicate union? This is not as easy as most people imagine (Fig. 24.5). Russe (1960) has pointed out that, when assessing radiographs of recent fractures of the scaphoid,

'in the absence of clearly visible osseous trabeculations bridging the former defect, one should look for increased density of the bone at the site of the former fracture cleft or on each side of the cleft. It is not generally known that these calcified bands in the fracture site or on both sides of the fracture site are signs of bone union in fresh fractures of the navicular. Such calcifications occur in about 40% of fresh fractures. (In old fractures, of course, these bands cannot be considered as signs of bone union).'

This is still not generally known, and in many centres such sclerotic lines would be interpreted as signs of developing non-union; these are, of course, the sort of cases in which an operation for 'non-union' will do well!

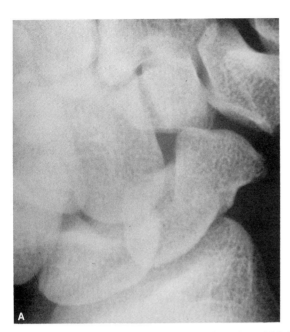
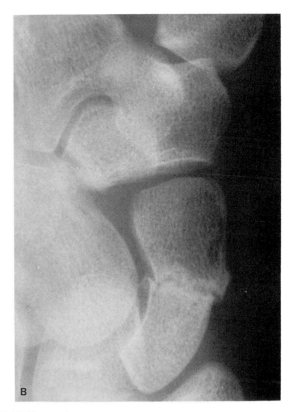

Fig. 24.5   Union and non-union of the scaphoid: but which is which? (See text)

A great deal depends on the exact angle of the fracture and whether this coincides with the exact angle of the X-ray beam. Scaphoid views are conventionally taken in PA, semi-pronated, semi-supinated, and lateral positions, these being achieved by rotating the forearm while the beam remains perpendicular. However the long axis of the scaphoid does not lie in the long axis of the arm, but flexed some 45° to it; the degree of flexion obviously changes with flexion or extension of the wrist but also alters with radial and ulnar deviation. To get the scaphoid as fully extended as possible (i.e. approaching the long axis of the arm) the pictures are taken with the wrist in ulnar deviation, but even then the scaphoid remains flexed to some extent. It follows that a fracture transverse to the long axis of the scaphoid on a lateral view will not be in the same plane as a perpendicular beam of X-rays (Lindgren 1949). To show such a fracture properly, it is necessary either to dorsiflex the wrist (most easily done by having the patient make a fist) or to tilt the X-ray machine so that as the beam passes posteriorly, it also passes some 25° or 30° distally (Fig. 24.6). A radiological view which combines this tilt with ulnar deviation of the wrist and pronation of the forearm has been described by Ziter (1973).

Now look up to Figure 24.5A which shows the radiograph of a patient discharged from the fracture clinic as having union of his scaphoid fracture. When he returned, complaining that his wrist still hurt, further films were taken with a tilted beam and these showed clearly (Fig. 24.7) that the fracture had failed to unite.

Conversely, most surgeons who have operated on many ununited scaphoid fractures have had the embarrassing experience of exposing the scaphoid and being unable to find any fracture, as I did in the patient whose radiograph forms Figure 24.5B: presumably it had united anteriorly (which is the surface one sees at operation) but it was still ununited posteriorly (accounting for the X-ray appearance).

Thus there are many pitfalls in the radiological

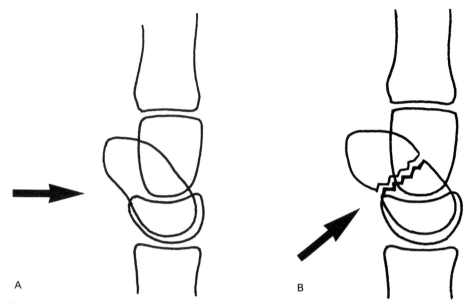

A   B

Fig. 24.6 Standard radiological views of the scaphoid, though they may be PA, lateral, or oblique, all are taken with the beam perpendicular to the long axis of the arm (A). Since the scaphoid is at an angle to the long axis of the arm, a transverse fracture of that bone will be better shown if the X-ray beam is tilted (B)

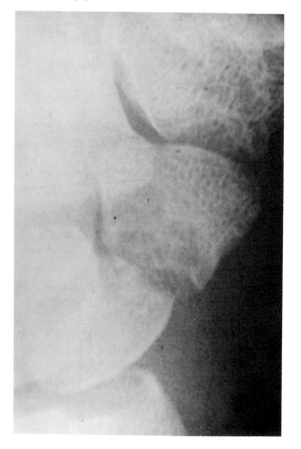

diagnosis of union of fractures of this bone, and one should beware of dogmatic statements about the incidence of non-union, and even more of statements about how many weeks the fracture takes to unite. Nevertheless it seems to this author that Leslie and Dickson's (1981) figure of 5% non-union of treated fractures is probably nearer the mark than the 50% suggested by Herbert and Fisher (1984).

At present we over-treat many fractures and sprains in order to avoid under-treating those few fractures likely to proceed to non-union. If we could pick out those with a bad prognosis, our treatment would be more rational. Unfortunately we cannot do this with much accuracy, but we can say that non-union is more likely in untreated fractures, in those due to violent forces such as motorcycle accidents, and in certain patterns of fracture (Fig. 24.8). Non-union is very rare in women, but this may just reflect the fact that scaphoid fractures are themselves uncommon in women; in addition they seldom ride motorbikes and may be more responsible about keeping a plaster cast on until the fracture has united.

Fig. 24.7 A tilted view of the same scaphoid as in Figure 24.5A, showing that in fact there is non-union

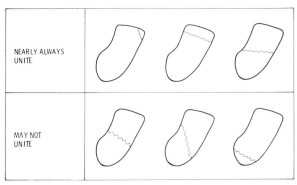

Fig. 24.8 Probability of union in different types of scaphoid fracture (but, as explained in the text, other factors are often more important than the shape of the fracture)

Management of the un-united scaphoid

Broadly speaking, there are three methods of management. One can treat it symptomatically by conservative means, one can try to make it unite, or one can accept that it is not going to unite and carry out some form of salvage operation.

Conservative measures. Patients who only get occasional mild ache may choose to grin and bear it. The argument for operating to obtain union is that degenerative changes will be prevented, and this has particular force in younger patients. The argument may be correct, but it lacks supporting evidence. Since this is such an important issue in deciding whether a patient with non-union but little or no pain should have an operation, it is worth studying what few facts are available.

London (1961) studied 60 patients with established non-union and his findings as to osteoarthritis are shown in Table 24.1. He concluded that 'In general the older the fracture, the greater the likelihood of osteoarthritis, but even after thirty years there may be none, and some badly degener-

Table 24.1 Incidence of osteoarthritis in patients with symptomatic non-union of the scaphoid, according to London (1961)

Age of fracture	Number of wrists	Osteoarthritis (number of wrists)
Less than 5 years	19 } 24	12
6–10 years	5	
11–20 years	3 } 11	7
Over 20 years	8	
Unknown	25	17

ative wrists are so free from symptoms as to be regarded as almost normal' clinically.

There are two papers entitled: 'The natural history of scaphoid non-union': both are interesting, but their title misleading since the patients were all complaining of pain in the wrist. Mack et al (1984), from the US navy, studied 47 sailors with non-union of from 5 to 53 years' duration. They concluded that, after 'between five and ten years, almost all non-unions showed cyst formation and resorptive changes within the scaphoid. Degenerative arthritis of the radioscaphoid joint was most common after ten years. Generalized arthritis of the wrist occurred frequently after twenty years' ... 35 patients had only mild or moderate symptoms and, 'in these patients, no correlation was seen between the symptoms and the roentgenographic findings or the duration of the non-union'.

Ruby et al (1985) analysed 55 patients all complaining of pain in the wrist. Of these 40% had been free of symptoms until a second injury, while 60% had apparently suffered pain ever since the fracture. In these patients, the incidence of degenerative changes on radiograph was found to be as shown in Table 24.2.

Lindstrom (1975) made a most interesting and important study of patients treated in Gothenburg and followed-up for at least seven years, the average period being ten years. Of 220 patients whose fractures united, 21 (9%) showed radiological evidence of osteoarthritic changes around the scaphoid, the changes being fairly mild in most cases. In contrast, of 57 patients with non-union, no less than 53 (93%) had radiological osteoarthritis and over half of these were advanced changes. His findings are summarized in Tables 24.3 and 24.4. Moreover, Lindstrom found that symptoms of pain and stiffness corresponded with radiological osteoarthritis. What is now needed is a similar study of patients who did have non-union but who

Table 24.2 Incidence of osteoarthritis in patients with symptomatic non-union of the scaphoid, according to Ruby et al (1985)

Years after fracture	Patients	O.A.
1–4	24	1
5–9	13	12
10+	19	19

Table 24.3 Incidence of OA in patients with healed scaphoid fractures from 7 to 13 years (av. 10.2 years)

Severity of OA changes	No. of patients	%
None	220	91.3
Osteophytes	12	5.0
Sclerosis	7	2.9
Reduced cartilage space	2	0.8
	241	100

After Lindstrom (1975)

Table 24.4 Incidence of OA in patients with non-union of scaphoid for 10–24 years (av. 11 years)

Severity of OA changes	No. of patients	%
None	4	7.0
Osteophytes	15	26.4
Sclerosis	8	14.0
Reduced cartilage space	30	52.6
	57	100

After Lindstrom (1975)

were successfully treated by a bone-grafting operation, and Lindstrom is currently making that study.

Unfortunately we do not know, and presumably never will, how many patients have ununited scaphoid fractures which cause no symptoms and have not been stirred up by some later injury. As Mack et al (1984) say, a prospective longitudinal study of individual patients would be required to determine this. 'It is possible, for example, that an undisplaced non-union in a sedentary patient is less likely to displace, slower to undergo degenerative change, and less likely to cause symptoms than our data suggest', though they doubt this. Moreover, we do not yet know the incidence or severity of degenerative changes in patients who have been treated successfully by bone grafting: we *hope* that the joints last longer but cannot be sure that this is the case, particularly with grafts of a type which may protrude into the joints around the scaphoid or methods of fixation (such as the Herbert screw) which involve damage to a previously normal joint in a young man. Non-union has also been reported as leading to rupture of flexor tendons (Mahring et al 1985). Nevertheless, the benefit of bone grafting in preventing the development of symptoms is unproved, though there is no doubt that a successful graft is effective in relieving symptoms which are already present. The other fact which may cause hesitation in recom-

mending surgical treatment in a patient with few symptoms is that the operation is by no means always successful and may have significant disadvantages, as will be discussed in the next section. The approach suggested by Mack et al (1984) seems wise: 'based on the high probability that degenerative changes will occur, we recommend that a scaphoid non-union that demonstrates displacement and instability be reduced and grafted before degenerative changes occur. An asymptomatic patient with an undisplaced non-union and no evidence of instability of the wrist should be advised of the possibility of late degenerative changes'.

The other factor in this equation is the likelihood of success. It is known that failure of bone-grafting is more likely in small proximal pole fragments (Russe 1960), with avascular necrosis (Green 1985, though he stresses that this can only be determined at operation) and in patients with psychiatric disorders (Kim et al 1983). The latter may range from total irresponsibility in care of the plaster cast to unrecognized paranoid schizophrenia: the surgeon who, one would think, should get to know his patient reasonably well is often unaware of the psychiatric abnormality.

Operations to achieve union. Internal fixation alone, regarded by some as the panacea for all traumatic ills, is one of the methods least likely to result in bony union, though it often relieves the symptoms by holding the two fragments together (Maudsley & Chen 1972) and, surprisingly, this relief may continue for many years even though union has not taken place (McLaughlin & Parkes 1969). Dehne, Deffer and Feighney (1964) simply transfixed the non-union with a Kirschner wire, after which they reported union in 19 of 23 patients (83%). Cosio and Camp (1986) using a similar method, but with several wires and followed by a thumb spica cast, claimed union in 10 out of 13 patients (77%), though they excluded patients with radiological pseudarthrosis indicated by densely sclerotic margins. They consider that this type of patient really has delayed union and that it will unite if immobilized; this is reminiscent of the teaching of Sir Reginald Watson-Jones (1943) who, in his famous textbook of fractures, wrote 'The wrist must be immobilized until the fracture is united whether this takes eight or ten weeks as in the average case, or any period up to eight or ten months as it may do in some cases'.

A quite different kind of operation is to insert electrodes as a means of applying electrical stimulation by direct current for a period of three months. This is combined with a plaster cast. Bora et al (1984) reported success by this means in 12 out of 17 cases, which is 71%, and Taylor et al (1985) in 6 out of 11: the latter group suggested that the method might have a role in the treatment of a very small proximal pole fragment, or as a salvage procedure after a failed bone graft.

The apparatus is expensive and most of it can only be used for one patient. The pins, which can be introduced percutaneously, cross the fracture site so they provide some immobilization, and the patient is also treated in a plaster cast. It could be said that the electricity makes no difference and the method is really the same as that described in the previous paragraph, but it does seem capable of achieving union in established pseudarthrosis.

An alternative method of electrical stimulation, not requiring the insertion of pins and therefore not open to the above criticism, is by the use of external electrodes producing a pulsed electromagnetic field. This avoids an operation altogether, though a plaster cast is used. The placing of the electrodes and the nature of the electrical impulses are very critical. Frykman et al (1986), using this method, reported union in 35 out of 44 patients (80%). It is interesting that the union rate was higher when an above-elbow plaster was used than a below-elbow plaster.

My experience of both methods has been small and unsuccessful; I feel it is too soon to say whether these methods will replace bone grafting, which must be regarded as the most effective proved way to achieve union. They should be considered in cases of failed grafting.

The first type of bone graft for ununited scaphoid fractures appears to have been that of Murray of Toronto who, about 1930, began using a peg-graft of cortical bone passed through a drill hole in the long axis of the bone, i.e. like a screw. He described his early results in 1935 and in 1946 reported 100 cases with bony union in 96, and 'excellent functional results'. He did not say how union was determined. This method has since fallen into disuse, as most surgeons found that their success

rate was more like 50% (Agner & Anderson 1970, Cooney et al 1980).

In 1936, Matti described, in a German journal, a dorsal inlay graft: the scaphoid was exposed from the back, a trough curetted in both fragments, and a cancellous iliac graft inserted. In 1960 Russe from Vienna reported 22 patients treated in 1956/7/8, also by cancellous iliac inlay graft, but put into the scaphoid from the front. (He did not mention Matti's method.) It was claimed that the anterior approach was less likely to damage the blood supply, and this has been supported by more recent anatomical studies (Gelberman & Menon 1980), but the relationship, if any, between avascular necrosis and non-union is far from clear. However, many workers consider that there is often a flexion deformity in the scaphoid, and this could be easier to correct by an anterior than a posterior graft. The essential features of the Russe technique, as described in that paper and as practised by most surgeons since then, are that 'the sclerotic bone ends are freshened with a small gouge, and a cavity formed, extending well into the adjacent fragments'. An oblong piece of cancellous bone taken from the iliac crest is then 'placed in the centre of the preformed cavity, and multiple small chips are firmly packed around it, completely obliterating the cavity. The process resembles that of a dentist filling a cavity in a tooth'. Since the publication of Russe's paper, many other series of his operation have been published and these are listed as Table 24.5. Symptomatic non-union of the scaphoid is actually an uncommon condition, and eleven of these series have less than 30 patients: it is remarkable that Mulder (1968) was able to report 100 cases, though he probably had patients referred from all over the Netherlands. Some may really have been cases of delayed union. He says that the operation was done as described by Russe, 'except that the cavity is filled with one snugly fitting piece of cancellous bone'. However, Mulder also says that he used the Matti-Russe method, and since the first cases in this series were done in 1955, whereas Russe did his first cases in 1956 and did not report the operation until 1960, it may be that Mulder's series includes both Matti and Russe procedures.

The reported rate of success in these series ranges from 40 to 100%, but in few of them are we

Table 24.5 Published series of results after conventional Russe grafting for non-union of the scaphoid

Russe grafting published series			Operations	Union	Union (%)
1960	RUSSE	Vienna, Austria	22	20	90
1968	DOOLEY	Melbourne, Australia	23	20	87
1968	VERDAN	Lausanne, Switzerland	45	44	98
1968	MULDER	Leiden, Netherlands	100	97	97
1969	UNGER	San Diego, USA	42	33	78
1969	CAMERON	Christchurch, New Zealand	11	9	82
1975	McDONALD	Toronto, Canada	20	17	85
1975	EDDELAND	Malmö, Sweden	23	20	87
1976	HULL	Minnesota, USA	22	16	73
1976	SEW HOY	Auckland, New Zealand	10	4	40
1977	HERNESS	New York, USA	40	40	100
1978	GLASS	New York, USA	23	22	96
1980	COONEY	Mayo Clinic, USA	44	38	86
1982	SCHNEIDER	Philadelphia, USA	10	9	90
1984	BOECKSTYNS	Hellerup, Denmark	28	24	85
1984	BARTON	Nottingham, England	23	15	65
1985	RASMUSSEN	Milwaukee, USA	28	20	71

told how bony union is defined and the value of those papers is therefore questionable.

In my own series, many of the earlier patients had been discharged from the clinic as 'successes', and it was only when they were brought back and radiographed again some years later that it was discovered that bony union had not in fact been achieved. I strongly suspect that this would also be true in many of the published series, and the very fact that few even mention the difficulty in deciding when and whether union has occurred suggests that they have not studied this aspect very carefully. I have learned that if there is one thing more difficult than deciding when a scaphoid fracture has united, it is deciding when a grafted scaphoid fracture has united: the graft bridges the fracture site, so one has to look for union between the two ends of the graft and their surrounding bone, and also peripheral union at the fracture site which takes a very long time indeed. A minimum follow-up of 6 months, with radiographs at the end of that time, is needed to make even a moderately assured statement about union; a year is preferable.

One honourable exception is the series reported by Cooney, Dobyns and Linscheid (1980) from the Mayo Clinic. The vast area of referral to that institution has enabled them to accumulate a large number of patients, and to compare the results of different methods. All patients were reviewed clinically and radiologically at 1–13 years (average 5 years). The five designated as 'uncertain' lend

credence to the results. However, it is possibly a mistake to put too much stress on the radiological results: the purpose is to relieve the symptoms and Rasmussen (1985) found 'no significant difference between united grafts and persistent non-unions when comparing postoperative pain level, grip strength or range of motion, except radial deviation'. I would not go as far as that, but would agree that radiological failures may be clinical successes, at least in the short term. However, Russe later changed his operation, presumably because he was dissatisfied with the results, though this was never published in English and surgeons throughout the world (including the present writer) continued doing the Mark 1 Russe procedure in the belief that they were doing what Russe had recommended. Green (1985) established that Russe's later operation, though still an anterior inlay graft, used two small corticocancellous struts, with the cortex outwards for maximum strength. With this Mark 2 Russe procedure, Green achieved a 75% union rate (34 of 45 cases), most of the failures being due to avascularity of the proximal pole, though he stresses that this could not be determined from the preoperative radiographs: increased density did not necessarily mean that the fragment was avascular, or normal density that it was vascular. He found that the best method of determining actual vascularity was by direct inspection of the bone during the operation for punctate bleeding points. Andrews, also in 1985, reported 14 cases treated by what seems to be a similar procedure, with union in 11 (70%).

Böhler and Ender (1986) use a graft similar to the Mark 1 Russe but then put a compression plate into the front of the scaphoid, with a hook which goes round the end of the proximal pole. They claim a success rate of 99% with this method, but of course the plate has to be removed later.

A third type of bone graft involves excision of the non-union and insertion of a wedge-shaped piece of bone (Fig. 24.9) taken from the iliac crest or the radial styloid, right across the defect. The wedge shape enables any flexion deformity within the scaphoid bone to be corrected and thus, in theory, a normal scapholunate angle to be restored. Fisk (1984) reported 41 operations of this type, after which the wrist was immobilized for 2–4 months. The clinical results were excellent in 17 and good in 13 (union but some restriction of movement): 11 failed to achieve bony union, but 7 of those had their symptoms largely relieved.

Herbert uses a similar graft, plus his screw to hold it in place and provide compression, and describes his indications and methods in Chapter 17 of this book.

The use of a wedge graft makes it even more difficult to obtain radiographs in which the beam passes through the correct plane: tilted views are necessary, and maybe two differently tilted views (*see* Fig. 24.8).

Thus there is no entirely satisfactory operation for non-union. In writing this chapter, I have been

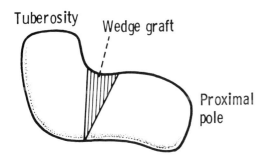

Fig. 24.9 Wedge graft to the scaphoid, to correct flexion deformity within the bone from old fracture

struck by how many series, using different methods, report success in 70 to 80% of patients, a success-rate not all that different from that achieved by placebos in trials of drug treatment. Even in the best recent series, one in ten patients fails to achieve bony union, and the operations have significant disadvantages. Conventional grafting without internal fixation requires 4 months in plaster (which is a second sentence, if the original injury was treated in plaster) which may prevent the patient from working, and is likely to result in some loss of movement. These disadvantages are eliminated if the graft is held with a Herbert screw, but this must be introduced through the scaphotrapezial joint and, although the end of the screw can be buried beneath the articular surface, the dissection and retraction necessary to obtain access cause some damage to the joint surface. One cannot feel happy to be violating a normal joint in a young patient, but only time will show if this creates any problems.

The conclusion from all this would appear to be that, since our methods of treating non-union are neither certain nor harmless, we must redouble our efforts to *prevent* non-union by early diagnosis and treatment of scaphoid fractures. As we have seen (p. 321), the type of immobilization probably makes little difference and the greatest scope for improvement lies in continued education of general practitioners and casualty officers on this subject. The responsibility for this falls upon the surgeons who have to treat the non-unions: nobody else is going to do it.

Palliative operations. Some of these, including excision of the radial styloid, have been considered in Chapter 17. An intriguing alternative is Bentzon's operation, based on the view that there is no harm in having nine carpal bones instead of eight, so long as the wrist does not hurt. To achieve this, a flap of soft-tissue is placed and anchored between the two fragments of the scaphoid to stop them rubbing together. Boeckstyns and Busch (1984) who compared the results of Bentzon's operation with those of Russe grafting, found that in terms of relief of symptoms, Bentzon's operation was just as good, in two groups of patients. However, as it often (though not always) leaves an unstable carpus, they therefore prefer bone grafting in the first instance; if grafting should fail, Bentzon's operation appears to be a good way out. Boeckstyns et al (1985) have also made a long-term review of 26 of Bentzon's patients studied 22–30 years after operation, confirming that very satisfactory relief of symptoms is obtained; as far as I know, we do not possess such long-term results for any other type of operation for non-union, and this provides a yardstick against which the newer methods will ultimately need to be judged. Among these is arthroplasty by replacement of the scaphoid with a silastic prosthesis (Swanson 1970b), but Kleinert et al (1985) found that this gave unsatisfactory results and failed to prevent post-traumatic arthrosis of the periscaphoid joints. Excision of the scaphoid is no longer favoured but Dwyer (1949) reported good results in 12 out of 19 patients, these 12 being able to carry out fairly strenuous work. The results were less good if, before the operation, there was established osteoarthritis or if there was what we now call dorsal intercalated segment instability.

Once more widespread degenerative changes are present, the operation must also involve more of the wrist. Neviaser (1983) favoured proximal row carpectomy. Total replacement of the wrist does not seem justifiable in young vigorous men whose other wrist is normal and likely to remain that way, so most surgeons have favoured either partial (Watson et al 1981) or complete arthrodesis of the wrist.

The hand

Non-union is a rare problem in the hand. Robins (page 311) states that it occurs most often in the proximal phalanx of the thumb (Fig. 24.10), but in my admittedly limited experience, it has been encountered more often in the middle phalanges of the fingers (Fig. 24.11). Of the eight cases I have treated, seven followed attempts at internal fixation which had succeeded only in holding the fragments apart and perhaps interfering with their blood supply. If Kirschner wires have been left sticking out of the skin, or have been passed across a joint, there is a natural and correct desire to remove the wire as soon as possible. However in the distal part of the middle phalanx, union may take as long as three months (Moberg, 1950) so premature removal of internal fixation may well lead to non-union (*see* Fig. 8.5); in such a situation, the fixation

should be of a type which can be left in place without harm.

Jupiter et al (1985) collected 25 cases of non-union in the hand, many doubtless referred from elsewhere, and their experience was different again: 16 were in the phalanges (four distal, one middle, and eleven proximal—only one of the latter being of the thumb); nine were in the metacarpals; 13 of the fractures were open ones; and 17 had been treated by internal fixation with Kirschner wires. In six of these, the wires were distracting the fracture and, in five, one or more of the wires did not enter both fracture fragments. This emphasizes that internal fixation in the hand is difficult, and that bad treatment produces bad results.

Internal fixation should not be condemned because of this, but it should be reserved for those fractures which really need it and it should be carried out by an expert. Obviously non-union is more likely after fractures of the severe type described in Chapters 13 and 14, and early bone grafting is often indicated in such injuries, particularly where there is loss of bone. Pathological fractures usually unite satisfactorily: it is the pathological condition preceding the fracture which may need treatment, as Chapter 12 explains.

Treatment of metacarpal non-union by plating and grafting can be expected to produce a good result. In the shafts of the phalanges, no treatment is entirely satisfactory. Bone grafting alone leads to union but a stiff finger. The same may be said of internal fixation because it is seldom possible to make this rigid, so a period of immobilization is often necessary. Non-union of fractures near the ends of bones can be treated by bone excision, arthrodesis, or arthroplasty.

MALUNION

As I said at the beginning of this chapter, the natural history of most fractures is to unite, but with deformity, and this deformity not only looks bad but often interferes with function. Whereas in the part of the body with which we are concerned, non-union is largely a carpal problem and even there is a comparatively rare event, malunion is a very common consequence of fractures in the hand

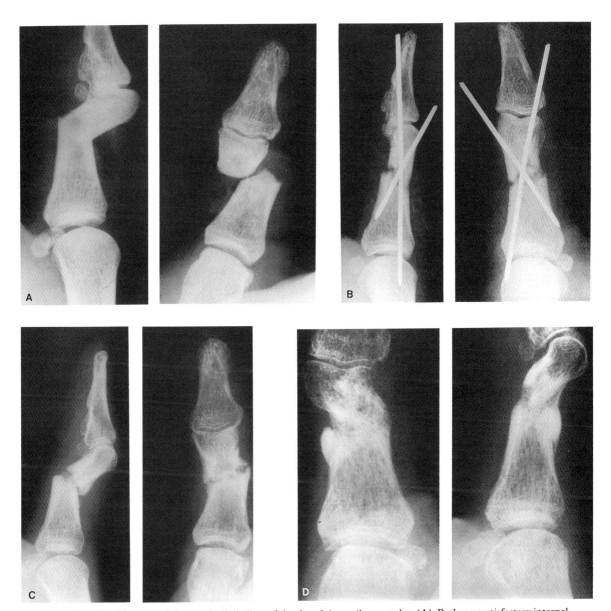

Fig. 24.10 Displaced fracture of the proximal phalanx of the thumb in a railway worker (A). Rather unsatisfactory internal fixation was carried out (B). Four months later, non-union and deformity (C). After bone grafting and further stabilization with wires, the deformity is decreased, the bone has united, and the patient is back at work which involves heavy lifting (D)

and of the distal end of the radius. The first purpose of treatment being to prevent malunion, any description of treatment—even in an undergraduate textbook—is essentially about how to obtain reduction and then retain it. Readers of this book do not need to be reminded of these basic methods, and the book itself describes the more complex techniques which may be necessary, but a few special points can be stressed.

The hand

Prevention of malunion

The most common error is failure to appreciate the extent of the deformity at the fracture site.

In the *metacarpals*, where the fracture nearly always flexes, considerable angulation may be compatible with good function, especially in fractures in the distal part of the metacarpal and of

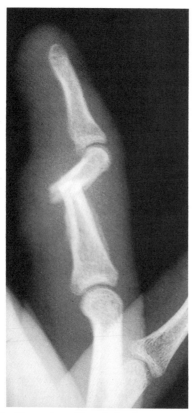

Fig. 24.11 Non-union of the middle phalanx following unsuccessful internal fixation

the fifth metacarpal, whose carpometacarpal joint allows some $30°$ of movement which can compensate for some flexion deformity. Lateral deformity of the metacarpals is uncommon because they are to some extent splinted by neighbouring metacarpals, but rotational deformity can easily occur and be overlooked. It is, of course, essential to examine the fingers end-on and check the plane of the fingernail in relation to those of the other fingers, and by comparison with the other hand.

In the *phalanges*, angulation is almost always in the opposite direction i.e. into extension. Older texts explain this, and the contrast with the flexion deformity of metacarpal fractures, in terms of muscle pull. It seems more likely that the difference is in the nature of the injury; metacarpal fractures usually result from a blow on the clenched fist or the back of the hand, whereas phalangeal fractures are generally caused by a fall on the outstretched hand or an object falling onto the finger. This angulation is readily visible both clinically and

radiologically where it occurs at the mid-shaft of the phalanx, and visible radiologically but not clinically at the neck of the phalanx, but it is more difficult to detect by either method when the fracture is at the base of the proximal phalanx (Coonrad & Pohlman 1969) because clinically it looks as though the MCP joint is extended and radiologically the phalanx is superimposed on the other phalanges on the lateral film. However, once the deformity has been detected, it is easily corrected by manipulation and the finger can then be splinted with the MCP joint flexed, which is the safe position for immobilization anyway.

Rotational deformity is again easy to miss. Radiographs such as that in Figure 24.12 should shriek out 'I am malrotated! Correct me!' but, as in this patient, the message is often not heard. Even without radiographs, the deformity should be

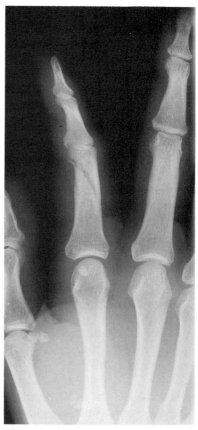

Fig. 24.12 Fracture of proximal phalanx of index finger with rotational deformity visible on X-ray examination. Often it can only be detected by clinical examination

observed by just looking at the finger, provided the end-on view of the finger has not been obscured by a splint or dressings. In stable fractures, the patient can be persuaded to flex the finger through a fair range and this often makes the torsion obvious. The deformity is easy to correct at the time of fracture, but much more difficult later.

Lateral angulation of phalangeal fractures is less common, except with epiphyseal injuries at the base of the proximal phalanx. Usually what seems at first sight like lateral angulation proves to be largely rotational deformity, though of course there may be an element of both. Even when angulation or rotation has been eliminated, there may be persistent malalignment of the phalanx, with a step at the fracture site. This may not cause visible deformity, but interferes with the gliding of the tendons which are closely applied to the front and back of the phalanx. Reduction by closed manipulation is often possible, but may be unstable and require retention by one of the methods described in Chapters 3, 4, 5 and 6, or by Ellis's traction-splintage method (Fitzgerald & Khan 1984).

Treatment of malunion

This can only be by osteotomy.

In the *metacarpals*, this can be followed by plating of the bone to achieve rigid fixation and maintenance of the bone in the corrected position, while allowing early movement to prevent the extensor tendons from sticking down.

In the *phalanges*, both correction and fixation are more difficult. An excellent account of these procedures is given by Reid (1974). Angular deformities require removal or insertion of a wedge of bone. Removal of a wedge can be done by osteotomy-osteoclasis, especially in children, but it tends to spring open again and must be well held in the corrected position, preferably by a short Kirschner wire. Insertion of a wedge is more difficult but may be indicated in certain circumstances (Coonrad & Pohlman 1969).

Correction of rotational deformity is particularly difficult to get right. An estimate should be made of the degree of rotation to be achieved, and Kirschner wires passed transversely across the bone on either side of, but not too close to, the proposed osteotomy site. These wires should not be parallel but at an angle equal to that to be corrected: after the bone has been divided the wires are then used as handles to rotate the two fragments until the wires are in the same plane. If the osteotomy is not exactly perpendicular to the long axis of the phalanx, then rotation will also introduce an angular deformity; moreover the cross section of a phalanx is more semi-circular than circular so increasing rotation decreases the area of contact between the two bone ends and fixation becomes more difficult. Before fixation is concluded, it is essential to check that the rotational position is now correct, by flexing the fingers and making sure the injured one goes down in the right position.

Several authors (Weckesser 1965, Pieran 1972, Botelheiro 1985) have suggested that the difficulty of correcting rotational deformity in the phalanx can be avoided by carrying out the correction at the metacarpal level in the same ray, where the bone is bigger, rounder, partly clothed in muscle, and rigid fixation can be achieved by plating. This sounds attractive, but in my limited experience has not worked out well: when the finger looked correct, the osteotomy did not, and vice-versa. Presumably this was because the osteotomy was not exactly transverse, but the more proximal osteotomy site must magnify the error. Gross and Gelberman (1985) studied this technique in 40 cadaveric hands and found that the deep transverse metacarpal ligament limited the rotation which can be achieved in this way to about $20°$.

DAMAGE TO OTHER TISSUES

With open fractures, important soft-tissue structures may be divided at the same time, but this is a complication of the injury or a part of the injury rather than a complication of the fracture. However in closed injuries the sharp ends of the broken bones may damage other tissues with important consequences.

Blood-vessels

In certain types of injury, the circulation can be restored by microvascular anastomosis (*see* Chapter

15) but with diffuse crushing injuries this is not applicable. In such circumstances, one can only reduce the fractures, elevate the hand high in hospital, and splint it in the correct position. Sometimes, as explained in Chapter 8, stabilization of the skeleton is the best way of protecting the soft tissues, but often surgery is best avoided except for the rare cases requiring fasciotomy to decompress a closed compartment syndrome affecting the muscles in the hand (Rowland 1982).

As with other acute closed compartment syndromes, if you wonder whether you should do a fasciotomy, then you should do it: no attempt should be made to close the skin, though a split skin graft may be taken for application later. In practice, ischaemia is most likely to be caused by tight or constricting dressings, especially on a finger after operation, when bleeding can change a soft dressing into something as hard as plaster of Paris.

Nerves

In closed fractures of the *hand*, associated injuries to the nerves are very uncommon. One example is shown in Figure 24.13 in which it became apparent later that the deep motor branch of the ulnar nerve had been injured; this could not be detected at the time of injury because the fractures made it impossible to test the function of the interossei and there was, of course, no sensory loss. Carpal fractures may also be associated with nerve injury, usually because a direct blow has injured them both rather than by a displaced fragment of bone pressing on the nerve. The best known example is disturbance of sensation in the superficial branches of the ulnar nerve accompanying a fracture of the hook of the hamate.

In closed fractures of the *distal radius*, some degree of median nerve damage is more common than is generally realized, and this is pointed out in Chapter 20. It is important to ask every patient with a lower radial fracture whether sensation in the fingers is normal and, if not, to be prepared to intervene at an early stage if simple reduction and elevation do not lead to a rapid improvement.

The *ulnar nerve* can also be compressed (Howard 1961, Joshi 1976). Stewart et al (1985) found that mild irritation of the terminal sensory branches of

the radial nerve developed quite often when a cast-brace was being used to treat a Colles's fracture.

Tendons

As with nerves, open injuries may damage tendon as well as bone, but closed injuries are more likely to result in adherence of tendons, as discussed earlier in this chapter.

Rupture of extensor pollicis longus is a well-recognized complication of Colles's fractures (Helal et al 1982), but rupture of the finger extensors (Sadr 1984) and of the flexor pollicis longus tendon and profundus to the index finger (Wong & Pho 1984) have also been reported. The latter has also resulted from attrition by an un-united scaphoid (Mahring et al 1984), simulating anterior interosseous nerve palsy.

Kirschner wires used in fixation of fractures probably quite often penetrate tendons; fortunately this seldom causes problems, but Rae and Finlayson (1984) described a case in which a Kirschner wire used to fix a Bennett's fracture–dislocation penetrated into the carpal tunnel and caused an attrition rupture of the flexor pollicis longus tendon.

OTHER COMPLICATIONS

Anything can happen, but the important complications have already been covered. Those listed below are included in an attempt at completeness, but even so do not cover every possibility.

Infection

This is rare (because of the good blood-supply of the hand) even after severely contaminated injuries, provided that basic principles are followed and adequate debridement performed. However Sloan et al (1987), in a prospective trial of 85 patients with compound fractures of the distal phalanx, all treated by conventional surgical toilet, found an infection rate of 30% where antibiotics were not used, but only 3% with antibiotics.

Infection is most likely to occur after a compound fracture, but is an occasional complication of operating on a closed fracture. It could also be a problem with a pathological fracture through an

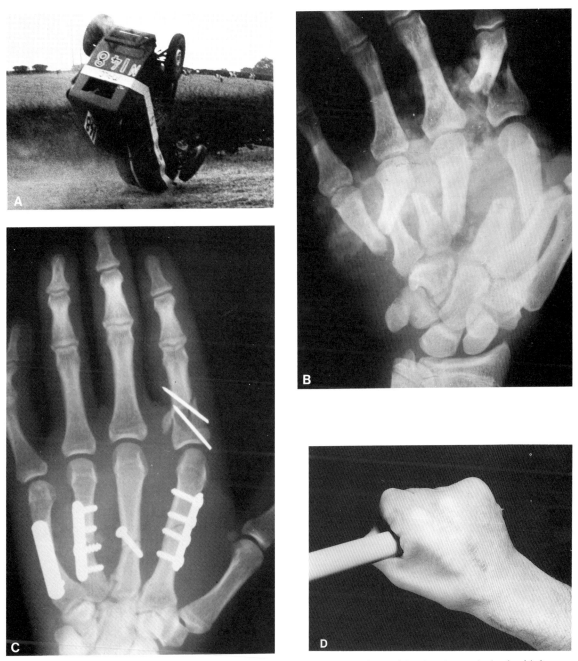

Fig. 24.13   This car crash (A) resulted in the fractures shown in B. Treatment by internal fixation; interestingly, the third metacarpal failed to unite until it was grafted and plated (C). Excellent recovery of movement, but it is now apparent that the injury caused a lesion of the deep branch of the ulnar nerve. There was no sensory disturbance and, at the time he was admitted, with the injury shown in (B), it was hardly possible to test the intrinsic muscles of the hand (D)

infected area. Antibiotics will seldom cure it once such infection is established and surgical removal of all infected tissue is necessary. Subsequent management may well involve the use of one of the external fixators described in Chapter 13.

Development of Dupuytren's disease

All hand surgeons have seen patients with Dupuytren's disease which seems to have appeared very soon after a fracture or some other injury. Chapter 20 shows that this occurs after Colles's fractures more often than has been realized in the past. Hueston (1963), noting that Dupuytren's disease also appears in limbs affected by a stroke, suggests that it is not so much the injury itself but the period of enforced inactivity afterwards which initiates the disease in individuals who have an hereditary susceptibility to Dupuytren's contracture.

Traumatic tenovaginitis

Drury (1960) claimed that tenovaginitis affecting the fifth dorsal compartment of the wrist (that containing the tendon of extensor digiti minimi)

occurs as a complication of approximately 5% of fractures and injuries in the wrist joint in adults, the most common precipitating cause being a Colles's fracture. No less an authority than Bunnell (1949) stated that tenovaginitis of the sixth compartment (through which passes the tendon of extensor carpi ulnaris) may follow a fracture of the ulnar styloid process.

Another fracture

Finsen et al (1986) have found that in patients who sustain a second fracture in the hand, it is more likely to be in the same hand, whereas patients who have a second Colles's fracture are much more likely to fracture the other wrist. The reason for this is not clear, but it seems not to be due to post-traumatic demineralization.

CONCLUSION

Complications are common after fractures of the hand and wrist, but most of them can be prevented by proper care and attention to detail.

REFERENCES

Agner O, Anderson K S 1970 Late results in non-united carpal scaphoid fractures treated with bone peg. Nordisk Medicin 12:1459 (in Danish, with English summary)

Alho A, Kankaanpää K 1975 Management of fractured scaphoid bone. A prospective study of 100 fractures. Acta Orthopaedica Scandinavica 46:737–743

Andrews J, Miller G, Haddad R 1985 Treatment of scaphoid non-union by volar inlay distal radius bone graft. Journal of Hand Surgery 10B:214–216

Barton N J 1979 Fractures of the shafts of the phalanges of the hand. The Hand 11:119–133

Barton N J 1984a Operative treatment of fractures of the hand. In: Birch R, Brooks D (eds) The Hand–Operative Surgery (4th edn). Butterworths, London

Barton N J 1984b Results of Russe grafting for non-union of the scaphoid. Journal of Bone and Joint Surgery 66B:276–277

Berlin D 1929 Position in the treatment of fractures of the carpal scaphoid. New England Journal of Medicine 201:574–579

Boeckstyns M E H, Busch P 1984 Surgical treatment of scaphoid pseudarthrosis: evaluation of the results after soft-tissue arthroplasty and inlay bone grafting. Journal of Hand Surgery 9A:378–382

Boeckstyns M E H, Kjäer L, Busch P, Holst-Nielsen F 1985 Soft tissue interposition arthroplasty for scaphoid non-union. Journal of Hand Surgery 10A:109–114

Böhler L 1935 The treatment of fractures (4th English edn) John Wright, Bristol p 247–252

Böhler V L, Trojan E, Jahna H 1954 Behandlungsergebnisse von 734 frischen einfachen Brüchen des Kahnbeinkörpers der Hand. Wiederherstellungschirurgie Und Traumatologie 2:86–111 (in German, with English summary)

Böhler J, Ender H G 1986 Die Pseudarthrose des Scaphoids. Orthopäde 15:109–120

Bora F W, Osterman A L, Woodbury D F, Brighton C T 1984 Treatment of non-union of the scaphoid by direct current. Orthopedic Clinics of North America 15:107–112

Botelheiro J C 1985 Overlapping of fingers due to malunion of a phalanx corrected by a metacarpal rotational osteotomy—report of two cases. Journal of Hand Surgery 10B:389–390

Broome A, Cedell L A 1964 High plaster immobilization for fracture of the carpal scaphoid bone. Acta Chirurgica Scandinavica 128:42–44

Bunnel S 1949 Surgery of the Hand (2nd edn). J. B. Lippincott, Philadelphia

Cameron S 1969 Non-union of carpal scaphoid fractures treated with cancellous bone grafting. Journal of Bone and Joint Surgery 51B:198

Cooney W P, Dobyns J H, Linscheid R L 1980 Non-union of the scaphoid: analysis of the results from bone grafting. Journal of Hand Surgery 5:343

Coonrad R W, Pohlman M H 1969 Impacted fractures in the

proximal portion of the proximal phalanx of the finger. Journal of Bone and Joint Surgery 51A:1291–1296

Cosio M Q, Camp R A 1986 Percutaneous pinning of symptomatic scaphoid non-unions. Journal of Hand Surgery, 11A:350–355

Dehne E, Deffer P A, Feighey R E 1964 Pathomechanics of the fracture of the carpal navicular. Journal of Trauma 4:96–114

Dias J J, Wray C C, Jones J M, Gregg P J 1987 The role of early mobilization in the treatment of Colles's Fractures. Journal of Bone and Joint Surgery 69B (in press)

Dooley B J 1968 Inlay bone grafting for non-union of the scaphoid bone by the anterior approach. Journal of Bone and Joint Surgery 50B:102

Drury B S 1960 Traumatic tendovaginitis of the fifth dorsal compartment of the wrist. Archives of Surgery 80:554–556

Dwyer F C 1949 Excision of the carpal schaphoid for ununited fracture. Journal of Bone and Joint Surgery 31B:572–577

Eddeland A, Eiken O, Hellgren E, Ohlssen N 1975 Fractures of the scaphoid. Scandinavian Journal of Plastic and Reconstructive Surgery 9:234–239

Finsen V, Benum P 1986 Regional bone mineral density changes after Colles' and forehand fractures. Journal of Hand Surgery 11B:357–359

Fisk G R 1970 Carpal instability and the fractured scaphoid. Annals of the Royal College of Surgeons of England 46:63–76

Fisk G R 1982 Injuries of the wrist. In: Wilson J N (ed) Watson-Jones—Fractures and joint injuries (6th edn). Churchill Livingstone, Edinburgh

Fisk G R 1984 Non-union of the carpal scaphoid treated by wedge grafting. Journal of Bone and Joint Surgery 66B:277

Fitzgerald J A W, Khan M A 1984 The conservative management of fractures of the shafts of the phalanges of the fingers by combined traction-splintage. Journal of Hand Surgery 9B:303–306

Frykman G, Taliesnik J, Peters G, Kaufman R, Helal B, Wood V E, Unsell R S 1986 Treatment of non-united scaphoid fractures by pulsed electromagnetic field and cast. Journal of Hand Surgery 11A:344–346

Gelberman R H, Menon J 1980 The vascularity of the scaphoid bone. Journal of Hand Surgery 5:508

Glass K S, Hochbery F 1978 Non-union of carpal navicular bone: comparison of two methods of treatment. Bulletin of the New York Academy of Medicine 54:865–868

Green D P 1985 The effect of avascular necrosis on Russe bone grafting for scaphoid non-union. Journal of Hand Surgery 10A:597–605

Gross M S, Gelberman R H 1985 Metacarpal rotational osteotomy. Journal of Hand Surgery 10A:105–108

Helal B, Chen S C, Iwegbu G 1982 Rupture of the extensor pollicis longus tendon in undisplaced Colles's type of fracture. The Hand 14:41–47

Herbert T J, Fisher W E 1984 Management of the fractured scaphoid using a new bone screw. Journal of Bone and Joint Surgery 66B:114–123

Herness D, Posner M A 1977 Some aspects of bone grafting for non-union of the carpal navicular. Analysis of 41 cases. Acta Orthopaedica Scandinavica 48:373–378

Hicks J H 1960 External splintage as a cause of movement in fractures. Lancet i:667–670

Howard F M 1961 Ulnar-nerve palsy in wrist fractures. Journal of Bone and Joint Surgery 43A:1197–1201

Hueston J R 1963 Dupuytren's Contracture. Livingstone, Edinburgh

Hull W J, Horse J H, Gustillo R B, Kleven L, Thompson W 1976 The surgical approach and source of bone graft for symptomatic non-union of the scaphoid. Clinical Orthopaedics 115:241–247

Joshi B B 1976 An unusual cause of ulnar nerve palsy associated with Colles's fracture. The Hand 9:76–78

Jupiter J B, Koniuch M P, Smith R J 1985 The management of delayed union and nonunion of the metacarpals and phalanges. Journal of Hand Surgery 10A:457–466

Kim W L, Shaffer J W, Idzikowski C 1983 Failure of treatment of ununited fractures of the carpal scaphoid. The role of non-compliance. Journal of Bone and Joint Surgery 65A:985–991

King R J, MacKenney R P, Elnur S 1982 Suggested method for closed treatment of fractures of the carpal scaphoid : hypothesis supported by dissection and clinical practice. Journal of the Royal Society of Medicine 75:860–867

Kleinert J M, Stern P J, Lister G D, Kleinhans R J 1985 Complications of scaphoid silicone arthroplasty. Journal of Bone and Joint Surgery 67A:422–427

Koch S L 1935 Disabilities of hand resulting from loss of joint function. Journal of the American Medical Association 104:30–35

Lamphier T A 1957 Improper reduction of fractures of the proximal phalanges of fingers. American Journal of Surgery 94:926–930

Leslie I J, Dickson R A 1981 The fractured carpal scaphoid. Journal of Bone and Joint Surgery 63B:225

Lindgren E 1949 Some radiological aspects on the carpal scaphoid and its fractures. Acta Chirurgica Scandinavica 98:538–548

Lindström G 1975 Scaphoideum-Fracturer. Thesis: University of Goteborg (in Swedish, with 5 pp English summary)

London P S 1961 The broken scaphoid bone. The case against pessimism. Journal of Bone and Joint Surgery 43B:237–244

London P S 1967 A practical guide to the care of the injured. E & S Livingstone, Edinburgh p 283–290

Mack G R, Bosse M J, Gelberman R H, Yu E 1984 The natural history of scaphoid non-union. Journal of Bone and Joint Surgery 66A:504–509

Mahring M, Semple C, Gray I C M 1985 Attritional flexor tendon rupture due to a scaphoid non-union imitating an anterior interosseous nerve syndrome : a case report. Journal of Hand Surgery 10B:62–64

Matti H 1936 Technik und Resultate meiner Pseudarthrosenoperation. Zentralblatt für Chirurgie 63:1442

Maudsley R H, Chen S C 1972 Screw fixation in the management of the fractured carpal scaphoid. Journal of Bone and Joint Surgery 54B:432

McCue F C, Honner R, Johnson M C, Greck J H 1970 Athletic injuries of the proximal interphalangeal joint requiring surgical treatment. Journal of Bone and Joint Surgery 52A:937–956

McDonald G, Petrie D 1975 Ununited fracture of the scaphoid. Clinical Orthopaedics 108:110–114

McGrouther D A, Ahmed M R 1981 Flexor tendon excursions in 'no-man's land'. The Hand 13:129–141

McLaughlin H L 1954 Fractures of the carpal navicular (scaphoid) bone. Journal of Bone and Joint Surgery 36A:765–774

McLaughlin H L, Parkes J C 1969 Fracture of the carpal navicular (scaphoid) bone: gradations in therapy based upon pathology. Journal of Trauma 9:311–319

Moberg E 1950 The use of traction treatment for fractures of phalanges and metacarpals. Acta Chirurgica Scandinavica, 99:341–352

Mulder J D 1968 The results of 100 cases of pseudarthrosis in the scaphoid bone treated by the Matti-Russe operation. Journal of Bone and Joint Surgery 50B:110

Murray G 1946 End results of bone grafting for non-union of the carpal navicular. Journal of Bone and Joint Surgery 28:749

Neviaser R J 1983 Proximal row carpectomy for post-traumatic disorders of the carpus. Journal of Hand Surgery 8:301–305

Pieran A P 1972 Correction of rotational malunion of a phalanx by metacarpal osteotomy. Journal of Bone and Joint Surgery 54B:516–519

Pool C 1973 Colles's fracture. A prospective study of treatment. Journal of Bone and Joint Surgery 55B:540–544

Rae P S, Finlayson D 1984 Closed rupture of flexor pollicis longus tendon associated with treatment of Bennett's fracture. Journal of Hand Surgery 9B:129–130

Rasmussen P, Schwab J P, Johnson R P 1985 Symptomatic scaphoid non-unions treated by Russe bone grafting. Orthopaedic Review 14:41–47

Reid D A C 1974 Corrective osteotomy in the hand. The Hand 6:50–57

Rowland S A 1982 Fasciotomy. In: Green D P (ed) Operative hand surgery, Churchill Livingstone, Edinburgh p 565–581

Ruby L K, Stinson J, Belsky M R 1985 The natural history of scaphoid non-union. Journal of Bone and Joint Surgery 67A:428–432

Russe O 1960 Fracture of the carpal navicular—diagnosis, non-operative treatment and operative treatment. Journal of Bone and Joint Surgery 42A:759–768

Sadr B 1984 Sequential rupture of extensor tendons after a Colles's fracture. Journal of Hand Surgery 9A:144–145

Schneider L H, Autoclinio P 1982 Non-union of the carpal scaphoid: the Russe procedure. Journal of Trauma 22:315–319

Sew Hoy A 1976 A review of surgical treatment of scaphoid fractures. Journal of Bone and Joint Surgery 58B:264

Sloan J P, Dove A F, Maheson M, Cope A, Welsh K R 1987 Antibiotics in open fractures of the distal phalanx? Journal of Hand Surgery 12B:123–124

Squire C M 1959 Letter. Journal of Bone and Joint Surgery 41B:210

Stener B 1962 Displacement of the ruptured ulnar collateral ligament of the metacarpophalangeal joint of the thumb. Journal of Bone and Joint Surgery 44B:869–879

Stener B, Stener I 1969 Shearing fractures associated with rupture of ulnar collateral ligament of metacarpophalangeal joint of thumb. Injury 1:12–16

Stewart H D, Innes A R, Burke F D 1985 The hand complications of Colles's fracture. Journal of Hand Surgery 10B:103–106

Swanson A B 1970a Fractures involving the digits of the hand. Orthopedic Clinics of North America 1:261–274

Swanson A B 1970b Silicone rubber implants for the replacement of the carpal scaphoid and lunate bones. Orthopedic Clinics of North America 1:299–309

Taylor L J, Simonis R B, Moschos N 1985 Non-union of the scaphoid: a prospective study of direct current stimulation. Journal of Bone and Joint Surgery 67B:493–494

Thomaidis V T 1973 Elbow-wrist-thumb immobilisation in the treatment of fractures of the carpal scaphoid. Acta Orthopaedica Scandinavica 44:679–689

Unger H S, Stryker W C 1969 Non-union of the carpal navicular: analysis of 42 cases treated by the Russe procedure. Southern Medical Journal 62:620

Van der Linden W, Ericson R 1981 Colles's fracture. How should its displacement be measured and how should it be immobilised? Journal of Bone and Joint Surgery 63A:1285–1288

Verdan C 1960 Fractures of the scaphoid. Surgical Clinics of North America 40:461–464

Verdan C, Narakas A 1968 Fractures and pseudarthroses of the scaphoid. Surgical Clinics of North America 48:1083–1095

Watson H K, Light T R, Johnson T R 1979 Checkrein resection for flexion contracture of the middle joint. Journal of Hand Surgery 4:67–71

Watson H K, Goodman M L, Johnson T R 1981 Limited wrist arthrodesis. Part II: intercarpal and radiocarpal combinations. Journal of Hand Surgery 6:223–233

Watson-Jones R 1943 Fractures and joint injuries (3rd edn). Livingstone, Edinburgh p 559

Weckesser E C 1965 Rotational osteotomy of the metacarpal for overlapping fingers. Journal of Bone and Joint Surgery 47A:751–756

Wong F Y H, Pho R W H (1984) Median nerve compression with tendon ruptures after Colles's fracture. Journal of Hand Surgery 9B:139–141

Ziter F M H 1973 A modified view of the carpal navicular. Radiology 108:766–767

Appendix: Kirschner wires

HISTORY

Martin Kirschner (1879–1942) was in a very real sense a general surgeon, his day to day work and his special interests encompassing the full spectrum of contemporary surgery. He studied under Trendelenburg, worked at first in Greifswald, and was subsequently Professor at Königsberg before moving to Tübingen and then Heidelberg. He became an innovator in several fields of surgery, publishing dozens of papers on numerous subjects. In 1909, he developed the use of fascia lata patches in the repair of abdominal hernia. In 1917, he wrote comparing the wounds produced by ordinary infantry bullets and dumdum bullets. In 1920, he described a thoraco-abdominal approach to the lower oesophagus and upper stomach. He was the first surgeon to successfully perform a Trendelenburg operation for the removal of an embolus from the pulmonary artery in 1924. However, he is probably best known for the 'Wires' which bear his name.

Interestingly enough, in his oft-quoted paper 'Ueber Nagelextension' (1909), Kirschner in fact described the use of much thicker pins, which he referred to as 'Steinmann's pins', measuring 3.5–6.0 mm in diameter. These were used to transfix the tibia or femur above and below a fracture, to provide traction and counter-traction through a form of External Fixator. He was unhappy with the soft-tissue damage that might be caused by these large pins and worked on reducing their diameter, eventually settling on chrome-plated piano-wires between 0.7 mm and 1.5 mm in diameter (Meals & Meuli 1985).

Schum has been credited (Mock & Ellis 1927) with the first use of Steinmann pins in the hand, in 1924. However, a number of other authors described the use of similar devices, used in a variety of different ways for the treatment of fractures in the hand, at about the same time. Mock and Ellis themselves describe the use of Steinmann pins inserted through the phalanges transversely, for the application of continuous traction to obstinate fractures. Lambotte (1925) described open trans-articular intra-medullary pinning of transverse fractures of the phalanges or metacarpals, using cabinet-maker's pins. The technique most frequently used nowadays was first described by Tennant (1924), who advocated the use of steel phonograph needles to transfix fractures in small bones, especially in the hand. He particularly recommended this for oblique displaced fractures, which he found could sometimes be reduced by closed manipulation and then transfixed percutaneously.

Kirschner wires as we know them were recommended specifically for internal splinting of metacarpal fractures by Bosworth (1937), and for a wide variety of fractures in the hand by Vom Saal (1953).

TERMINOLOGY

Although most authors refer to Kirschner wires, some prefer the term pins. The most frequent relevant dictionary definitions are as follows:

1. WIRE. n. Metal that has been drawn out into a long thread, or slender flexible rod.

   v.t. To furnish, connect, bind etc. with wire.

2. PIN. n. A small pointed peg of metal, used to fasten things together.

v.t. To transfix, attach, confine etc. with a pin.

It is clear that either noun quite satisfactorily describes the item, but used as a transitive verb, PIN is perhaps the more precise. Since malleable wire is employed in hand surgery, for example in interosseous wiring, it would perhaps give rise to less confusion if the term 'pin' were used for these more rigid transfixing pins. The term 'wire' is, however, well established and would clearly be difficult to eradicate.

MATERIALS

Most 'K' wires are made out of stainless steel, but there are also vitallium and titanium wires available, and these have slightly different properties. The stainless steel wires tend to be highly polished, which has the advantage of giving rise to less friction, and therefore less heat, during insertion, especially when using a powered driver at moderate speeds. The polished surface has the theoretical disadvantage of leading to loosening more easily than the matt finish on the other types of wire.

If the wire is to be left in for a long time, as in the case of interphalangeal fusion, the relative lack of tissue reaction produced by vitallium may make its use desirable.

POINTS

The commonly found points are the trocar point (Fig. A1) and the bayonet point (Fig. A2).

On engineering grounds, one would expect the bayonet point to be more efficient, since it has an angled cutting surface and also the ability to clear away swarf, at least from the direct vicinity of that cutting surface. While this may apply when drilling into a flat surface at or close to a right-angle, other factors become more important when drilling into small tubular structures at angles determined by circumstances. As can be seen in Figure A2, the bayonet point is not truly pointed, since the leading edge is an oblique line. To prevent 'skating', such a drill should normally be started using a pointed

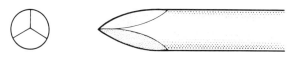

Fig. A.1 Trocar point

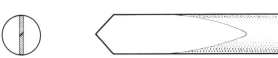

Fig. A.2 Bayonet point

nail starter, but this may not be practical at operation. Furthermore, the shoulders and obtuse included angle on the bayonet point mean that small alterations in angle of approach may lead to the shoulder striking the edge of a drill hole, giving rise to 'skating'.

Wires with pencil points also exist, but are unsatisfactory because of their even less efficient drilling characteristics.

For these reasons, the trocar point is to be preferred despite its theoretically inferior drilling characteristics. The trocar point was also found to be superior in practical terms by Semple (personal communication 1986) who compared the ease of insertion of different wires under standardized conditions.

If a bayonet point is to be used, it is important to be aware that some of them are made with their cutting edge marginally wider than the diameter of the shaft. This is an undesirable feature, since it ensures that the wire lies in a channel which is too wide for it and is therefore loose. Kirschner specifically warned against this in his paper 'Ueber Nagelextension'.

Frequently it is useful to be able to advance a wire through a fracture surface into one fragment and then reduce the fracture and pass the wire in the opposite direction back into the other fragment. For this purpose, many wires are made with points at each end and use of these is far more satisfactory than attempting to achieve the same effect by cutting a single-point wire obliquely to sharpen the other end.

DIAMETERS

A wide variety of diameters is available. Surprisingly, the diameters are still often described in

Table A1 Kirschner wires

Diameter (mm)	Diameter (inches)	Threaded	Smooth	Bayonet-tipped (Single ended)	Bayonet-tipped (Double ended)	Trocar-tipped (Single ended)	Trocar-tipped (Double ended)	Length
0.6	0.025		√					
0.6	0.025		√				√	S
0.8	0.030		√	√	√			L
0.8	0.030		√				√	S
0.9	0.035	√	√	√	√			S+M+L
0.9	0.035	√	√			√	√	S
1.0	0.040		√	√	√			S+M+L
1.0	0.040		√			√		M
1.1	0.045	√	√	√	√			S+M+L
1.1	0.045	√	√			√	√	S+M
1.25	0.050		√	√				L
1.25	0.050		√			√		M
1.5	0.060		√	√	√			S+L
1.5	0.060		√					
1.6	0.0625	√	√	√	√			S+M+L
1.6	0.0625	√				√	√	S+M
2.0	0.078	√	√	√	√			M+L
2.0	0.078	√	√			√	√	S+M
2.4	0.095	√	√	√	√			M
2.4	0.095	√	√			√	√	M
2.5	0.1		√			√		M+L
3.0	0.12		√			√		M+L

S = short = 2–5 inches (5–12 cm); M = medium = 5–9 inches (12–23 cm); and L = long = 10–12 inches (25–30 cm)
Two rows shown for each diameter since different tips not always available in same range of lengths

thousandths of an inch. Table A1 shows these sizes with their metric equivalents. For most purposes in the field of hand surgery, a selection between 0.8 mm and 2 mm should be adequate; thicknesses of up to 3 mm may be useful in less common circumstances, for example for fixation following wrist centralization for radial club hand.

As can be seen from the table, some diameters are available in almost any length, with a variety of points. Thinner wires tend to be available only in short lengths (2–5 inches or 5–12 cm).

Some threaded wires are available which can be used, for example, in tetraplegic patients to provide a potentially reversible interphalangeal fusion simply by transfixing the joint (Newman 1977).

LENGTHS

Many different lengths of wire are available, but broadly speaking they can be simplified into short (less than 5 inches or 12 cm), medium (5–9 inches or 12–23 cm) and long (10–12 inches or 23–30 cm). This is mainly of significance in double-ended wires, where circumstances may dictate the space available for advancing the wires in each direction. It is also important when certain types of introducer are used, since some have a limited capacity for wire length.

INTRODUCERS

The type of introducer used is most important. Hand-driven introducers are, by and large, difficult to use satisfactorily, especially in hand surgery, since the drilling movement used inevitably also results in a degree of circumduction which may cause the wire to wander.

Powered introducers of various types are available and completely eliminate the problem of circumduction. These have the disadvantage that the high speed drilling may give rise to excessive heat production, and speed of drilling should therefore be as low as possible and irrigation may be helpful.

Although bulky, a pistol-grip on the introducer gives excellent control of direction while drilling. The better adjustable chucks allow insertion of the wire to begin without too much wire protruding, but still allow this to be adjusted while inserting the wire, without using both hands. This minimizes any tendency of the wire to deviate or bend, especially when fine wires are used.

The least satisfactory chucks are those which require both hands to release and adjust them, which means that the surgeon is unable to control the instrument and the part being operated on at the same time.

A motorized introducer is indispensable when inserting wires obliquely; if they are put in by hand the obliquity causes them to skid off the bone or, in an attempt to prevent this, the wires are inserted too transversely.

A special instrument has been designed which assists in the reduction and pinning of phalangeal fractures (Blalock et al 1975). This instrument not only allows reduction of the fracture, but also holds the reduction and is cannulated to allow wires to be inserted through it while it is applied to the finger.

REFERENCES

Blalock H S, Pearce H L, Kleinert H, Kutz J 1975 An instrument designed to help reduce and percutaneously pin fractured phalanges. Journal of Bone and Joint Surgery 57A : 792–794

Bosworth D M 1937 Internal splinting of fractures of the fifth metacarpal Journal of Bone and Joint Surgery 19 : 826–827

Kirschner M 1909 Ueber Nagelextension. Beitrage zur Klinischen Chirurgie 64 : 266–279

Lambotte A 1925 L'Ostéosynthèse par Clouage Trans-articulaire. Paris Chirurgical. Avril-Mai 1925

Meals R A, Meuli H C 1985 Carpenter's nails, phonograph needles, piano wires and safety pins : The history of operative fixation of metacarpal and phalangeal fractures.

Journal of Hand Surgery 10A : 144–150

Mock H E, Ellis J D 1927 The treatment of fractures of the fingers and metacarpals with a description of the authors' finger caliper. Surgery, Gynaecology and Obstetrics 15 : 551–556

Newman J H 1977 The use of the Key-Grip procedure for improving hand function in quadriplegia. The Hand 9 : 215–220

Tennant C E 1924 Letter. Journal of the American Medical Association 83 : 193

Vom Saal F H 1953 Intramedullary fixation in fractures of the hand and fingers. Journal of Bone and Joint Surgery 35A : 5–16

Index